CUISINART

WOOD PELLET GRILL AND SMOKER

COOKBOOK FOR BEGINNERS

550 BBQ RECIPES TO MAKE STUNNING MEALS WITH YOUR FAMILY AND TO SHOW YOUR SKILLS AT THE BARBECUE!

JAMES OSBORNE

Copyright © 2021 by James Osborne All rights reserved worldwide.

No part of this book may be reproduced or transmitted in any form or by any means, electronic or mechanical, including photo- copying, recording or by any information storage and retrieval system, without written permission from the publisher, except for the inclusion of brief quotations in a review.

Warning-Disclaimer: The purpose of this book is to educate and entertain. The author or publisher does not guarantee that anyone following the techniques, suggestions, tips, ideas, or strategies will become successful. The author and publisher shall have neither liability or responsibility to anyone with respect to any loss or damage caused, or alleged to be caused, directly or indirectly by the information contained in this book.

CONTENTS

INTRODUCTION..11
What the Cuisinart Wood Pellet Grill is 11
How Does the Cuisinart Wood Pellet Grill Work? 11
The Pros of the Cuisinart Wood Pellet Grill..11
Better to Use Your Cuisinart Wood Pellet Grill.......................................13
Cleaning Approaches for Your Cuisinart Wood Pellet Grill......................14

SEAFOOD RECIPES 15
Grilled Salmon 15
Bacon Wrapped Scallops.....................................15
Grilled Lemon Salmon...15
Mango Rice Wine Thai Shrimp 15
Garlic Grilled Shrimp Skewers 16
Vodka Brined Smoked Wild Salmon.....................16
Grilled Albacore Tuna With Potato-tomato Casserole 17
Baked Steelhead 17
Grilled Garlic Shrimp With Cajun Dip.................17
Smoked Salmon Candy 18
Smoky Crab Dip 18
Spicy Lime Shrimp...18
Swordfish With Sicilian Olive Oil Sauce 19
Dijon-smoked Halibut 19
Spicy Shrimp Skewers 19
Shrimp Cabbage Tacos With Lime Cream 20
Oysters In The Shell 20
Grilled Trout With Citrus & Basil 20
Planked Trout With Fennel, Bacon & Orange 21
Moules Marinières With Garlic Butter Sauce 21
Smoked Lobster Scampi..22
Cajun-blackened Shrimp.......................................22
Simple Glazed Salmon Fillets 23
Alder Smoked Scallops With Citrus & Garlic Butter Sauce...23
Traeger Jerk Shrimp 23
Lobster Tail...24
Lemon Shrimp Scampi 24
Cider Hot-smoked Salmon 24
Delicious Smoked Trout 25
Flavour Fire Spiced Shrimp...................................25

Pacific Northwest Salmon 26
Grilled Maple Syrup Salmon 26
Bacon Wrapped Shrimp 26
Grilled Pepper Lobster Tails 27
Bbq Roasted Salmon..27
Traeger Smoked Salmon..28
Grilled Artichoke Cheese Salmon 28
Garlic Bacon Wrapped Shrimp 29
Kimi's Simple Grilled Fresh Fish 29
Roasted Halibut With Spring Vegetables 29
Mezcal Shrimp With Salsa De Molcajete 30
Grilled Tuna Steaks With Lemon & Caper Butter 31
Bbq Oysters...31
Citrus-smoked Trout 32
Lime Mahi Mahi Fillets 32
Smoke-roasted Halibut With Mixed Herb Vinaigrette 32
Baked Tuna Noodle Casserole...............................33
Grilled Lobster Tails With Smoked Paprika Butter 33
Smoked Honey Salmon 34
Smoked Trout...34
Lemon Lobster Rolls 34
Mexican Mahi Mahi With Baja Cabbage Slaw...........35
Salmon Cakes With Homemade Tartar Sauce 35
Cold-smoked Salmon Gravlax................................36
Sweet Mandarin Salmon.......................................36
Grilled Tilapia With Blistered Cherry Tomatoes 36
Hot-smoked Salmon...37
Prosciutto-wrapped Scallops.................................38
Barbecued Shrimp..38
Garlic Pepper Shrimp Pesto Bruschetta 38
Grilled Mussels With Lemon Butter.......................39

Smoked Mango Shrimp 39
Smoked Crab Legs 39
Traeger Crab Legs..40
Grilled Whole Steelhead Fillet 40
Florentine Shrimp Al Cartoccio......................40
Seared Bluefin Tuna Steaks............................41
Seared Ahi Tuna Steak With Soy Sauce.........41
Honey Balsamic Salmon 41
Grilled Blackened Saskatchewan Salmon 42
Thai-style Swordfish Steaks With Peanut Sauce..........42

Lemon Herb Grilled Salmon............................43
Barbecued Scallops...43
Teriyaki Smoked Honey Tilapia.......................43
Grilled Fresh Fish...43
Grilled Oysters With Mignonette 44
Garlic Blackened Catfish 44
Wood-fired Halibut...45
Smoked Fish Chowder 45
Traeger Baked Rainbow Trout.........................45

PORK RECIPES..47

Pickle Brined Grilled Pork Chops 47
Simple Smoked Baby Backs 47
Smoked Baby Back Ribs 47
Honey Pork Belly Burnt Ends 47
Smoky Pork Tenderloin 48
Smoked Traeger Pulled Pork 48
Spicy Ribs...49
Competition Style Bbq Pork Ribs...................49
Smoked Bacon Roses 50
Pulled Pork Sliders Hawaiian Rolls 50
Smoked Pork Tomato Tamales.........................50
Pineapple-pepper Pork Kebabs 51
Traeger Pulled Pork Sandwiches......................51
St Louis Style Bbq Ribs With Texas Spicy Bbq Sauce.52
Hanging St. Louis-style Grilled Ribs...............52
Kodiak Cakes Candied Bacon Crumble Brownies 53
Orange & Maple Baked Ham..........................53
Bacon Wrapped Pickles....................................54
Bbq Pork Belly 54
Pulled Pork Stew 54
Spiced Orange Ribs 55
Smoked Porchetta 55
Pulled Pork Taquitos With Sour Cream..........56
Baked Sage & Sausage Stuffing 56
Grilled Pork Tacos Al Pastor 57
Stuffed Pork Crown Roast 57
Apple-smoked Pork Tenderloin........................58
Apple & Bourbon Glazed Ham 58
Jamaican Jerk Pork Chops...............................58
First-timer's Pulled Pork..................................59
Maple Baby Backs 59

Grilled Dr. Pepper Ribs...................................60
Cajun Double-smoked Ham 60
Bacon-draped Injected Pork Loin Roast 61
Pulled Pork Corn Tortillas 61
Classic Pulled Pork 61
Pulled Pork Shoulder And Chicken 61
Baked German Pork Schnitzel With Grilled Lemons . 62
Balsamic Brussels Sprouts With Bacon 62
Smoked Pork Spare Ribs 63
Bbq Pulled Pork With Sweet & Heat Bbq Sauce 63
Bacon Wrapped Asparagus...............................63
Smoked Spare Ribs 64
Smoked Rack Of Pork......................................64
Bbq Pork Shoulder Steaks 65
Beer Pork Belly Chili Con Carne 65
Bbq Brown Sugar Bacon Bites.........................66
Grilled German Sausage With A Smoky Traeger
Twist 66
Bbq Pork Short Ribs..67
Beer Braised Garlic Bbq Pork Butt 67
Home-cured Picnic Ham With Mustard Caviar..........67
Smoke-roasted Beer-braised Brats....................68
Smoked Ham 68
Unique Carolina Mustard Ribs........................69
Home-cured Hickory-smoked Bacon................69
Apple-smoked Bacon..70
Baked Honey Glazed Ham...............................70
Whiskey- & Cider-brined Pork Shoulder 70
Pig On A Stick With Buffalo Glaze.................71
Barbecued Tenderloin.......................................71
Egg Bacon French Toast Panini.......................72

Pork Tenderloin With Bourbon Peaches 72
Leftover Pulled Pork With Eggs.................................73
Bbq Rib Sandwich...73
Hawaiian Pulled Pig..74
Maple Syrup Bacon Wrapped Tenderloin 74
Hot & Fast Smoked Baby Back Ribs..........................74
Traeger Cajun Broil...75
Grilled Lasagna With Cold-smoked Mozzarella..........75
Roasted Bacon Weave Holiday Ham..........................76
Double-decker Pulled Pork Nachos With Smoked
Cheese 76

Cocoa-crusted Pork Tenderloin 77
Delicious Smoked Bone-in Pork Chops.....................77
Smoked Apple Pork Belly..77
Bacon Stuffed Onion Rings.......................................78
Grilled Ham & Egg Cups 78
Baby Back Ribs With Mustard Slather 78
Bbq Pork Chops 79
Traeger Roasted Easter Ham 79
Bbq Bacon-wrapped Water Chestnuts 79
Bbq Pulled Pork Grilled Cheese Sandwich 80

BEEF LAMB AND GAME RECIPES 81

Smoked Beef Back Ribs 81
Smoked Texas Bbq Brisket 81
Flavour Smoked Corned Beef Brisket Hash 81
Beer Chili Bratwurst...82
Perfect Roast Prime Rib..82
Vietnamese Beef Jerky..83
Smoked Spiced Pulled Beef Chuck Roast...................83
Grilled Bell Pepper Flank Steak Fajitas 84
Cucumber Beef Kefta 84
Carne Asada Recipe 84
Hot Coffee-rubbed Brisket 85
Bbq Brisket Tacos 85
Smoked Red Wine Beef Roast...................................86
Cheesy Skillet Shepherd's Pie 86
Steak Tips With Mashed Potatoes 87
Savory Chili Mac And Cheese....................................87
Salt & Pepper Dinosaur Bones 88
Jalapeno Pepper Jack Cheese Bacon Burgers 88
The Boss Beef Burger..89
Lemon Tomahawk Steak 89
Teriyaki Bbq Beef Skewers..90
Chorizo Cheese Stuffed Burgers................................90
Smoked Black Pepper Beef Back Ribs 90
Sweet And Spicy Beef Sirloin Tip Roast 91
Bacon-swiss Cheesesteak Meatloaf............................91
Savory Cheese Steak Rolls With Puff Pastry 92
Smoked Corned Beef & Cabbage 92
Kansas City Cheese Brisket Burger............................93
Traditional Tomahawk Steak......................................93
Smoked Beef Ribs 93

Grilled Skirt Steak Quesadillas..................................94
Bbq Bacon Meatballs..94
Roasted Duck..95
Flavour Reverse Seared T-bone Steak 95
Smoked Meatball Egg Sandwiches.............................95
Citrus Grilled Lamb Chops 96
Smoked Chicken Steak Sandwiches 96
Flavour Texas Smoke Beef...97
Pulled Beef 98
Grilled Bison Rib Eye Kabobs 98
Slow Smoked Spiced Beef 98
Smoked Beer Corned Beef 99
Greek Leg Of Lamb 99
Irish Pasties 100
Spicy Beer Beef Jerky 100
Savory Whiskey Grilled Elk Steaks 100
Bistecca Alla Fiorentina With Mushroom Ragout.....101
Garlic Standing Rib Roast 101
Smoked New York Steaks...102
Smoked Bourbon Jerky 102
Grilled Rosemary Rack Of Lamb 103
Duck Fat Fries (confit) 103
Texas-style Smoked Beef Brisket By Doug Scheiding104
Grilled Garlic Tomahawk Steak..................................104
Italian Beef Pinwheels...105
Rosemary-smoked Lamb Chops 105
Spatchcocked Quail With Smoked Fruit.....................105
Santa Maria Tri-tip..106
Reverse Sear Tomahawk Chop...................................106
Smoked Burgers 107

Grilled Lemon Skirt Steak 107
3-2-1 Bbq Beef Cheeks......................................107
Smoked Beer Brisket...107
Bbq Burnt End Sandwich 108
Grilled Loco Moco Burger..................................108
Grilled Tomahawk Steak 109
Flavour Bbq Brisket Burnt Ends.........................109
Korean Style Bbq Prime Ribs.............................109
Smoked Longhorn Brisket 110
Smoked Garlic Prime Rib Roast..........................110
Kalbi-style Steak Wraps.....................................110

Grilled Garlic Tri Tip...111
Bbq Burnt Ends 112
Tuscan Cheesesteaks 112
Smoked Bacon Brisket Flat 113
Braised Onion Chuck Roast Beef Sandwiches 113
Smoked Corned Beef Brisket 113
Beef Brisket With Chophouse Steak Rub 114
Smoked Cheese Beef Burgers 114
Pastrami 114
Grilled Lemon Steak Pinwheels 115

APPETIZERS AND SNACKS 116

Chicken Wings With Teriyaki Glaze 116
Bacon-wrapped Jalapeño Poppers 116
Bacon Pork Pinwheels (kansas Lollipops)...............117
Bayou Wings With Cajun Rémoulade.....................117
Pulled Pork Loaded Nachos 118
Citrus-infused Marinated Olives..........................118
Chorizo Queso Fundido.....................................118
Grilled Guacamole 119
Pigs In A Blanket...120
Simple Cream Cheese Sausage Balls.....................120
Deviled Eggs With Smoked Paprika 120

Smoked Cashews 121
Pig Pops (sweet-hot Bacon On A Stick) 121
Chuckwagon Beef Jerky.....................................122
Smoked Cheese..122
Roasted Red Pepper Dip 123
Delicious Deviled Crab Appetizer 123
Smoked Turkey Sandwich 124
Sriracha & Maple Cashews.................................124
Jalapeño Poppers With Chipotle Sour Cream..........124
Cold-smoked Cheese...125

POULTRY RECIPES 126

Smoked Chicken With Apricot Bbq Glaze 126
Roasted Tin Foil Dinners...................................126
Buffalo Chicken 126
Roasted Duck With Cherry Salsa 127
Loaded Chicken Fries..128
Duck Breast With Pomegranate Sauce 128
Thai Chicken Satays..129
Chile Chicken Thighs..129
Smoked Chicken Vermicelli Noodles 130
Garlic Sriracha Buffalo Chicken Wings..................130
Whole Roasted Chicken 131
Wood-fired Chicken Breasts................................131
Buffalo Chicken Wings 131
Oktoberfest Pretzel Mustard Chicken 132
Savory Smoked Turkey Legs...............................132
Grilled Honey Garlic Wings 132
Savory-sweet Turkey Legs..................................133
Smoked Whiskey Peach Pulled Chicken 133

Roasted Honey Bourbon Glazed Turkey 134
Bourbon Chicken Waffles 134
Bbq Chicken Breasts...135
Easy Grilled Chicken Shawarma 135
Cranberry Turkey Breast 135
Dry Brine Traeger Turkey 136
Roasted Chicken With Wild Rice & Mushrooms 136
Chicken On A Throne 137
Cajun Spatchcock Turkey...................................137
Bbq Spatchcocked Chicken 137
Smoked Thanksgiving Turkey..............................138
Bbq Pulled Turkey Sandwiches 138
Yucatán-spiced Chicken Thighs...........................139
Lemon Rosemary Beer Can Chicken 139
Chicken Tenders...139
Smoked Pulled Chicken 140
Smoked Maple Syrup Thanksgiving Turkey..............140
Lemon Parmesan Chicken Wings.........................140

County Fair Turkey Legs 141
Baked Prosciutto-wrapped Chicken Breast With
Spinach And Boursin 141
Smoked Whole Chicken 142
Roasted Stuffed Turkey Breast....................142
Bacon Wrapped Chicken Wings 142
Carrot Celery Chicken Drumsticks...............143
Spiced Smoked Chicken Quarters 143
Fried Chicken Sliders 143
Kansas City Hot Fried Chicken 144
Bacon Weaved Stuffed Turkey Breast 144
Smoked Avocado Turkey Tamale Pie 145
Savory Cajun Bbq Chicken 145
Cajun Brined Maple Smoked Turkey Breast 146
Grilled Cheesy Chicken 146
Turkey & Bacon Kebabs With Ranch-style Dressing 147
Mini Turducken Roulade................................147
Skinny Smoked Chicken Breasts 148
Italian Grilled Barbecue Chicken Wings 148
Sweet Cajun Wings 148
Bbq Breakfast Sausage.................................149
Smoke Roasted Chicken With Herb Butter 149
Chicken Parmesan Sliders With Pesto Mayonnaise ...150

Spatchcocked Chicken With Toasted Fennel &
Garlic 150
Smoked Wings...150
Bourbon-brined Turkey Thighs 151
Traeger Bbq Half Chickens...........................151
Teriyaki Apple Cider Turkey..........................152
Spatchcocked Chicken With White Barbecue Sauce. 152
Spicy Bbq Whole Chicken 153
Green Chile Chicken Enchiladas 153
Bacon-wrapped Chicken Breasts 154
Nashville Spiced Smoked Chicken 154
Smoked Cheesy Chicken Quesadilla 154
Cider-brined Turkey......................................155
Bbq Chicken Tostada 156
Smoked Quarters 156
Hot Turkey Sandwich With Gravy 156
Chicken Breast Calzones 157
Bacon Wrapped Turkey Legs 157
Whole Smoked Honey Chicken.....................158
Grilled Honey Chicken Wings........................158
Apricot Glazed Ham 158
Smoked Honey Chicken Drumsticks 159
Smoke-roasted Chicken Thighs 159

COCKTAILS RECIPES 160

Smoked Berry Cocktail 160
Smoking Gun Cocktail 160
Traeger Smoked Daiquiri...............................160
In Traeger Fashion Cocktail 161
Smoked Apple Cider 161
Grilled Blood Orange Mimosa 161
Sunset Margarita 161
Ryes And Shine Cocktail 162
Grilled Peach Sour Cocktail...........................162
Zombie Cocktail Recipe 163
Smoked Hot Buttered Rum 163
Strawberry Mule Cocktail 163
Garden Gimlet Cocktail..................................164
Grilled Hawaiian Sour 164
Smoked Pomegranate Lemonade Cocktail 164
Smoked Mulled Wine 165
Batter Up Cocktail 165
Smoked Ice Mojito Slurpee............................165

Grilled Frozen Strawberry Lemonade 165
Smoked Sangria 166
Smoked Pumpkin Spice Latte 166
Fig Slider Cocktail 167
Bacon Old-fashioned Cocktail 167
Smoked Salted Caramel White Russian 167
Smoky Scotch & Ginger Cocktail 168
A Smoking Classic Cocktail 168
Cran-apple Tequila Punch With Smoked Oranges ... 168
Smoked Cold Brew Coffee 169
Smoked Hibiscus Sparkler.............................169
Smoked Jacobsen Salt Margarita 170
Smoked Barnburner Cocktail 170
Smoked Pineapple Hotel Nacional Cocktail 170
Dublin Delight Cocktail..................................171
Grilled Peach Mint Julep 171
Smoked Irish Coffee 172
Smoked Texas Ranch Water 172

Traeger Old Fashioned 172
Traeger Boulevardier Cocktail 173
Grilled Rabbit Tail Cocktail 173
Traeger Paloma Cocktail................................173
Smoked Grape Lime Rickey 174
Honey Glazed Grapefruit Shandy Cocktail 174
Smoked Plum And Thyme Fizz Cocktail.................174

Grilled Peach Smash Cocktail....................175
Smoked Eggnog...175
Traeger Gin & Tonic....................................176
Smoke And Bubz Cocktail 176
Smoked Raspberry Bubbler Cocktail................176
Smoky Mountain Bramble Cocktail.................176

VEGETABLES RECIPES..................................178

Smoked & Loaded Baked Potato....................178
Grilled Cabbage Steaks With Warm Bacon
Vinaigrette 178
Braised Creamed Green Beans 178
Carolina Baked Beans 179
Stuffed Jalapenos 179
Roasted Jalapeno Cheddar Deviled Eggs 180
Roasted Green Beans With Bacon 180
Butternut Squash...180
Roasted New Potatoes With Compound Butter 180
Baked Sweet Potato Casserole With Marshmallow
Fluff..181
Whole Roasted Cauliflower With Garlic Parmesan
Butter..182
Roasted Sheet Pan Vegetables.........................182
Smoked Macaroni Salad.................................182
Baked Heirloom Tomato Tart 183
Baked Kale Chips 183
Grilled Broccoli Rabe 183
Roasted New Potatoes....................................184
Steak Fries With Horseradish Creme 184
Baked Bacon Green Bean Casserole 184
Baked Stuffed Avocados.................................185
Roasted Sweet Potato Steak Fries 185
Grilled Chili-lime Corn 185
Roasted Vegetable Napoleon 186
Spicy Asian Brussels Sprouts..........................186
Parmesan Roasted Cauliflower........................186
Baked Winter Squash Au Gratin 186
Roasted Beet & Bacon Salad..........................187
Grilled Corn On The Cob With Parmesan And
Garlic..187
Chef Curtis' Famous Chimichurri Sauce 188
Roasted Mashed Potatoes 188

Broccoli-cauliflower Salad 188
Roasted Do-ahead Mashed Potatoes...............188
Grilled Asparagus And Hollandaise Sauce 189
Green Bean Casserole 189
Smoked Beet-pickled Eggs.............................190
Double-smoked Cheese Potatoes....................190
Grilled Fingerling Potato Salad 191
Traeger Smoked Coleslaw 191
Grilled Asparagus And Spinach Salad.............191
Portobello Marinated Mushroom....................192
Smoked Mushrooms 192
Smoked Pickled Green Beans 192
Baked Loaded Tater Tots 193
Grilled Zucchini Squash Spears......................193
Christmas Brussel Sprouts 193
Grilled Ratatouille Salad 194
Roasted Fall Vegetables 194
Butter Braised Green Beans 194
Bacon Wrapped Corn On The Cob 194
Roasted Garlic Herb Fries 195
Grilled Asparagus & Honey-glazed Carrots 195
Potluck Salad With Smoked Cornbread 196
Baked Breakfast Mini Quiches 196
Smoked Jalapeño Poppers...............................197
Traeger Grilled Whole Corn 197
Smoked Mashed Potatoes...............................197
Grilled Beer Cabbage.....................................198
Tater Tot Bake...198
Salt Crusted Baked Potatoes...........................198
Roasted Hasselback Potatoes By Doug Scheiding 199
Roasted Jalapeño Poppers...............................199
Red Potato Grilled Lollipops..........................200
Blt Pasta Salad 200
Sweet Potato Marshmallow Casserole..............200

Grilled Street Corn 201
Smoked Parmesan Herb Popcorn 201
Traeger Baked Potato Torte 201
Roasted Pickled Beets 202
Cast Iron Potatoes 202
Roasted Potato Poutine 203
Baked Garlic Duchess Potatoes 203
Roasted Olives 203
Mashed Red Potatoes 204

Smoked Bbq Onion Brussels Sprout 204
Roasted Tomatoes 204
Baked Sweet And Savory Yams By Bennie Kendrick. 205
Roasted Asparagus 205
Roasted Pumpkin Seeds 205
Smoked Asparagus Soup 205
Roasted Red Pepper White Bean Dip 206
Skillet Potato Cake 206

BAKING RECIPES 208

Baked Cast Iron Berry Cobbler 208
Double Chocolate Chip Brownie Pie...........208
Vanilla Chocolate Bacon Cupcakes.............209
Baked Cheesy Parmesan Grits 209
Smoked Sweet Beer Bread 209
Smoked Lemon Cheesecake.........................210
Smoked, Salted Caramel Apple Pie 210
Green Bean Casserole Circa 1955...............211
Blueberry Pancakes....................................211
Pull-apart Dinner Rolls 212
Savory Beaver Tails 212
Smoked Blackberry Pie 212
Pizza Bites 213
Savory Cheesecake With Bourbon Pecan Topping 214
Baked Chocolate Brownie Cookies With Egg Nog ...214
Basil Margherita Pizza 215
Grilled Beer Cheese Dip 215
Quick Baked Dinner Rolls 216
Smoked Vanilla Apple Pie 216
Chocolate Almond Cake.............................216
Marbled Brownies With Amaretto & Ricotta 217
Baked Peach Cobbler Cupcakes 217
Carrot Cake 218
Delicious Pellet Grill Cornbread 218
Garlic Lemon Pepper Chicken Wings.........218
Beer Bread 219
Sourdough Pizza.......................................219
Baked Molten Chocolate Cake 220
Easy Smoked Cornbread.............................220
Smoky Pimento Cheese Cornbread 220
Chicken Pot Pie 221
Butternut Squash Macaroni And Cheese.....221

Smokin' Lemon Bars 221
Spiced Lemon Cherry Pie...........................222
Donut Bread Pudding.................................222
Baked Pumpkin Pie 223
Baked Green Chile Mac & Cheese By Doug
Scheiding...223
Dark Chocolate Brownies With Bacon-salted
Caramel 224
Onion Cheese Nachos 224
Smoked Lemon Tea 224
Eyeball Cookies 225
Baked Irish Creme Cake.............................225
Cake With Smoked Berry Sauce 225
Delicious Peanut Butter Cookies................226
Crème Brûlée 226
Pretzel Rolls 227
Baked Bourbon Monkey Bread 227
Crescent Rolls 228
Bananas Rum Foster 228
Zucchini Bread 228
Maple Syrup Pancake Casserole 229
Chicken Pizza On The Grill 229
Sweet And Spicy Baked Pork Beans............230
Eggs Ham Benedict....................................230
Cinnamon Pull-aparts................................230
Pumpkin Bread 231
Baked Buttermilk Biscuits 231
Sopapilla Cheesecake By Doug Scheiding.................232
Mexican Black Bean Cornbread Casserole 232
Skillet Buttermilk Cornbread 232
Vanilla Chocolate Chip Cookies 233
Chili Cheese Fries......................................233

Italian Herb & Parmesan Scones 234
Cornbread Chicken Stuffing 234
Blueberry Sour Cream Muffins 235
Smoky Apple Crepes 235
Traeger Baked Protein Bars 236
Baked Brie 236
Baked Wood-fired Pizza 236
Anzac Coconut Biscuits 237

Blueberry Bread Pudding 237
Mint Butter Chocolate Chip Cookies 238
The Dan Patrick Show Pull-apart Pesto Bread 238
Smoker Wheat Bread 238
Focaccia 239
Grilled Apple Pie 240
Garlic Cheese Pull Apart Bread 240

RECIPE INDEX **241**

INTRODUCTION

What the Cuisinart Wood Pellet Grill is

A wood pellet grill — also known as a wood pellet smoker — is a special type of grill that uses indirect, pellet-generated heat and smoke to cook food in several different ways. With a pellet grill, you can enjoy traditionally grilled favorites or leave the meat to cook slowly on low smoke throughout the day. You can also use a pellet grill like a type of outdoor oven.

Like other grills, a pellet smoker makes an excellent addition to a campout, tailgating party and your own backyard.

How Does the Cuisinart Wood Pellet Grill Work?

So now you know what they do, but how do pellet grills work?

Much of what a pellet grill does is automated, meaning there's a very small learning curve on figuring out how to operate it correctly. Wood pellets are loaded into a storage chamber called the hopper, where a motor and combustion fan ignite the pellets and circulate that smoky wood flavor throughout the main cooking chamber.

Once they're going, pellet grills work basically like a gas grill or kitchen oven, trapping heat under the hood to cook your food, all while the hopper continues to circulate the aroma and flavor of your choice of wood pellets. Air fans ensure that heat and smoke are evenly dispersed during the cook time, and temperature control dials give you the option to cook either low and slow or hard and fast, depending on the taste and texture that you're trying to achieve.

The Pros of the Cuisinart Wood Pellet Grill

1. Laid-Back Approach

If you're not the type of person to babysit your grill, opting for a pellet grill can be a far better option. Compared to gas, pellet grills cook slowly and thoroughly with minimal intervention and safety concerns. You'll even find that many have easy-to-use features that allow you to monitor the cooking process remotely.

For example, some pellet grills are equipped with digital controllers that allow you to set specific cook times. You can even use a smartphone app to adjust the grill settings. The only maintenance you'll have to consider with a wood pellet grill vs propane grill is making sure the hopper has enough pellets.

2. Minimal Maintenance

Because pellet grills typically cook for longer, most of the fats and grease will be burnt away, compared to gas grills. At most, you'll have to clean the firepot and any juices and drippings that are collected. You could also opt to season the smoker after cooking to burn away any traces of food.

3. Superior Flavor

The number one reason why people suggest pellet grills are better than gas grills is their flavor profiles. With pellet grills, you will have a diverse selection of different types of wood that you can cook with. Instead of using regular flavorless gas, these appliances allow you to inject different flavors into the meat. A few of the most popular flavored pellets on the market include pecan, mesquite, hickory, and apple. There are plenty of manufacturers that have an extensive product list of fabulously flavored wood pellets. If you buy them in bulk, you're likely to get better discounts than you would with gas canisters.

Another exciting aspect of the flavors from wood pellets is you can customize them to your liking. You could mix apple and mesquite pellets for a unique flavor for ribs and brisket.

4. Versatility

Interestingly enough, pellet grills are far more versatile than gas grills because they give you several different ways to cook. You can easily set the temperature low, close the lid for smoking, or use it as a traditional grill. Some of the higher-end models even allow you to sear and braise, as well.

5. Enhanced Moisture and Meat Quality

Most people who opt for gas grills search for a quick and efficient outdoor appliance for everyday meals. With a pellet smoker, you have more control over how your meat cooks, especially if you want juicier cuts.

Since this appliance cooks for longer times and at lower temperatures, you'll find the inside of meat will be more moist. You might also find that it's a preferable option for higher-quality cuts of meat that need more attention.

Better to Use Your Cuisinart Wood Pellet Grill

1. Use Lighter-Flavored Wood

Switching up your hardwood changes the flavor of what you're cooking.

You'll want to leave the big smoke flavors for meat and veggies and use a lighter-flavored wood for your baked goods.

You simply want the wood flavor to lightly touch your baked goods. Go ahead and experiment to see which flavors you like the best. Go ahead and combine them, too.

2. Prep Your Ingredients

Just like with baking in the house, you want to prep your ingredients ahead of time. Then, put it all together so it's ready to cook when you are.

For example, if you're having an evening party, put your dessert together in the morning, so you just have to slip it into your grill when you're ready to cook.

3. Keep It Simple

Whether you're a novice baker or a seasoned expert, let the flavor of your hardwood season your baked goods and give it a light smoky flavor.

So, keep your dessert simple and let the grill do the work. There's no reason to over complicate your dessert. After all, the fun of having a party is hanging out with friends and family.

Think cookies, cake, crumbles, and even fruit. Grilled fruit is delightful and refreshing when you put some cool whip on the side.

4. Use a Recipe You Know

A great tip is to use a recipe you know and are comfortable with. You can basically make anything you'd like on your pellet grill. So, pull out your favorite cookie, brownie, cake, pie, or cheesecake recipe. You don't really have to make any modification to cook on your grill.

Do note, though, that recipes may cook a bit faster, so you'll want to check often for doneness.

Cleaning Approaches for Your Cuisinart Wood Pellet Grill

To prove to you just how easy it can be let's review the common methods of cleaning.

1. The Obvious Approach: Brushing

This method works best if it is done immediately after grilling while the grate is still hot. Before the grates cool off, scrape each grate with a brush, both top and bottom sides. You can also dip the brush in water which will create a steam that loosens the grease. Not only will this make cleaning time shorter, but it will discourage insects from hanging around your grill. Depending on your grate you may need to wipe them down with a cloth after scrapping.

2. The Lazy Approach: Burning

The idea behind this method is simple, get the grate super hot (550° F) until all the caked on grease burns up. You can throw the grates in a self-cleaning oven or simply place some aluminum foil down on top of the grate, close the lid and light up the grill. After about 10-15 minutes all of the grease should be a white powder, simply brush it off and you're done.

3. The Neat Freak Approach: Soaking

Although, brushing and burning are the standard methods for cleaning, all grates should be soaked at least a couple times a year.

Just fill up the sink or a large bucket with water and a bunch of dish soap. Add a little baking soda and let the grates soak for an hour. Afterward, scrub and rinse.

4. The DIY Approach

You can easily make your own scrubber with a block of hardwood. Use the block to scrub the grates after grilling, eventually, you will carve grooves into the block that fit perfectly onto your grate.

Aluminum foil is another easy DIY scrubber and also a lifesaver if you have to use a lazy person's grill. Simply heat up the grates, then wad up some foil and scrub away. Let's jump into some do-it-yourself methods to cleaning up those nasty grates.

SEAFOOD RECIPES

Grilled Salmon

Servings: 4
Cooking Time: 25 Minutes

Ingredients:

- 1 (2-pound) half salmon fillet
- 3 tablespoons mayonnaise
- 1 batch Dill Seafood Rub

Directions:

1. Supply your smoker with wood pellets and follow the start-up procedure. Preheat the grill, with the lid closed, to 325°F.
2. Using your hands, rub the salmon fillet all over with the mayonnaise and sprinkle it with the rub.
3. Place the salmon directly on the grill grate, skin-side down, and grill until its internal temperature reaches 145°F. Remove the salmon from the grill and serve immediately.

Bacon Wrapped Scallops

Servings: 8
Cooking Time: 20 Minutes

Ingredients:

- 24 jumbo deep sea diver scallops, dry-packed
- 1/2 Cup butter
- salt
- freshly ground black pepper
- 1 Clove garlic, minced
- 12 Slices thin-cut bacon, cut in half crosswise
- lemon wedges, for serving

Directions:

1. Remove the small, crescent-shaped muscle from the side of each scallop, if still attached. Dry the scallops thoroughly on paper towels, then transfer to a medium bowl.
2. Melt butter in a small saucepan, add garlic and cook for 1 minute. Let cool slightly then pour over the scallops. Season with salt and pepper and gently toss to coat.

3. Wrap a piece of bacon around each scallop and secure with a toothpick.
4. Supply your smoker with wood pellets and follow the start-up procedure. Preheat the grill, with the lid closed, to 400° F.
5. Arrange the scallops directly on the grill grate. Grill for 15 to 20 minutes, or until the scallop is opaque and the bacon has begun to crisp. If desired, you can turn the scallops on their side, bacon-side down, turning occasionally to crisp the bacon. Do not overcook. Grill: 400 °F
6. Transfer the scallops to a platter and serve with lemon wedges.

Grilled Lemon Salmon

Servings: 4
Cooking Time: 60 Minutes

Ingredients:

- Dill, Fresh
- 1 Lemon, Sliced
- 1 1/2 - 2 Lbs Salmon, Fresh

Directions:

1. Supply your smoker with wood pellets and follow the start-up procedure. Preheat the grill, with the lid closed, to 225° F.
2. Place the salmon on a cedar plank. Lay the lemon slices along the top of the salmon. Smoke in your Grill for about 60 minutes.
3. Top with fresh dill and serve.

Mango Rice Wine Thai Shrimp

Servings: 4
Cooking Time: 15 Minutes

Ingredients:

- 2 Tablespoons Brown Sugar
- 2 Tablespoons Mango Magic Seasoning
- 1 Pinch (Optional) Red Pepper Flakes
- 1/2 Tablespoons Rice Wine Vinegar
- 1 Pound Raw Tail-On, Thaw And Deveined Shrimp, Uncooked

- 2 Tablespoons Soy Sauce
- 1 Teaspoon Sriracha Hot Sauce
- 1/2 Cup Sweet Chili Sauce

Directions:

1. Supply your smoker with wood pellets and follow the start-up procedure. Preheat the grill, with the lid closed, to 425° F. Rinse shrimp off in sink with cold water. Place in bowl and put in all of the ingredients listed above. Let marinade for 2 - 4 hours.

2. Thread several shrimp onto a skewer, so that they are all just touching each other. Repeat with other skewers and remaining shrimp.

3. Grill shrimp for 2 - 3 minutes on each side, or until pink and opaque all the way through. Remove from grill and serve immediately.

Garlic Grilled Shrimp Skewers

Servings: 3
Cooking Time: 6 Minutes

Ingredients:

- 1 pound large shrimp
- 1/4 cup olive oil
- 1/4 cup fresh cilantro, finely chopped
- 1/4 cup fresh parsley, finely chopped
- 4 cloves garlic, minced
- 1 tablespoon lemon juice
- 1/2 teaspoon salt
- 1/4 teaspoon black pepper
- Pinch cayenne pepper, adjust to spice preference

Directions:

1. Add the olive oil, herbs, and spices to a small mixing bowl and whisk together.

2. Place the shrimp in a bowl and pour 3/4 of the marinade on top of the shrimp. Mix together gently to coat the shrimp evenly.

3. Cover the bowl and marinate the shrimp for 30 minutes to an hour.

4. Thread the shrimp on the skewers and make sure to get all the good garlic and herbs from the bowl and spread on to the shrimp.

5. Supply your smoker with wood pellets and follow the start-up procedure. Preheat the grill, with the lid closed, to medium high heat.

6. Once the grill is hot, arrange the shrimp skewers on the grill and cook for 2-3 minutes per side, or until they turn pink and opaque.

7. Remove the shrimp skewers to a plate and spoon the remaining marinade on top before serving.

Vodka Brined Smoked Wild Salmon

Servings: 4
Cooking Time: 60 Minutes

Ingredients:

- 1 Cup brown sugar
- 1 Tablespoon black pepper
- 1/2 Cup coarse salt
- 1 Cup vodka
- 1 (1-1/2 to 2 lb) wild caught salmon
- 1 lemon wedges
- capers

Directions:

1. In a small bowl, whisk together brown sugar, pepper, salt and vodka.

2. Place the salmon in a large resealable bag. Pour in marinade and massage into the salmon. Refrigerate for 2 to 4 hours.

3. Remove from bag, rinse and dry with paper towels.

4. Supply your smoker with wood pellets and follow the start-up procedure. Preheat the grill, with the lid closed, to 180° F.

5. Smoke the salmon, skin-side down for 30 minutes.

6. Increase grill temperature to 225°F and continue to cook salmon for an additional 45 to 60 minutes or until the internal temperature in the thickest part of the fish reaches 140°F or the fish flakes easily when pressed with a finger or fork. Grill: 225 °F Probe: 140 °F

7. Serve with lemons and capers. Enjoy!

Grilled Albacore Tuna With Potato-tomato Casserole

Servings: 8
Cooking Time: 20 Minutes

Ingredients:

- 6 Tuna Steaks, 6oz
- 1 Whole lemon zest
- 1 chile de árbol, thinly sliced
- 1 Tablespoon thyme
- 1 Tablespoon fresh parsley

Directions:

1. To make the fish: Season the fish with the lemon zest, chile, thyme, and parsley. Cover and refrigerate at least 4 hours.
2. Remove fish from the refrigerator 30 minutes before cooking to come to room temperature.
3. Season the fish with salt and pepper on both sides. Grill 2-3 minutes per side (next to the cast iron with the casserole) rotating it once or twice. The tuna should be well seared but still rare.

Baked Steelhead

Servings: 4
Cooking Time: 20 Minutes

Ingredients:

- 1 steelhead fillet
- 16-oz bottle Italian dressing
- 3 Tablespoon unsalted butter
- Blackened Saskatchewan Rub
- 1/2 shallot, minced
- 2 Clove garlic, minced
- 1 lemon

Directions:

1. Supply your smoker with wood pellets and follow the start-up procedure. Preheat the grill, with the lid closed, to 350° F.
2. Put butter in a small cast iron pan and place inside Traeger while preheating to soften. Pour Italian dressing over fillet to evenly coat.
3. Shake Traeger Blackened Saskatchewan rub evenly in a thin layer to cover dressing. Mince shallot and garlic.

4. Remove butter from pre-heated grill, careful as the cast iron will be hot. Stir in shallots and garlic.
5. Spread a nice thick layer of mixture on the top-middle of the fillet. Cut lemon into thin slices and place on top of butter mix.
6. Place steelhead on the grill and cook for 20 to 30 minutes, until fish is flaky, being careful not to over cook.
7. Remove fillet from the grill. Enjoy!

Grilled Garlic Shrimp With Cajun Dip

Servings: 4
Cooking Time: 15 Minutes

Ingredients:

- 1 Grated Garlic Cloves, Peeled
- 1 Tsp Lemon Juice
- ½ Cup Mayonnaise
- 2 Tbsp Olive Oil
- 1 ½ Tbsp Hickory Bacon Rub
- Scallions
- ½ Lb Shelled And Deveined Shrimp
- 1 Cup Sour Cream

Directions:

1. Supply your smoker with wood pellets and follow the start-up procedure. Preheat the grill, with the lid closed, to 350° F. If you're using a gas or charcoal grill, set it to medium heat.
2. In a glass mixing bowl, add mayonnaise, sour cream, Cajun seasoning, garlic, lemon juice, hot sauce, and Hickory Bacon. Whisk together until well combined.
3. Cajun shrimp: In a small bowl, add shrimp, olive oil, Cajun-style seasoning and Hickory Bacon seasoning and toss to combine. Set aside.
4. Transfer dip mixture into cast iron ramekin or small Dutch oven and cover with foil. Place on preheated grill and cook for 10-15 minutes, or until dip begins to bubble along the edges. At the same time, place cast iron pan on grill and add shrimp. Cook for about 3-5 minutes on each side or until shrimp are opaque.
5. Remove dip from grill and top with Cajun shrimp and scallions. Serve warm alongside garlic toast squares and enjoy!

Smoked Salmon Candy

Servings: 4
Cooking Time: 180 Minutes

Ingredients:

- 2 Cup gin
- 1 Cup dark brown sugar
- 1/2 Cup kosher salt
- 1 Cup maple syrup
- 1 Tablespoon black pepper
- 3 Pound salmon
- vegetable oil
- dark brown sugar

Directions:

1. In a large bowl, combine all ingredients for the cure.
2. Cut the salmon into 2 ounce pieces and place in the cure.
3. Cover and refrigerate overnight.
4. Supply your smoker with wood pellets and follow the start-up procedure. Preheat the grill, with the lid closed, to 180° F.
5. Spray foil with vegetable oil. Place salmon on foil and sprinkle with additional brown sugar.
6. Place foil directly on the grill grate. Close the lid and smoke the salmon for 3 to 4 hours or until fully cooked. Grill: 180 °F
7. Serve hot or chilled. Enjoy!

Smoky Crab Dip

Servings: 6
Cooking Time: 20 Minutes

Ingredients:

- 1/3 Cup mayonnaise
- 3 Ounce sour cream
- 1 Teaspoon smoked paprika
- 1/4 Teaspoon cayenne pepper
- 1 1/2 Pound Crab meat, lump
- salt and pepper
- scallions, chopped
- butter crackers

Directions:

1. Supply your smoker with wood pellets and follow the start-up procedure. Preheat the grill, with the lid closed, to 350° F.
2. Meanwhile, in a large bowl gently stir together all of the ingredients except the crackers, garnish scallions and the crab meat until thoroughly combined. Gently fold in the crab meat, being careful not to break it up too much.
3. Season to taste and transfer to an oven-safe serving dish.
4. Bake for 20 to 25 minutes, until bubbly and golden on top. Grill: 350 °F
5. Garnish with the additional chopped scallions and serve warm with butter crackers. Enjoy!

Spicy Lime Shrimp

Servings: 4
Cooking Time: 10 Minutes

Ingredients:

- 2 Tsp Chili Paste
- 1/2 Tsp Cumin
- 2 Cloves Garlic, Minced
- 1 Large Lime, Juiced
- 1/4 Tsp Paprika, Powder
- 1/4 Tsp Red Flakes Pepper
- 1/2 Tsp Salt

Directions:

1. In a bowl, whisk together the lime juice, olive oil, garlic, chili powder, cumin, paprika, salt, pepper, and red pepper flakes.
2. Then pour it into a resealable bag, add the shrimp, toss the coat, let it marinate for 30 minutes.
3. Supply your smoker with wood pellets and follow the start-up procedure. Preheat the grill, with the lid closed, to 400° F.
4. Next place the shrimp on skewers, place on the grill, and grill each side for about two minutes until it's done. One finished, remove the shrimp from the grill and enjoy!

Swordfish With Sicilian Olive Oil Sauce

Servings: 4
Cooking Time: 10 Minutes

Ingredients:
- 1/2 Cup extra-virgin olive oil, plus 2 tablespoons for oiling the fish
- 1 Whole lemon, juiced
- 2 Clove garlic, minced
- 3 Tablespoon finely chopped fresh parsley
- 1 Tablespoon finely chopped fresh oregano or 1 teaspoon dried oregano
- 1 Tablespoon brined capers, drained (optional)
- 4 (6 to 8 oz) swordfish, halibut, tuna or salmon steaks, 1 inch thick
- salt and pepper

Directions:
1. Put 1/2 cup of olive oil in a small saucepan and warm over low heat.
2. Whisk in lemon juice and 2 tablespoons hot water. Stir in garlic, parsley, oregano, capers (if using), and salt and pepper to taste (go easy on the salt if you're using capers). Keep warm.
3. Supply your smoker with wood pellets and follow the start-up procedure. Preheat the grill, with the lid closed, to 400° F.
4. Brush the fish steaks with 2 tablespoons of olive oil and season with salt and pepper. Grill: 400 °F
5. Arrange on the grill grate and grill until the fish is opaque and flakes easily when pressed with a fork, about 18 minutes. (If you prefer your tuna or salmon on the rare side, cook them for less time.) Grill: 400 °F
6. Transfer the fish steaks to a platter or plates and drizzle with the warm olive oil sauce.
7. Serve the remaining sauce on the side. Enjoy!

Dijon-smoked Halibut

Servings: 6
Cooking Time: 120 Minutes

Ingredients:
- 4 (6-ounce) halibut steaks
- ¼ cup extra-virgin olive oil
- 2 teaspoons kosher salt
- 1 teaspoon freshly ground black pepper
- ½ cup mayonnaise
- ½ cup sweet pickle relish
- ¼ cup finely chopped sweet onion
- ¼ cup chopped roasted red pepper
- ¼ cup finely chopped tomato
- ¼ cup finely chopped cucumber
- 2 tablespoons Dijon mustard
- 1 teaspoon minced garlic

Directions:
1. Rub the halibut steaks with the olive oil and season on both sides with the salt and pepper. Transfer to a plate, cover with plastic wrap, and refrigerate for 4 hours.
2. Supply your smoker with wood pellets and follow the start-up procedure. Preheat, with the lid closed, to 200°F.
3. Remove the halibut from the refrigerator and rub with the mayonnaise.
4. Put the fish directly on the grill grate, close the lid, and smoke for 2 hours, or until opaque and an instant-read thermometer inserted in the fish reads 140°F.
5. While the fish is smoking, combine the pickle relish, onion, roasted red pepper, tomato, cucumber, Dijon mustard, and garlic in a medium bowl. Refrigerate the mustard relish until ready to serve.
6. Serve the halibut steaks hot with the mustard relish.

Spicy Shrimp Skewers

Servings: 4
Cooking Time: 6 Minutes

Ingredients:
- 2 Pound shrimp, peeled and deveined
- 6 Thai chiles
- 6 Clove garlic
- 2 Tablespoon Winemaker's Napa Valley Rub
- 1 1/2 Teaspoon sugar
- 1 1/2 Tablespoon white vinegar
- 3 Tablespoon olive oil

Directions:

1. If using bamboo skewers, place them in cold water to soak for 1 hour before grilling.

2. Place shrimp in a bowl and set aside. Combine all remaining ingredients in a blender and blend until a coarse-textured paste is reached. Note: if a milder flavor is preferred, feel free to adjust amount of chiles to taste.

3. Add chile-garlic mixture to the shrimp and place in fridge to marinate for at least 30 minutes.

4. Remove from fridge and thread shrimp onto bamboo or metal skewers.

5. Supply your smoker with wood pellets and follow the start-up procedure. Preheat the grill, with the lid closed, to 450° F.

6. Place shrimp on grill and cook for 2 to 3 minutes per side or until shrimp are pink and firm to touch. Enjoy! Grill: 450 °F

Shrimp Cabbage Tacos With Lime Cream

Servings: 4
Cooking Time: 10 Minutes

Ingredients:
- 1/4 Cabbage, Shredded
- 2 Tsp Cilantro, Chopped
- Corn Tortillas
- 1/2 Lime, Wedges
- 1/4 Cup Mayonnaise
- Blackened Sriracha Rub
- 1/4 Red Bell Pepper, Chopped
- 1 Lb Shrimp, Peeled & Deveined
- 1/4 Cup Sour Cream
- 2 Tsp Vegetable Oil
- 1/2 White Onion, Chopped

Directions:
1. Place shrimp In a medium bowl. Season with Blackened Sriracha Rub, then drizzle with vegetable oil. Toss by hand to coat well then set aside.

2. In a small mixing bowl, stir together mayonnaise, sour cream, and fresh lime juice. Season to taste with Blackened Sriracha. Set aside.

3. In a small mixing bowl, combine jalapeño, onion, red bell pepper, and cilantro. Set aside.

4. Supply your smoker with wood pellets and follow the start-up procedure. Preheat the grill, with the lid closed, till over medium heat. If using a grill, preheat a cast iron skillet over medium-heat.

5. Place tortillas on the griddle to warm each side, then turn off the burner below.

6. Transfer shrimp to the hot griddle, and cook for 4 to 6 minutes, tossing occasionally, until opaque. For spicier shrimp, season with additional Blackened Sriracha.

7. Assemble tacos: shredded cabbage, shrimp, pepper mixture, then drizzle with sauce. Serve warm with fresh lime wedges.

Oysters In The Shell

Servings: 4
Cooking Time: 20 Minutes

Ingredients:
- 8 medium oysters, unopened, in the shell, rinsed and scrubbed
- 1 batch Lemon Butter Mop for Seafood

Directions:
1. Supply your smoker with wood pellets and follow the start-up procedure. Preheat the grill, with the lid closed, to 375°F.

2. Place the unopened oysters directly on the grill grate and grill for about 20 minutes, or until the oysters are done and their shells open.

3. Discard any oysters that do not open. Shuck the remaining oysters, transfer them to a bowl, and add the mop. Serve immediately.

Grilled Trout With Citrus & Basil

Servings: 4
Cooking Time: 10 Minutes

Ingredients:
- 6 Whole Trout
- 2 Teaspoon Blackened Saskatchewan Rub
- 10 Sprig fresh basil
- 2 Lemons, cut in half
- extra-virgin olive oil

Directions:

1. Supply your smoker with wood pellets and follow the start-up procedure. Preheat the grill, with the lid closed, to 450° F.

2. Season the center cavity of the trout with the Traeger Blackened Saskatchewan. Place two sprigs of Basil in each cavity, then add 4 lemon halves.

3. Next tie the fish closed using the Butchers twine, and then rub with olive oil.

4. Place the trout on the hot grill and cook 5 minutes on each side. Enjoy! Grill: 450 °F

Planked Trout With Fennel, Bacon & Orange

Servings: 4

Cooking Time: 40minutes

Ingredients:

• 4 whole trout, each about 14 to 16oz (400 to 450g), cleaned and gutted, fins removed

• coarse salt

• freshly ground black pepper

' for the filling

1 large navel orange

4 slices of thick-cut bacon, diced

1 large fennel bulb, trimmed, halved, decored, and ed, green fronds reserved

4oz (110g) baby spinach, about 6 cups

coarse salt

freshly ground black pepper

ctions:

upply your smoker with wood pellets and follow tart-up procedure. Preheat the grill, with the lid !, to 450° F. Place 4 cedar planks on the grate and them to singe slightly on both sides. Remove them he grill and place them on a heatproof surface to

wer the temperature to 300°F (149°C).

ce 4 thin rounds from the center of the orange en slice each in half for 8 pieces total. Zest the der of the orange and set aside.

a cold skillet on the stovetop over medium heat, e bacon, until the fat has rendered and the bacon n brown, about 6 to 8 minutes, stirring frequently.

Use a slotted spoon to transfer the bacon to paper towels to drain. Add the fennel to the fat in the skillet and cook until tender crisp, about 5 minutes. Add the spinach and stir until it wilts, about 1 to 2 minutes. Squeeze the juice of one of the reserved orange ends over the mixture. Add the drained bacon. Season with salt and pepper and then stir. Remove the skillet from the stovetop and set aside.

5. Rinse each trout inside and out under cold running water and pat dry with paper towels. Place three 12-inch (30.5cm) pieces of butcher's twine on each plank and place a trout on top. Season the inside of each fish with salt and pepper. Place two half-rounds of orange in each belly, rind side facing out. Top with some of the filling. Tie the trout with the butcher's twine and trim any ends. Repeat with the remaining trout.

6. Place the planks on the grate and cook the trout until they're cooked through, about 30 to 40 minutes.

7. Remove the planks from the grill and remove the twine. Top each trout with a few curls of orange zest and some reserved fennel fronds. Serve the trout on the planks.

Moules Marinières With Garlic Butter Sauce

Servings: 4

Cooking Time: 12 Minutes

Ingredients:

• 3lb (1.4kg) fresh mussels, scrubbed under cold running water and debearded

• lemon wedges

• crusty bread (optional)

• for the sauce

• 6 tbsp unsalted butter

• 3 garlic cloves, peeled and minced

• 1 cup dry white wine or hard cider

• 1 tbsp freshly squeezed lemon juice

• 2 tsp hot sauce, plus more

• coarse salt

• freshly ground black pepper

• 2 tbsp chopped fresh curly parsley or tarragon

Directions:

1. Supply your smoker with wood pellets and follow the start-up procedure. Preheat the grill, with the lid closed, to 450° F.

2. In a small saucepan on the stovetop over medium-low heat, make the sauce by melting the butter. Add the garlic and sauté for 1 to 2 minutes. Add the wine, lemon juice, and hot sauce. Season with salt and pepper to taste. Simmer for 5 minutes. Remove the saucepan from the heat and stir in the parsley. Keep warm.

3. Discard any mussels that are cracked or don't snap shut when tapped. Place the mussels in a large aluminum foil roasting pan and cover tightly with heavy-duty aluminum foil.

4. Place the pan on the grate and steam the mussels until the shells open, about 10 to 12 minutes. Remove the pan from the grill and use long-handled tongs to remove the foil from the pan. (Be careful of escaping steam.) Use the tongs to discard any mussels that don't open.

5. Pour the reserved garlic butter sauce over the mussels. Serve from the pan or transfer the mussels to a shallow serving bowl. Serve immediately with lemon wedges, additional hot sauce, and crusty bread (if using) to sop up the juices.

Smoked Lobster Scampi

Servings: 2
Cooking Time: 30 Minutes

Ingredients:
- 1 Lobster Tail
- 1 Handful Pasta, Angel Hair
- 2 Tablespoon butter
- 1 Teaspoon garlic, minced
- 1/2 Teaspoon lemon juice
- 2 Teaspoon Parmesan cheese, grated
- 2 Tablespoon Sun Dried Tomato Pesto
- fresh parsley

Directions:
1. Supply your smoker with wood pellets and follow the start-up procedure. Preheat the grill, with the lid closed, to 180° F.

2. Use kitchen shears to cut along the top of the lobster on both sides to expose the meat. Place the lobster directly on the grill for 20-25 minutes, depending on the size of the lobster. Grill: 180 °F

3. While lobster smokes, cook pasta according to packaged directions.

4. After 20-25 minutes, take lobster off the grill and remove the meat from the tail. Cut meat into chunks.

5. While the pasta is boiling, melt butter over medium high heat. Once butter starts to brown, add the garlic and lobster chunks. Toss in pan a few times then add lemon and parmesan. Set aside.

6. When pasta has finished, place 1 tbsp of the sun dried tomato pesto on the bottom of a bowl or plate. Top with pasta, then finish with the lobster scampi. Garnish with parsley. Enjoy!

Cajun-blackened Shrimp

Servings: 4
Cooking Time: 20 Minutes

Ingredients:
- 1 pound peeled and deveined shrimp, with tails on
- 1 batch Cajun Rub
- 8 tablespoons (1 stick) butter
- ¼ cup Worcestershire sauce

Directions:
1. Supply your smoker with wood pellets and follow the start-up procedure. Preheat the grill, with the lid closed, to 450°F and place a cast-iron skillet on the grill grate. Wait about 10 minutes after your grill has reached temperature, allowing the skillet to get hot.

2. Meanwhile, season the shrimp all over with the rub.

3. When the skillet is hot, place the butter in it to melt. Once the butter melts, stir in the Worcestershire sauce.

4. Add the shrimp and gently stir to coat. Smoke-braise the shrimp for about 10 minutes per side, until opaque and cooked through. Remove the shrimp from the grill and serve immediately.

22

Simple Glazed Salmon Fillets

Servings: 2

Cooking Time: 25 Minutes

Ingredients:

- 4 (6-8 oz) center-cut salmon fillets, skin on
- Fin & Feather Rub
- 1/2 Cup mayonnaise
- 2 Tablespoon Dijon mustard
- 1 Tablespoon fresh lemon juice
- 1 Tablespoon fresh chopped tarragon or dill
- lemon wedges

Directions:

1. Season the fillets with the Traeger Fin & Feather Rub.
2. Make the Glaze: Combine the mayonnaise and mustard in a small bowl. Stir in the lemon juice and dill or tarragon.
3. Spread the flesh-side of the fillets with the glaze.
4. Supply your smoker with wood pellets and follow the start-up procedure. Preheat the grill, with the lid closed, to 350° F.
5. Arrange the salmon fillets on the grill grate, skin-side down. Grill for 25 to 30 minutes, or until the salmon is opaque and flakes easily with a fork. Grill: 350 °F
6. Transfer to a platter or plates, garnish with sliced lemons and chopped dill and serve immediately. Enjoy!

Alder Smoked Scallops With Citrus & Garlic Butter Sauce

Servings: 4

Cooking Time: 35 Minutes

Ingredients:

- 2 Pound large dry sea scallops
- kosher salt
- freshly ground black pepper
- 8 Tablespoon salted butter, melted
- 1 Clove garlic, minced
- 1 Small orange
- 1/4 Teaspoon Worcestershire sauce
- 1 1/2 Teaspoon fresh chopped parsley or tarragon

- flat-leaf parsley, for serving

Directions:

1. Wash the scallops under cold running water and thoroughly pat dry on paper towels. Remove any tags of abductor muscle tissue you find on the sides of the scallops.
2. Arrange the scallops on a baking sheet fitted with a cooling rack, and season with salt and pepper.
3. Supply your smoker with wood pellets and follow the start-up procedure. Preheat the grill, with the lid closed, to 165° F.
4. Place the baking sheet with the scallops on the grill grate and smoke for 20 minutes.
5. While your scallops are smoking, make your sauce. Melt the butter in a small saucepan over medium-low heat. Add a pinch of salt, garlic, Worcestershire sauce, zest and juice from half of the orange, and parsley. Simmer for 5 minutes. Keep warm.
6. Remove the baking sheet with the scallops from the grill and set aside. Increase the temperature to 400°F and preheat, lid closed. Optional: Place an oyster bed or oyster pan in the grill to preheat. These heavy iron pans are a great way to sear the scallops. Grill: 400 °F
7. Return the baking sheet with the scallops to the grill, brush with the butter sauce, reserving some for serving. Roast until just opaque and tender, 10 to 15 minutes. The time will depend on how thick the scallops are. Do not overcook. If you are using an oyster pan, brush each compartment lightly with olive oil to prevent sticking. Spoon butter sauce on each of the scallops, reserving some for serving.
8. Serve the scallops hot with a little more orange zest, fresh parsley and the the warm citrus and garlic butter sauce. Enjoy!

Traeger Jerk Shrimp

Servings: 8

Cooking Time: 10 Minutes

Ingredients:

- 1 Tablespoon brown sugar
- 1 Tablespoon smoked paprika
- 1 Teaspoon garlic powder

- 1/4 Teaspoon Thyme, ground
- 1/4 Teaspoon ground cayenne pepper
- 1 Teaspoon sea salt
- 1 lime zest
- 2 Pound shrimp in shell
- 3 Tablespoon olive oil

Directions:

1. Combine spices, salt, and lime zest in a small bowl and mix. Place shrimp into a large bowl, then drizzle in the olive oil, Add the spice mixture and toss to combine, making sure every shrimp is kissed with deliciousness.

2. Supply your smoker with wood pellets and follow the start-up procedure. Preheat the grill, with the lid closed, to 450° F.

3. Arrange the shrimp on the grill and cook for 2 – 3 minutes per side, until firm, opaque, and cooked through. Grill: 450 °F

4. Serve with lime wedges, fresh cilantro, mint, and Caribbean Hot Pepper Sauce. Enjoy!

Lobster Tail

Servings: 2
Cooking Time: 25 Minutes

Ingredients:

- 2 lobster tails
- Salt
- Freshly ground black pepper
- 1 batch Lemon Butter Mop for Seafood

Directions:

1. Supply your smoker with wood pellets and follow the start-up procedure. Preheat the grill, with the lid closed, to 375°F.

2. Using kitchen shears, slit the top of the lobster shells, through the center, nearly to the tail. Once cut, expose as much meat as you can through the cut shell.

3. Season the lobster tails all over with salt and pepper.

4. Place the tails directly on the grill grate and grill until their internal temperature reaches 145°F. Remove the lobster from the grill and serve with the mop on the side for dipping.

Lemon Shrimp Scampi

Servings: 3
Cooking Time: 10 Minutes

Ingredients:

- 2 Tsp Blackened Sriracha Rub Seasoning
- 1/2 Cup Butter, Cubed, Divided
- 1/2 Tsp Chili Pepper Flakes
- 3 Garlic Cloves, Minced
- To Taste, Lemon Wedges, For Serving
- 1 Lemon, Juice & Zest
- Linguine, Cooked
- 3 Tbsp Parsley, Chopped
- 1 1/2 Lbs Shrimp, Peeled & Deveined
- Toasted Baguette, For Serving

Directions:

1. Supply your smoker with wood pellets and follow the start-up procedure. Preheat the grill, with the lid closed, to medium-high heat. If using a gas or charcoal grill, set it up for medium-high heat.

2. Add half of the butter to the griddle, then sauté the garlic, Blackened Sriracha, and chili flakes for 1 minute, until fragrant.

3. Add the shrimp, turning occasionally for 2 minutes, until opaque.

4. Add the remaining butter, parsley, lemon zest and juice. Toss the shrimp to coat in lemon butter, then remove from the griddle, and transfer to a serving bowl.

5. Serve immediately, with fresh lemon wedges, and toasted baguette. Serve over linguine, spaghetti or zucchini noodles, if desired.

Cider Hot-smoked Salmon

Servings: 4
Cooking Time: 60 Minutes

Ingredients:

- 1 1/2 Pound Wild Caught Salmon Fillet, skinned, pin bones removed
- 12 Ounce apple juice or cider
- 4 Pieces juniper berries
- 1 Pieces Star Anise, Broken
- 1 Pieces bay leaf, coarsely crumbled
- 1/2 Cup kosher salt

- 1/4 Cup brown sugar
- 2 Teaspoon Blackened Saskatchewan Rub
- 1 Teaspoon coarse ground black pepper, divided

Directions:

1. Rinse the salmon fillet under cold running water and check for pin bones by running a finger over the fleshy part of the fillet. If you feel a bone, remove it with kitchen tweezers or a needle-nose pliers.

2. In a sturdy resealable plastic bag, combine the cider, crushed juniper berries, star anise, and bay leaf. Add the salmon fillet and put the bag in a bowl or pan in the refrigerator. Let sit for at least 8 hours, or overnight.

3. Remove the salmon from the bag and discard the cider mixture. Dry the salmon well on paper towels. Make the cure: In a small mixing bowl, combine the kosher salt, brown sugar, and Traeger rub.

4. Pour half into a shallow plate, or baking dish. Put the salmon fillet, skin-side down, on top of the cure. Generously sprinkle the top with the remaining cure, cover with plastic wrap, and refrigerate for 1 to 1-1/2 hours. Any longer, and the fish will get too salty.

5. Remove the salmon from the cure and pat dry with paper towels. Sprinkle the black pepper on top of the fillet.

6. Supply your smoker with wood pellets and follow the start-up procedure. Preheat the grill, with the lid closed, to 200° F.

7. Lay the salmon skin-side down on the grill grate. Cook for 1 hour, or until the internal temperature in the thickest part of the fish reaches 150 or the fish flakes easily when pressed with a finger or fork. Grill: 200 ˚F Probe: 150 ˚F

8. Let cool slightly. Turn the fillet over and remove the skin; it should come off in one piece.

9. If not serving immediately, let the salmon cool completely, then wrap in plastic wrap and refrigerate for up to 2 days. Transfer to a platter and serve with some or all of the suggested accompaniments. Enjoy!

Delicious Smoked Trout

Servings: 8
Cooking Time: 120 Minutes

Ingredients:

- 6 rainbow trout fillets
- Brine:
- 2 Tablespoons kosher salt
- 2 Tablespoons brown sugar
- 4 cups cool water

Directions:

1. For the brine, dissolve the kosher salt and brown sugar in water.

2. Place the trout fillets in the brine, skin side up, and brine the fillets for 15 minutes.

3. Supply your smoker with wood pellets and follow the start-up procedure. Preheat the grill, with the lid closed, to 180° F.

4. Remove the trout from the brine and transfer it to the grill grates.

5. Smoke the trout for 1.5 to 2 hours with the lid closed, depending on the thickness of your fillets.

6. Smoke until the trout reaches an internal temperature of 145 ˚F, or until the trout flakes easily.

7. Remove the trout from the smoker and serve warm, or let it cool completely and serve chilled with your favorite accouterments.

Flavour Fire Spiced Shrimp

Servings: 2
Cooking Time: 8 Minutes

Ingredients:

- 1 pound of extra large raw whole wild shrimp
- 1 tablespoon vegetable oil
- 1 tablespoon chili powder
- 1 teaspoon garlic powder
- 1/2 teaspoon onion powder
- 1/2 teaspoon cayenne pepper
- 1/4 teaspoon paprika
- 1/4 teaspoon dried oregano
- Pinch of Kosher salt

Directions:

1. Supply your smoker with wood pellets and follow the start-up procedure. Preheat the grill, with the lid closed, to High heat.

2. While grill is preheating, remove the shrimp shells, leaving the heads.

3. Butterfly shrimp by using a knife to cut each shrimp down the middle, from the head down to the tail.

4. Remove the vein, rinse off the shrimp and lightly dry off with paper towels.

5. Place the shrimp in a large bowl, sprinkle with all the seasonings and the oil.

6. Mix together, ensuring the mixture evenly covers each shrimp.

7. Using a skewer, impale the whole body of a shrimp, from head to tail. (Wrap them in aluminum foil if using wooden skewers).

8. Place the whole shrimp on the grill and cook for 3-4 minutes on each side (Or until shells turns pink and the shrimp is opaque).

9. Serve with your favorite sauce or condiment.

Pacific Northwest Salmon

Servings: 4
Cooking Time: 75 Minutes

Ingredients:
- 1 (2-pound) half salmon fillet
- 1 batch Dill Seafood Rub
- 2 tablespoons butter, cut into 3 or 4 slices

Directions:
1. Supply your smoker with wood pellets and follow the start-up procedure. Preheat the grill, with the lid closed, to 180°F.

2. Season the salmon all over with the rub. Using your hands, work the rub into the flesh.

3. Place the salmon directly on the grill grate, skin-side down, and smoke for 1 hour.

4. Place the butter slices on the salmon, equally spaced. Increase the grill's temperature to 300°F and continue to cook until the salmon's internal temperature reaches 145°F. Remove the salmon from the grill and serve immediately.

Grilled Maple Syrup Salmon

Servings: 6
Cooking Time: 30 Minutes

Ingredients:
- 1 large salmon fillet (around 3 pounds)
- 1/2 cup salted butter (melted)
- 2 tablespoons soy sauce
- Salt and pepper
- 1/4 cup maple syrup

Directions:
1. Supply your smoker with wood pellets and follow the start-up procedure. Preheat the grill, with the lid closed, to 400° F.

2. Place the salmon fillet in a baking pan lined with parchment paper.

3. Sprinkle the fish with salt and pepper.

4. Add half of the melted butter to the salmon and place the baking pan on the grill.

5. Grill for 15-20 minutes or until fish is roughly 70% cooked. It will feel still gelatinous in the thickest parts of the salmon.

6. Combine the remaining melted butter, soy sauce, and maple syrup and pour over the salmon.It will run off the sides so use a spoon to pour it back over the fish. It's also perfectly fine that some will be left on the sides of the pan.

7. Cook for 5 to 10 additional minutes or until the fish is cooked through. The fish should be firm to the touch but still moist and soft when pressed on,and the ridges will flake or pull apart if pressed on.

Bacon Wrapped Shrimp

Servings: 6
Cooking Time: 20 Minutes

Ingredients:
- 1 1/2 Pound Jumbo Shrimp, Peeled And Deveined
- 10 Strips Bacon
- Cheesy Grits, For Serving
- 1/4 Cup extra-virgin olive oil
- 2 Tablespoon lemon juice
- 1 Teaspoon Fresh Chopped Parsley
- 1 Tablespoon lemon zest
- 1 Teaspoon garlic, minced
- 1 Teaspoon salt
- 1/2 Teaspoon black pepper

Directions:

1. Rinse the shrimp under cold running water and dry thoroughly on paper towels.
2. Transfer to a re-sealable plastic bag or a bowl.
3. For the marinade: Combine the olive oil, lemon juice, lemon zest, garlic, salt, pepper, and parsley in a small jar with a tight-fitting lid and shake vigorously until combined.
4. Pour over the shrimp and refrigerate for 30 minutes to 1 hour.
5. Supply your smoker with wood pellets and follow the start-up procedure. Preheat the grill, with the lid closed, to 400° F.
6. Lay the bacon strips diagonally on the grill grate and grill for 10 to 12 minutes, or until the bacon is partially cooked but still very pliable.
7. Cut each strip in half width-wise. Leave the grill on.
8. Drain the shrimp, discarding the marinade. Wrap a strip of bacon around the body of each shrimp, securing with a toothpick. Grill for 4 minutes per side, turning once. Enjoy! Grill: 400 °F
9. Wrap a strip of bacon around the body of each shrimp, securing with a toothpick.
10. Grill for 4 minutes per side, turning once. Serve over cheesy grits, if desired. Enjoy!

Grilled Pepper Lobster Tails

Servings: 3
Cooking Time: 10 Minutes

Ingredients:

- Tt Black Pepper
- 3/4 Stick Butter, Room Temp
- 2 Tablespoons Chives, Chopped
- 1 Clove Garlic, Minced
- Lemon, Sliced
- 3 (7-Ounce) Lobster, Tail
- Tt Salt, Kosher

Directions:

1. Start your Grill on "SMOKE" with the lid open until a fire is established in the burn pot (3-7 minutes).
2. Supply your smoker with wood pellets and follow the start-up procedure. Preheat the grill, with the lid closed, to 350° F.

3. Blend butter, chives, minced garlic, and black pepper in a small bowl. Cover with plastic wrap and set aside.
4. Butterfly the tails down the middle of the softer underside of the shell. Don't cut entirely through the center of the meat. Brush the tails with olive oil and season with salt, to your liking.
5. Grill lobsters cut side down about 5 minutes until the shells are bright red in color. Flip the tails over and top with a generous tablespoon of herb butter. Grill for another 4 minutes, or until the lobster meat is an opaque white color.
6. Remove from the grill and serve with more herb butter and lemon wedges.

Bbq Roasted Salmon

Servings: 4
Cooking Time: 15 Minutes

Ingredients:

- 1/3 Cup honey
- 3 Tablespoon Mustard, whole-grain
- 1 Cup ketchup
- 1/2 Cup dark brown sugar
- 1 Teaspoon Cider Vinegar
- 1/2 Teaspoon Thyme Leaves, finely chopped
- 1/8 Teaspoon Jacobsen Salt Co. Pure Kosher Sea Salt
- 1/8 Teaspoon freshly ground black pepper
- 4 Whole Salmon Fillets, 6oz each, skin-on

Directions:

1. Combine all sauce ingredients in a large bowl, preferably one day prior to making the salmon.
2. Rub salmon fillets on both sides with sauce. Reserve any extra, unused sauce.
3. Supply your smoker with wood pellets and follow the start-up procedure. Preheat the grill, with the lid closed, to 350° F.
4. Place fillets on grill, skin-side down, and cook for 15 minutes. Grill: 350 °F
5. Let the fish rest for about 3-5 minutes. Serve with extra sauce. Enjoy!

Traeger Smoked Salmon

Servings: 6
Cooking Time: 240 Minutes

Ingredients:

- 1 (2-1/2 to 3 lb) salmon fillet
- 1/2 Cup kosher salt
- 1 Cup brown sugar, firmly packed
- 1 Tablespoon ground black pepper

Directions:

1. Remove all pin bones from salmon.
2. In a small bowl, combine salt, sugar and black pepper. Lay a large piece of plastic wrap on a flat surface that is at least 6 inches longer than the fillet. Spread 1/2 of the mixture on top of the plastic and lay the fillet skin side down on top of the cure. Top with the other 1/2 of the cure spreading it evenly over the top of the fillet. Fold up the edges of the plastic and wrap tightly.
3. Place the wrapped salmon fillet in the bottom of a flat, rectangle baking dish or hotel pan. Place another identical pan on top of the fillet. Place a couple of cans or something heavy inside the top pan to weigh it down making sure the weight is distributed evenly.
4. Transfer the weighted salmon to the refrigerator and cure for 4 to 6 hours.
5. Remove the salmon from the plastic wrap and rinse the cure thoroughly (not rinsing thoroughly will result in a salty finished product). Place skin side down on a wire rack atop a sheet tray and pat dry. Place the sheet tray in the refrigerator and allow the salmon to dry overnight. This allows a tacky film called a pellicle to form on the surface of the salmon. The pellicle helps smoke adhere to the fish.
6. Supply your smoker with wood pellets and follow the start-up procedure. Preheat the grill, with the lid closed, to 180° F.
7. Place the salmon skin side down directly on the grill grate and smoke for 3 to 4 hours or until the internal temperature of the fish registers 140°F. Enjoy warm or chilled. Grill: 180 °F Probe: 140 °F

Grilled Artichoke Cheese Salmon

Servings: 12

Cooking Time: 270 Minutes

Ingredients:

- 28 Oz Artichoke Hearts, Whole, Canned
- 1/2 Cup Breadcrumbs
- 1/2 Cup Brown Sugar
- 8 Oz Cream Cheese
- 1 Tbsp Garlic Powder
- 1 Cup Italian Cheese Blend, Shredded
- 1/4 Cup Kosher Salt
- 1 Cup Mayonnaise
- 2 Tsp Olive Oil
- 1 Tbsp Onion Powder
- 1/2 Cup Parmesan Cheese
- 2 Tbsp Parsley, Chopped
- Blackened Sriracha Rub
- 1 1/4 Lbs Salmon, Fillet, Scaled And Deboned
- Sour Cream
- 1/2 Tsp White Pepper, Ground

Directions:

1. In a small mixing bowl, whisk together the brown sugar, salt, garlic powder, onion powder, and white pepper. This will make twice the cure needed, so be sure and place the remaining half in a resealable plastic bag and save for smoking fish at a later date.
2. Lay a sheet of plastic wrap on a sheet tray and sprinkle a thin layer of the cure on it. Place the salmon skin-side down on top of the cure, then sprinkle a couple tablespoons of cure on top. Gently press the cure on top of the salmon flesh, then wrap in plastic wrap.
3. Refrigerate for 8 hours, or overnight.
4. Remove salmon from the refrigerator and wash off the cure in the sink, under cold water.
5. Blot salmon with a paper towel, then set salmon skin side on a wire rack. Dry at room temperature for two hours, or until a yellowish shimmer appears on the salmon.
6. Supply your smoker with wood pellets and follow the start-up procedure. Preheat the grill, with the lid closed, to 250° F. If using a gas, charcoal or other grill, set it to low, indirect heat.
7. Place the salmon in the upper cabinet. Smoke for 2 hours, then increase the grill temperature to 350° F to

maintain a cabinet temperature of 225°F and smoke another 1 to 2 hours, until salmon reaches an internal temperature of 145° F.

8. Remove salmon from the cabinet and set aside to rest for 15 minutes, then flake apart. Reserve ½ cup to top dip after grilling.

9. While the salmon is resting, drain the artichokes, then skewer onto metal skewers (if using wooden skewers, make sure to soak in water for 1 hour prior to grilling, or you can use a grill basket as well).

10. Season with Blackened Sriracha, then set on the grill. Grill for 2 to 3 minutes, until lightly browned.

11. Remove from the grill, cool slightly, then roughly chop. Set aside.

12. In a mixing bowl, combine shredded Italian cheese, grated parmesan, breadcrumbs and parsley. Set aside.

13. Place cream cheese, mayonnaise, and sour cream in a cast iron skillet. Stir frequently, with a wooden spoon, for about 5 minutes, until the mixture is smooth.

14. Carefully fold in flaked salmon and grilled artichoke hearts, then spread breadcrumb mixture over dip.

15. Drizzle with olive oil, then close the grill lid and bake for 25 to 30 minutes, until dip begins to bubble around the edges, and cheese begins to caramelize on top.

16. Remove dip from the grill, top with reserved salmon and a pinch of parsley. Serve warm with bagel chips, crackers, or crusty bread.

Garlic Bacon Wrapped Shrimp

Servings: 4
Cooking Time: 11 Minutes

Ingredients:

- 8 Bacon, Strip
- 1/4 Cup Butter Style Shortening (Melted)
- 1 Clove Garlic, Minced
- 1 Tsp Lemon, Juice
- Pepper
- Salt
- 16 (Peeled And Veined) Shrimp, Jumbo

Directions:

1. Supply your smoker with wood pellets and follow the start-up procedure. Preheat the grill, with the lid closed, to 450° F.

2. Take one slice of bacon, and wrap it around each piece of shrimp, and lock it in place with a wooden toothpick.

3. Place the shortening into a mixing bowl and whisk in the garlic and lemon juice. Brush each shrimp with the sauce on both sides.

4. Place on the grill, and barbecue for 11 minutes.

5. Turn the grill off, remove the shrimp, serve and enjoy!

Kimi's Simple Grilled Fresh Fish

Servings: 2
Cooking Time: 45 Minutes

Ingredients:

- 1 Cup soy sauce
- 1/3 Cup extra-virgin olive oil
- 1 Tablespoon garlic, minced
- 2 lemons, juiced
- fresh basil
- 4 Pound Fresh Fish, cut into portion-sized pieces

Directions:

1. Mix all ingredients to create sauce and cover fish in marinade for 45 minutes.

2. Supply your smoker with wood pellets and follow the start-up procedure. Preheat the grill, with the lid closed, to 140° F. Grill the marinated fish on the grill until it reaches an internal temperature of 140-145°F. Serve immediately, enjoy! Grill: 350 °F Probe: 145 °F

Roasted Halibut With Spring Vegetables

Servings: 4
Cooking Time: 20 Minutes

Ingredients:

- 4 thick-cut halibut fillets
- 2 Tablespoon Fin & Feather Rub
- Butcher Paper

- 1 Pound Carrots, Peeled and Cut into 3/4" Inch Slices
- 1 Pound asparagus, ends trimmed
- 1/2 Pound Oyster Mushrooms
- 2 Tablespoon butter
- salt and pepper
- 1/2 Cup white wine

Directions:

1. Season the halibut fillets with Traeger Fin and Feather Rub.

2. To build the packets: Start with four sheets of parchment paper about twenty inches long. Fold in half, then open it back up.

3. Divide the carrots, asparagus, and mushrooms between the four pieces of parchment and top each with a little bit of butter. Season with salt and pepper. Place a halibut fillet on top of the vegetables in each packet.

4. Next, fold the paper over so the two ends meet, enclosing the food. Beginning at either end of the center crease, make small, overlapping diagonal folds around the filling, sealing the packet tight. Before finishing the final fold, pour a little bit of wine in each packet then seal completely.

5. Supply your smoker with wood pellets and follow the start-up procedure. Preheat the grill, with the lid closed, to 500° F.

6. Place all four packets on a sheet tray and place in the grill. Cook for 7-10 minutes or until the internal temperature of the fish reaches 145°F. Remove from the grill and place packet on a serving dish. Grill: 500 °F Probe: 145 °F

7. Using a knife or scissors, cut open each packet and fold the edges back. Finish with a little bit of lemon juice if desired. Enjoy!

Mezcal Shrimp With Salsa De Molcajete

Servings: 4
Cooking Time: 14 Minutes

Ingredients:

- 18 to 24 jumbo shrimp, about 1½lb (680g) total, peeled and deveined
- ⅓ cup mezcal
- juice of ½ lime
- 2 tbsp extra virgin olive oil
- 2 tsp coarse salt
- 1 tsp ground cumin
- lime wedges
- for the salsa
- 2 Roma tomatoes
- 2 tomatillos, husked and washed
- 2 garlic cloves, peeled and impaled on a toothpick
- 1 jalapeño or serrano pepper
- 1 small white onion, halved
- ½ tsp coarse salt, plus more
- juice of ½ lime
- ¼ cup loosely packed fresh cilantro leaves

Directions:

1. Supply your smoker with wood pellets and follow the start-up procedure. Preheat the grill, with the lid closed, to 450° F.

2. In a large bowl, combine the shrimp, mezcal, lime juice, olive oil, salt, and ground cumin. Toss with your hands to mix thoroughly. Set aside for 15 minutes and then toss once more.

3. Begin to make the salsa by placing the tomatoes, tomatillos, garlic, jalapeño, and onion on the grate. Grill until they begin to char, about 3 minutes for the garlic and about 6 to 8 minutes for the other vegetables, turning as needed. Transfer the vegetables to a rimmed sheet pan. Remove the skewers from the garlic. Let everything cool. Coarsely chop the vegetables and leave them in separate piles.

4. Place the garlic in the molcajete and add the salt. Mash the garlic to a purée using the temolote. Add the onion and grind it into the garlic paste. Stir in the jalapeño (deseeded for a milder salsa), tomatoes, and tomatillos. Stir in the lime juice and cilantro leaves. Taste, adding salt. (If you don't own a molcajete or temolote, prepare the salsa using a small food processor.)

5. Drain the shrimp and discard the marinade. Thread the shrimp on wood or bamboo skewers. Place the shrimp on the grate and grill until they're white and opaque, about 4 to 6 minutes, tossing with tongs.

6. Transfer the shrimp to a platter. Serve with the salsa and lime wedges.

Grilled Tuna Steaks With Lemon & Caper Butter

Servings: 4
Cooking Time: 8 Minutes

Ingredients:

- 4 tuna steaks, each about 8oz (225g) and 1 inch (2.5cm) thick
- extra virgin olive oil
- coarse salt
- freshly ground black pepper
- for the butter
- 6 tbsp unsalted butter, chilled, divided
- 1 garlic clove, peeled and minced
- 3 tbsp brined capers, drained and coarsely chopped
- 1 tbsp freshly squeezed lemon juice, plus more
- 1 tsp lemon zest
- 1 tbsp minced fresh chives or flat-leaf parsley

Directions:

1. Supply your smoker with wood pellets and follow the start-up procedure. Preheat the grill, with the lid closed, to 450° F.
2. In a small saucepan on the stovetop over medium-low heat, begin making the butter by melting 1 tablespoon of butter. (Cut the remaining butter into ½-inch (1.25cm) cubes and keep them cold.) Add the garlic and capers. Cook until the garlic is softened, about 3 minutes. Stir in the lemon juice and zest. Remove the saucepan from the heat and set aside.
3. Lightly brush the tuna steaks with olive oil. Season with salt and pepper. Place the steaks on the grate and grill until seared, about 3 to 4 minutes per side. (The tuna will be quite rare in the center, almost like sashimi. If you prefer your tuna more well done, add 4 to 6 minutes to the grilling time.)
4. Transfer the steaks to a platter and let rest for 5 minutes.
5. Reheat the butter and caper mixture over low heat. Whisk in the chilled butter one or two cubes at a time until the sauce has emulsified. Stir in the chives. Ladle the sauce over the tuna. Serve immediately.

Bbq Oysters

Servings: 4
Cooking Time: 6 Minutes

Ingredients:

- 1 Pound unsalted butter, softened
- 1 Tablespoon Meat Church Holy Gospel BBQ Rub
- 1 Bunch green onions, chopped
- 2 Clove garlic, minced
- 12 oysters
- 1/4 Cup seasoned breadcrumbs
- 8 Ounce shredded pepper jack cheese
- Sweet & Heat BBQ Sauce
- 1/2 Bunch green onions, minced

Directions:

1. Supply your smoker with wood pellets and follow the start-up procedure. Preheat the grill, with the lid closed, to 375° F.
2. For the compound butter: Combine butter, garlic, onion and Meat Church Rub thoroughly.
3. Lay the butter on parchment paper or plastic wrap. Roll it up to form a log and tie each end with butcher's twine. Place in the freezer for an hour to solidify. You can use this butter on any grilled meat to enhance the flavor. You can also use a high-quality butter to replace the compound butter.
4. Shuck the oysters, keeping all of the juice in the shell. Sprinkle the oysters with breadcrumbs and place directly on the Traeger. Cook them for 5 minutes. You will be looking for the edge of the oyster to start to curl slightly.
5. After 5 minutes, place a spoonful of compound butter in the oysters. After the butter melts, add a pinch of pepper jack cheese.
6. Remove the oysters after 6 minutes on the grill total. Top oysters with a squirt of Traeger Sweet & Heat BBQ Sauce and a few chopped onions. Allow to cool for 5 minutes, then enjoy!

Citrus-smoked Trout

Servings: 6
Cooking Time: 120 Minutes

Ingredients:

- 6 to 8 skin-on rainbow trout, cleaned and scaled
- 1 gallon orange juice
- ½ cup packed light brown sugar
- ¼ cup salt
- 1 tablespoon freshly ground black pepper
- Nonstick spray, oil, or butter, for greasing
- 1 tablespoon chopped fresh parsley
- 1 lemon, sliced

Directions:

1. Fillet the fish and pat dry with paper towels.
2. Pour the orange juice into a large container with a lid and stir in the brown sugar, salt, and pepper.
3. Place the trout in the brine, cover, and refrigerate for 1 hour.
4. Cover the grill grate with heavy-duty aluminum foil. Poke holes in the foil and spray with cooking spray (see Tip).
5. Supply your smoker with wood pellets and follow the start-up procedure. Preheat, with the lid closed, to 225°F.
6. Remove the trout from the brine and pat dry. Arrange the fish on the foil-covered grill grate, close the lid, and smoke for 1 hour 30 minutes to 2 hours, or until flaky.
7. Remove the fish from the heat. Serve garnished with the fresh parsley and lemon slices.

Lime Mahi Mahi Fillets

Servings: 4
Cooking Time: 8 Minutes

Ingredients:

- 3/4 cup extra-virgin olive oil
- 1 clove garlic, minced
- 1/8 teaspoon ground black pepper
- 1/2 teaspoon cayenne pepper
- 2 tablespoons dill weed.
- 1 pinch salt
- 2 tablespoons lime juice

- 1/8 teaspoon grated lime peel
- 2 (4 ounce) mahi mahi fillets

Directions:

1. Supply your smoker with wood pellets and follow the start-up procedure. Preheat the grill, with the lid closed, to 325° F.
2. Lightly oil the grate.
3. Combine in a bowl the extra-virgin olive oil, minced garlic, black pepper, cayenne pepper, salt, lime juice, and grated lime zest.
4. Wisk to prepare the marinade.
5. Place the mahi mahi fillets in the marinade and turn to coat.
6. Allow to marinate at least 15 minutes.
7. Cook on preheated grill until fish flakes easily with a fork and is lightly browned (Typically 3 to 4 minutes per side).
8. Garnish with the twists of lime zest to serve.

Smoke-roasted Halibut With Mixed Herb Vinaigrette

Servings: 4
Cooking Time: 12 Minutes

Ingredients:

- 4 halibut fillets, each about 6 to 8oz (170 to 225g)
- for the vinaigrette
- 2 tbsp white wine vinegar or sherry vinegar, plus more
- ¼ tsp coarse salt, plus more
- ¼ tsp freshly ground black pepper, plus more
- ½ cup extra virgin olive oil
- 2 tbsp minced fresh herbs, such as dill, flat-leaf parsley, or oregano
- for serving
- 4 cups loosely packed baby arugula, spinach, or other mixed greens
- 1 lemon, cut lengthwise into 4 wedges

Directions:

1. Supply your smoker with wood pellets and follow the start-up procedure. Preheat the grill, with the lid closed, to 400° F.

2. In a small bowl, make the vinaigrette by whisking together the vinegar, and salt and pepper. Whisk until the salt dissolves. Continue to whisk while slowly adding the olive oil. Whisk until the vinaigrette is emulsified. Stir in the herbs. Taste, adding vinegar or salt and pepper to taste. Pour 1/3 of the vinaigrette into a separate container. Reserve the remainder.

3. Place the fillets on a rimmed sheet pan. Lightly brush both sides with the smaller portion of vinaigrette. (Dividing the vinaigrette into two containers prevents cross-contamination.) Lightly season with salt and pepper.

4. Place the fillets on the grate at an angle to the bars. Grill until the edges begin to look opaque, about 4 to 6 minutes. Gently turn and grill until the fish is cooked through, about 4 to 6 minutes more. (A fillet will break into clean flakes when pressed with a fork when it's done.)

5. Remove the fish from the grill. Place the greens in a large bowl and toss them with 2 to 3 tablespoons of the reserved vinaigrette (you want the greens lightly coated) and divide between 4 plates. Place a fillet on the greens on each plate. Drizzle a bit more of the vinaigrette over the top. Serve with lemon wedges.

Baked Tuna Noodle Casserole

Servings: 4
Cooking Time: 45 Minutes

Ingredients:

- 1 Whole Wheat Pasta, Box (13.25oz)
- 2 Cup Yogurt
- 1 Cup almond milk
- 1 Teaspoon ground mustard
- 1/2 Teaspoon celery salt
- 1 Cup Button Mushrooms, Sliced
- 10 Ounce Tuna, Cooked
- 1 Cup Peas, canned
- 1 Cup Cheese, Colby/Cheddar

Directions:

1. Bring a large pot of salted water to a boil over high heat. Add pasta and cook according to manufacturer's directions. Drain and set aside.

2. In a medium bowl mix yogurt, milk, ground mustard, and celery salt. Fold in mushrooms, tuna, peas and cooked pasta. Fold in half the cheese.

3. Transfer the mixture to a greased 13" x 9" baking dish and top with remaining cheese.

4. Supply your smoker with wood pellets and follow the start-up procedure. Preheat the grill, with the lid closed, to 350° F.

5. Place casserole dish directly on grill grate and cook for 45 minutes or until warmed through and cheese is melted. Enjoy! Grill: 350 °F

Grilled Lobster Tails With Smoked Paprika Butter

Servings: 4
Cooking Time: 10-12 Minutes

Ingredients:

- 4 lobster tails, each about 8 to 10oz (225 to 285g), thawed if frozen
- 3 lemons, 1 quartered lengthwise, 2 halved through their equators
- for the butter
- 1¼ cup unsalted butter, at room temperature
- 2 garlic cloves, peeled and finely minced
- 3 tbsp chopped fresh parsley
- 2 tbsp chopped fresh chives
- 1 tbsp freshly squeezed lemon juice
- 2 tsp finely chopped lemon zest
- 2 tsp smoked paprika
- 1 tsp coarse salt

Directions:

1. Supply your smoker with wood pellets and follow the start-up procedure. Preheat the grill, with the lid closed, to 450° F.

2. In a medium bowl, make the paprika butter by combining the ingredients. Beat with a wooden spoon until well blended.

3. Use a sharp, heavy knife or sturdy kitchen shears to cut lengthwise through the top shell of each lobster tail in a straight line toward the tail fin. Gently loosen the meat from the bottom shell and sides. Lift the meat through the slit you just made so the meat sits on top of

the shell. Slip a lemon quarter underneath the meat (between the meat and the bottom shell) to keep it elevated. Spread 1 tablespoon of paprika butter on top of each lobster. Melt the remaining butter and keep it warm.

4. Place the lobster tails flesh side up and lemon halves cut sides down on the grate. Grill the lobsters until the flesh is white and opaque and the internal temperature of the lobster meat reaches 135 to 140°F (57 to 60°C), about 10 to 12 minutes, basting at least once with some of the melted butter. (Don't overcook or the lobster will become unpleasantly rubbery.)

5. Transfer the lobsters and the lemon halves to a platter. Divide the remaining melted butter between 4 ramekins before serving.

Smoked Honey Salmon

Servings: 2
Cooking Time: 25 Minutes

Ingredients:

- 1 lb. salmon fillets
- 1/2 tsp. pepper
- 1/4 tsp. salt
- 2 tbsp. sriracha
- 2 tsp. honey
- 2 tsp. chili sauce
- 1 tsp. lime juice
- 1/2 tsp. fish sauce

Directions:

1. Supply your smoker with wood pellets and follow the start-up procedure. Preheat the grill, with the lid closed, to 350° F.

2. Sprinkle the salmon with salt and pepper.

3. In a bowl, whisk together the sriracha, honey, chili sauce, lime juice, and fish sauce.

4. Once the grill is hot, place the salmon on the grill and leave for 15 minutes.

5. After 15 minutes, brush the salmon with the sriracha chili sauce and keep cooking for 5-10minutes. The salmon should be firm to the touch and crispy on the edges.

6. Serve hot!

Smoked Trout

Servings: 6
Cooking Time: 120 Minutes

Ingredients:

- 8 rainbow trout fillets
- 1 Gallon water
- 1/4 Cup salt
- 1/2 Cup brown sugar
- 1 Tablespoon black pepper
- 2 Tablespoon soy sauce

Directions:

1. Clean the fresh fish and butterfly them.

2. For the Brine: Combine one gallon water, brown sugar, soy sauce, salt and pepper and stir until salt and sugar are dissolved. Brine the trout in the refrigerator for 60 minutes.

3. Supply your smoker with wood pellets and follow the start-up procedure. Preheat the grill, with the lid closed, to 225° F.

4. Remove the fish from the brine and pat dry. Place fish directly on grill grate for 1-1/2 to 2 hours, depending on the thickness of the trout. Fish is done when it turns opaque and starts to flake. Serve hot or cold. Enjoy! Grill: 225 °F

5. Fish is done when it turns opaque and starts to flake. Serve hot or cold. Enjoy!

Lemon Lobster Rolls

Servings: 4
Cooking Time: 35 Minutes

Ingredients:

- 1/2 Cup Butter
- 4 Hot Dog Bun(S)
- 1 Lemon, Whole
- 4 Lobster, Tail
- 1/4 Cup Mayo
- Pepper

Directions:

1. Supply your smoker with wood pellets and follow the start-up procedure. Preheat the grill, with the lid closed, to 300° F.

2. Using kitchen shears, cut the shell of the tail and crack in half so that the meat is exposed. Pour in butter and season with pepper. Place the tails meat side up on the grill and cook until the shell has turned red and the meat is white, about 35 minutes.

3. Remove from the grill and separate the shell from the meat. Place the meat in a bowl with mayo, lemon juice and rind and season with pepper. Stir to combine and evenly distribute into the hot dog buns.

Mexican Mahi Mahi With Baja Cabbage Slaw

Servings: 4
Cooking Time: 10 Minutes

Ingredients:
- 1½lb (680g) skinless mahi mahi, cod, or other firm white fish fillets
- coarse salt
- freshly ground black pepper
- chili powder
- lime wedges
- for the slaw
- 2 cups finely shredded green cabbage
- 2 cups finely shredded purple cabbage
- 4 tbsp reduced-fat mayo
- 2 tsp hot sauce, plus more
- 2 tsp freshly squeezed lime juice
- ½ tsp coarse salt
- for the marinade
- ¼ cup freshly squeezed orange juice
- ¼ cup freshly squeezed lime juice
- 2 tbsp extra virgin olive oil

Directions:
1. In a medium bowl, make the slaw by combining the ingredients. Stir well. Transfer to a serving bowl. Cover and refrigerate until ready to serve.

2. Place the fish fillets in a baking dish and pour the orange and lime juices and olive oil over them. Turn the fillets to coat thoroughly. Cover and refrigerate for 15 to 20 minutes.

3. Supply your smoker with wood pellets and follow the start-up procedure. Preheat the grill, with the lid closed, to 450° F.

4. Drain the fish and pat dry with paper towels. (Discard the marinade.) Season the fillets on both sides with salt and pepper and chili powder. Place the fillets on the grate and grill until golden brown, about 4 to 5 minutes per side, turning with a thin-bladed spatula.

5. Transfer the fish to a platter. Serve with the slaw and lime wedges.

Salmon Cakes With Homemade Tartar Sauce

Servings: 4
Cooking Time: 15 Minutes

Ingredients:
- 1 1/2 Cups Breadcrumb, Dry
- 1/2 Tablespoon Capers, Diced
- 1/4 Cup Dill Pickle Relish
- 2 Eggs
- 1 1/4 Cup Mayonnaise, Divided
- 1 Tablespoon Mustard, Grainy
- 1/2 Tablespoon Olive Oil
- 1/2 Red Pepper, Diced Finely
- 1/2 Tablespoon Sweet Rib Rub
- 1 Cup Cooked Salmon, Flaked

Directions:
1. In a large bowl, mix together the salmon, eggs, ¼ cup mayonnaise, breadcrumbs, red bell pepper, Sweet Rib Rub, and mustard. Allow the mixture to sit for 15 minutes to hydrate the breadcrumbs.

2. Supply your smoker with wood pellets and follow the start-up procedure. Preheat the grill, with the lid closed, to 350° F.

3. In a small bowl, mix together the remaining mayonnaise, dill pickle relish, and diced capers. Set aside.

4. Place the baking sheet on the grill to preheat. Once the baking sheet is hot, drizzle the olive oil over the pan and drop rounded tablespoons of the salmon mixture onto the sheet pan. Press the mixture down into a flat patty with a spatula. Allow to grill for 3 to 5 minutes, then flip and grill for 1 to 2 more minutes. Remove from the grill and serve with the reserved tartar sauce.

Cold-smoked Salmon Gravlax

Servings: 6
Cooking Time: 30 Minutes

Ingredients:

* 1 Cup kosher salt
* 1 Cup sugar
* 1 Tablespoon freshly ground black pepper
* 2 Pound Sushi-Grad Salmon Fillet, Skin-on, Pin Bones Removed
* 2 Bunch Dill Weed, fresh
* capers, drained
* red onion, sliced
* cream cheese
* lemons

Directions:

1. In a bowl stir together the salt, sugar and black pepper until thoroughly combined. On a work surface, turn salmon skin side up and sprinkle about half of salt mixture all over and rub in.
2. Arrange half the dill on the bottom of a baking dish large enough to hold the salmon. Set salmon skin side down on bed of dill.
3. Rub remaining salt mixture all over top and sides of salmon, then top with remaining dill. Cover with plastic, then top with a weight on a smaller baking dish or a plate with cans of beans on top, then place in refrigerator and allow to cure for 2 days.
4. Remove salmon from refrigerator, rinse under cold water and pat dry with paper towels. Allow to sit at room temperature on the counter for 1 hour
5. Supply your smoker with wood pellets and follow the start-up procedure. Preheat the grill, with the lid closed, to 180° F. Place salmon onto a baking pan. Fill another baking pan with ice and place baking pan with salmon over ice. Place onto grill and smoke for 30 minutes.
6. Remove from grill and slice thin. Serve with capers, red onion, dill, cream cheese, and lemon. Enjoy!

Sweet Mandarin Salmon

Servings: 2
Cooking Time: 10 Minutes

Ingredients:

* 1 Whole lime juice
* 1 Teaspoon sesame oil
* 1 1/2 Cup Mandarin Orange Sauce
* 1 1/2 Tablespoon soy sauce
* 2 Tablespoon cilantro, finely chopped
* Freshly cracked black pepper
* 1 Whole (4 oz) wild salmon fillets

Directions:

1. Supply your smoker with wood pellets and follow the start-up procedure. Preheat the grill, with the lid closed, to 375° F.
2. For the glaze, combine Mandarin orange sauce, lime juice, sesame oil, soy sauce, cilantro and fresh cracked black pepper. Mix together.
3. Cut the salmon into 4 fillets. Brush with glaze and place directly on the grill grate, skin side down.
4. Cook until salmon reaches an internal temperature of 155 degrees F (about 15-20 minutes). Half way through cook time, brush salmon again with the glaze.
5. Remove the salmon from the grill and serve with remaining glaze if desired. Enjoy!

Grilled Tilapia With Blistered Cherry Tomatoes

Servings: 4
Cooking Time: 15 Minutes

Ingredients:

* 1½lb (680g) tilapia fillets or other mild white fish fillets
* chopped fresh curly or flat-leaf parsley
* for the marinade
* ½ cup extra virgin olive oil
* 1 garlic clove, peeled and smashed with a chef's knife
* 3 tbsp freshly squeezed lemon juice
* 1 tsp smoked paprika
* ½ tsp coarse salt
* ¼ tsp freshly ground black pepper
* for the tomatoes
* 2 tbsp extra virgin olive oil
* 2 pints (1 liter) cherry tomatoes (red, yellow, or heirloom varieties)

- coarse salt
- freshly ground black pepper

Directions:

1. Place a cast iron skillet on the grate. Supply your smoker with wood pellets and follow the start-up procedure. Preheat the grill, with the lid closed, to 400° F.

2. In a jar with a tight-fitting lid, make the marinade by combining the ingredients. Shake the jar vigorously to emulsify the ingredients.

3. Place the fillets in a single layer in a nonreactive baking dish. Pour half the marinade over them and turn the fillets to thoroughly coat. Cover with plastic wrap and refrigerate for 15 minutes. (Refrigerate no more than 30 minutes or the acid in the marinade will begin to cook the fish.)

4. Place the olive oil in the skillet. Add the tomatoes and season with salt and pepper. Stir to coat. Cook the tomatoes until they begin to blister and collapse, about 5 minutes, stirring once or twice. Remove the skillet from the grill and transfer the tomatoes to a bowl.

5. Carefully lift each fish fillet from the marinade and let the excess drip off. Place the fillets on the grate at a slight angle to the bars. Lightly season with salt and pepper. Grill until the fish flakes easily when pressed with a fork, about 4 to 5 minutes per side, turning carefully with a thin-bladed spatula.

6. Transfer the fillets to a warmed platter. Top with some of the tomatoes. (Place the remaining tomatoes in a serving bowl.) Scatter the parsley around the platter. Drizzle some of the remaining marinade over the top. Serve immediately.

Hot-smoked Salmon

Servings: 4
Cooking Time: 180minutes

Ingredients:

- 1½lb (680g) skinless center-cut salmon fillet, preferably wild caught
- for the brine
- 1 quart (1 liter) distilled water
- ¼ cup coarse salt
- ¼ cup light brown sugar or low-carb equivalent
- ¼ cup gin (optional)

Directions:

1. In a saucepan on the stovetop over medium-high heat, make the brine by combining the water, salt, brown sugar, and gin (if using). Bring the mixture to a boil. Stir until the salt and sugar dissolve. Remove the pan from the stovetop and let the brine cool to room temperature. Refrigerate until cool.

2. Run your fingers over the salmon fillet, feeling for bones. Remove any with kitchen tweezers or needle-nosed pliers. Rinse the salmon under cold running water. Place the salmon in a resealable plastic bag and pour the brine over it. Refrigerate for 4 to 8 hours.

3. Place a wire rack on a rimmed sheet pan. Remove the salmon from the brine and rinse under cold running water. Pat dry with paper towels and then place the salmon on the wire rack. Place the pan in a cool area with good air circulation (such as near a fan). In 2 to 4 hours, you'll notice the salmon has developed a pellicle— a kind of sticky skin or coating that will help the smoke adhere to the fish. (Don't skip this step.)

4. Supply your smoker with wood pellets and follow the start-up procedure. Preheat the grill, with the lid closed, to 150° F.

5. Place the salmon on the grate and smoke until the fish flakes easily when pressed with a fork and the internal temperature reaches 140°F (60°C), about 3 hours. If albumin (a harmless white protein) appears on top of the fillet as it smokes, gently remove it with a paper towel.

6. Remove the salmon from the grill and let rest for 10 minutes. (You can also transfer the fish to a clean wire rack and let it cool to room temperature. Cover and refrigerate if not using immediately. The salmon will keep for up to 5 days.)

7. Serve the salmon with eggs, on salads, with Mustard Caviar, or with its traditional accompaniments: cream cheese, capers, chopped hard-boiled eggs, diced red onion, and dark bread.

Prosciutto-wrapped Scallops

Servings: 4
Cooking Time: 10 Minutes

Ingredients:
- 1½lb (680g) jumbo sea or diver scallops (size U-10)
- 8 to 10 thin slices of prosciutto, each halved lengthwise
- coarse salt
- freshly ground black pepper
- for the butter
- 8oz (225g) unsalted butter
- 2 tsp minced fresh curly or flat-leaf parsley
- 1½ tsp finely grated orange zest
- 1 tbsp freshly squeezed orange juice
- 1 tsp finely grated lemon zest
- 1 tsp finely grated lime zest
- ½ tsp coarse salt

Directions:
1. Supply your smoker with wood pellets and follow the start-up procedure. Preheat the grill, with the lid closed, to 450° F.
2. In a small saucepan on the stovetop over medium-low heat, make the citrus butter by melting the butter. Add the remaining ingredients and simmer for 3 to 5 minutes to blend the flavors. Keep warm.
3. Rinse the scallops under cold running water and dry with paper towels. Place each scallop on its side at the end of a piece of prosciutto and wrap the prosciutto around the scallop. Secure with a toothpick. Season the exposed sides of the scallop with salt and pepper.
4. Place the scallops exposed sides down on the grate and grill until the edges of the prosciutto begin to frizzle and the scallop is warm inside, about 3 to 5 minutes per side.
5. Transfer the scallops to a platter. Brush with some of the warm citrus butter before serving. Serve the remaining butter on the side.

Barbecued Shrimp

Servings: 4
Cooking Time: 10 Minutes

Ingredients:

- 1 pound peeled and deveined shrimp, with tails on
- 2 tablespoons olive oil
- 1 batch Dill Seafood Rub

Directions:
1. Soak wooden skewers in water for 30 minutes.
2. Supply your smoker with wood pellets and follow the start-up procedure. Preheat the grill, with the lid closed, to 375°F.
3. Thread 4 or 5 shrimp per skewer.
4. Coat the shrimp all over with olive oil and season each side of the skewers with the rub.
5. Place the skewers directly on the grill grate and grill the shrimp for 5 minutes per side. Remove the skewers from the grill and serve immediately.

Garlic Pepper Shrimp Pesto Bruschetta

Servings: 12
Cooking Time: 15 Minutes

Ingredients:
- 12 Slices Bread, Baguette
- 1/2 Tsp Chili Pepper Flakes
- 1/2 Tsp Garlic Powder
- 4 Cloves Garlic, Minced
- 2 Tbsp Olive Oil
- 1/2 Tsp Paprika, Smoked
- 1/4 Tsp Parsley, Leaves
- Pepper
- Pesto
- Salt
- 12 Shrimp, Jumbo

Directions:
1. Supply your smoker with wood pellets and follow the start-up procedure. Preheat the grill, with the lid closed, to 350° F. Place the baguette slices on a baking sheet lined with foil. Stir together the olive oil, and minced garlic, then brush both sides of the baguette slices with the mix. Place the pan inside the grill, and bake for about 10-15 minutes.
2. In a skillet, add a splash of olive oil, shrimp, chili powder, garlic powder, smoked paprika, salt pepper, and grill on medium-high heat for about 5 minutes (until the

shrimp is pink). Be sure to stir often. Once pink, remove pan from heat. Once the baguettes are toasted, let them cool for 5 minutes, then spread a layer of pesto onto each one, then top with a shrimp, and serve.

Grilled Mussels With Lemon Butter

Servings: 4
Cooking Time: 15 Minutes

Ingredients:
- 2 Pound Mussels, debearded, washed
- 5 Quart water
- 1/3 Cup salt
- 2 Clove garlic, minced
- 1/3 Cup white wine
- 1 Whole lemon juice
- 3 Tablespoon parsley, chopped
- 1 loaf French country bread

Directions:
1. Supply your smoker with wood pellets and follow the start-up procedure. Preheat the grill, with the lid closed, to 375° F.
2. Scrub mussels well in running water making sure to remove all dirt and barnacles.
3. Place clean mussels in a large bowl with 5 quarts (5 L) water and 1/3 cup (91 g) of salt for about 15 minutes.
4. Drain, rinse and repeat soaking method two more times to purge and remove all sand.
5. Melt butter in a saute pan over medium high heat. Add garlic and cook for 1 minute until fragrant. Add wine and bring to a simmer. Add mussels and lemon juice to the pan and toss to coat.
6. Cover with a tight fitting lid and transfer to the grill. Let the mussels steam 8-10 minutes. Remove from the grill and discard any unopened mussels.
7. Sprinkle with chopped parsley and transfer to a serving dish. Serve with sliced bread. Enjoy!

Smoked Mango Shrimp

Servings: 4
Cooking Time: 5 Minutes

Ingredients:
- 2 Tablespoon Olive Oil

- 1 Pound Raw Tail-On, Thawed And Deveined Shrimp, Uncooked

Directions:
1. Supply your smoker with wood pellets and follow the start-up procedure. Preheat the grill, with the lid closed, to 425° F. Rinse shrimp off in sink with cold water. Place in bowl and season generously with Mango Magic seasoning and olive oil. Toss well in bowl.
2. Thread several shrimp onto a skewer, so that they are all just touching each other. Repeat with other skewers and remaining shrimp.
3. Grill shrimp for 2 - 3 minutes on each side, or until pink and opaque all the way through. Remove from grill and serve immediately.

Smoked Crab Legs

Servings: 4
Cooking Time: 30 Minutes

Ingredients:
- 4 Whole crab legs
- 4 Tablespoon butter, melted
- 1/2 Cup Texas Spicy BBQ Sauce
- salt and pepper
- 1 Tablespoon Fin & Feather Rub

Directions:
1. Supply your smoker with wood pellets and follow the start-up procedure. Preheat the grill, with the lid closed, to 250° F.
2. Place the crab legs directly on the grill grate and smoke for 20 minutes. Grill: 250 °F
3. While the crab is smoking, make the sauce. In a medium bowl, combine melted butter, Traeger Texas Spicy BBQ sauce, salt, pepper and Traeger Fin & Feather Rub.
4. After 20 minutes of cooking, brush the crab legs with the BBQ sauce mixture. Continue to cook for another 10 minutes reserving the remaining sauce to serve. Remove crab legs from the grill, and serve with melted butter and BBQ sauce mixture. Enjoy!

Traeger Crab Legs

Servings: 4
Cooking Time: 30 Minutes

Ingredients:

- 3 Pound crab legs, thawed and halved
- 1 Cup butter, melted
- 2 Tablespoon fresh lemon juice
- 2 Clove garlic, minced
- 1 Tablespoon Fin & Feather Rub or Old Bay Seasoning, plus more to taste
- lemon wedges
- Italian Parsley, chopped

Directions:

1. If the crab legs are too long to fit in the roasting pan, break them down at the joints by twisting, or use a heavy knife or cleaver. Split the shells open lengthwise. Transfer to the roasting pan.

2. Combine the butter, lemon juice and garlic; whisk to mix. Pour mixture over the crab legs, turning the legs to coat. Sprinkle the Traeger Fin & Feather Rub or Old Bay Seasoning over the legs.

3. Supply your smoker with wood pellets and follow the start-up procedure. Preheat the grill, with the lid closed, to 350° F.

4. Cook the crab legs, basting once or twice with the butter sauce from the bottom of the pan, for 20 to 30 minutes (depending on the size of the crab legs) or until warmed through. Grill: 350 °F

5. Transfer the crab legs to a large platter and divide the sauce and accumulated juices between 4 dipping bowls. Enjoy!

Grilled Whole Steelhead Fillet

Servings: 6
Cooking Time: 30 Minutes

Ingredients:

- (2-1/2 to 3 lb) steelhead or salmon fillet, skin-on
- 2 Tablespoon Montana Mex Sweet Seasoning
- 1 Teaspoon Montana Mex Jalapeño Seasoning Blend
- 1 Teaspoon Montana Mex Mild Chile Seasoning Blend

- 2 Tablespoon Montana Mex Avocado Oil
- 2 Tablespoon freshly grated ginger
- 1 lemon, thinly sliced

Directions:

1. Coat fillet evenly with all three dry seasonings, avocado oil, grated ginger and thinly sliced lemon.

2. Supply your smoker with wood pellets and follow the start-up procedure. Preheat the grill, with the lid closed, to 380° F.

3. Place the fish skin-side down on the grill grate and cook for 20 minutes. Grill: 380 °F

4. Remove fillet from grill and let rest for 5 minutes. Enjoy!

Florentine Shrimp Al Cartoccio

Servings: 4
Cooking Time: 13 Minutes

Ingredients:

- 6 tbsp unsalted butter, melted
- ½ cup heavy whipping cream
- ½ cup grated Parmesan cheese
- 2 garlic cloves, peeled and minced
- 1 cup thinly sliced button mushrooms, cleaned and destemmed
- 1 cup baby spinach leaves
- 2 tbsp chopped sun-dried, oil-packed tomatoes
- ½ tsp dried oregano
- ½ tsp dried basil
- ½ tsp crushed red pepper flakes, plus more
- ½ tsp coarse salt
- ½ tsp freshly ground black pepper
- 20 to 24 jumbo shrimp, about 1lb (450g) total, peeled and deveined
- sprigs of fresh rosemary, basil, thyme, or oregano

Directions:

1. Supply your smoker with wood pellets and follow the start-up procedure. Preheat the grill, with the lid closed, to 400° F.

2. In a large bowl, combine the butter and whipping cream. Stir in the Parmesan, garlic, mushrooms, spinach, tomatoes, oregano, basil, red pepper flakes, and salt and pepper. Add the shrimp and stir gently to coat.

3. Place four 12-inch (30.5cm) sheets of wide heavy-duty aluminum foil on a workspace and pull up the sides. Divide the shrimp mixture evenly between the sheets of foil. Roll and crimp the top and sides of the foil to create sealed packages.

4. Place the packets seam side up on the grate and grill until the shrimp are cooked through, about 10 to 13 minutes. (You can carefully open one package to check on the shrimp.)

5. Transfer the packets to plates. Carefully open the packets to avoid any steam. Scatter fresh herbs over the shrimp before serving.

Seared Bluefin Tuna Steaks

Servings: 2
Cooking Time: 5 Minutes

Ingredients:
- 3 Whole Tuna, steak
- olive oil
- salt and pepper
- soy sauce
- Sriracha

Directions:
1. Lightly baste both sides of tuna steaks in olive oil; sprinkle sea salt and ground pepper on each side.
2. Supply your smoker with wood pellets and follow the start-up procedure. Preheat the grill, with the lid closed, to High heat.
3. Grill tuna steaks on each side for 2 to 2-1/2 minutes.
4. Remove tuna from grill and allow to cool slightly.
5. Cut into 1/2 - 3/4" pieces. Serve with a mixture of Soy Sauce and Sriracha. Enjoy!"

Seared Ahi Tuna Steak With Soy Sauce

Servings: 2
Cooking Time: 60 Minutes

Ingredients:
- 1/2 Cup Gluten Free Soy Sauce
- 1 Large Sushi Grade Ahi Tuna Steak, Patted Dry
- 1/4 Cup Lime Juice
- 2 Tablespoons Rice Wine Vinegar
- 2 Tablespoons Sesame Oil, Divided

- 2 Tablespoons Sriracha Sauce
- 4 Tablespoons Sweet Heat Rub
- 2 Cups Water

Directions:
1. Supply your smoker with wood pellets and follow the start-up procedure. Preheat the grill, with the lid closed, to 400° F. If using gas or charcoal, set it up for high heat over direct heat.

2. In the glass baking dish, pour in the water, soy sauce, lime juice, rice wine vinegar, 1 tablespoon sesame oil, sriracha sauce, and mirin. Whisk the marinade together with the whisk until everything is well combine. Place the ahi steak into the marinade and place the glass baking dish with the ahi steak in the refrigerator for 30 minutes. After 30 minutes, flip the ahi steak over so that the ahi has the chance to fully marinate on all sides, and allow to marinate for 30 more minutes.

3. After the tuna steak has finished marinating, drain off the marinade and pat the steak dry with paper towels on all sides. Pour the Sweet Heat Rub onto the plate and rub the remaining tablespoon of sesame oil generously on all sides of the tuna steak, and then gently place the tuna steak into the seasoning on the plate, turning on all sides to coat evenly.

4. Insert a temperature probe into the thickest part of the ahi steak and place the steak on the hottest part of the grill. Grill the ahi tuna steak for 45 seconds on each side, or just until the outside is opaque and has grill marks. Flip the steak and allow it to grill for another 45 seconds until the outside is just cooked through. The ahi tuna steak's internal temperature should be just at 115°F.

5. Remove the steak from the grill once it reaches 115°F, and immediately slice and serve. The inside of the steak should still be cool and ruby pink.

Honey Balsamic Salmon

Servings: 2
Cooking Time: 25 Minutes

Ingredients:
- 1 Medium salmon fillet
- Fin & Feather Rub
- 1/2 Cup balsamic vinegar

- 1 Tablespoon minced garlic
- 2 Tablespoon honey

Directions:

1. Season the fillet with the Traeger Fin & Feather Rub.

2. Make the glaze: Combine the vinegar, garlic and honey in a small saucepan. Simmer over medium heat until reduced by half. Usually 10 to 15 minutes. The glaze will be properly reduced when it coats the back of a spoon. Using a basting brush, coat the fillet with the glaze.

3. Supply your smoker with wood pellets and follow the start-up procedure. Preheat the grill, with the lid closed, to 350° F.

4. Arrange the salmon fillet on the grill grate. Grill for 25 to 30 minutes, or until the salmon is opaque and flakes easily with a fork. Grill: 350 °F

5. Transfer to a platter or plates and serve immediately. If desired, heat any remaining glaze to a boil and drizzle over top of the salmon. Enjoy!

Grilled Blackened Saskatchewan Salmon

Servings: 4
Cooking Time: 30 Minutes

Ingredients:

- 1 salmon fillets
- zesty Italian dressing
- Blackened Saskatchewan Rub
- lemon wedges

Directions:

1. Brush salmon with Italian dressing and season with Traeger Blackened Saskatchewan Rub.

2. Supply your smoker with wood pellets and follow the start-up procedure. Preheat the grill, with the lid closed, to 325° F.

3. Place salmon on the grill and cook for 20 to 30 minutes, until it reaches an internal temperature of 145°F and flakes easily. Remove salmon from grill. Serve with lemon wedges. Enjoy! Grill: 325 °F Probe: 145 °F

Thai-style Swordfish Steaks With Peanut Sauce

Servings: 4
Cooking Time: 8 Minutes

Ingredients:

- 4 center-cut swordfish steaks, each about 6oz (170g) and 1 inch (2.5cm) thick
- Peanut Sauce
- lime wedges
- for the marinade
- ½ cup light Thai-style unsweetened coconut milk
- 2 garlic cloves, peeled and smashed with a chef's knife
- juice and zest of 1 lime
- 1-inch (2.5cm) piece of fresh ginger, peeled and roughly chopped
- ½ Thai bird's eye chili pepper or serrano pepper, deseeded and thinly sliced, plus more
- 2 tbsp fresh cilantro leaves, coarsely chopped
- 1 tbsp Asian fish sauce
- 1 tbsp light soy sauce or liquid aminos
- 1 tbsp light brown sugar or low-carb substitute
- 1 tsp ground coriander
- ½ tsp ground turmeric

Directions:

1. In a medium bowl, make the marinade by whisking together the ingredients. Whisk until the brown sugar dissolves.

2. Place the swordfish steaks in a single layer in a nonreactive baking dish and pour the marinade over them, turning the steaks to coat thoroughly. Refrigerate for 1 hour.

3. Supply your smoker with wood pellets and follow the start-up procedure. Preheat the grill, with the lid closed, to 450° F.

4. Remove the swordfish from the marinade and scrape off any solids. (Discard the marinade.) Place the steaks on the grate and grill until the fish easily flakes when pressed with a fork, about 3 to 4 minutes per side, turning with a thin-bladed spatula.

5. Transfer the swordfish steaks to a platter. Serve with the peanut sauce and lime wedges.

Lemon Herb Grilled Salmon

Servings: 4
Cooking Time: 25 Minutes

Ingredients:

- 1 1/2 pounds salmon with skin
- 1/2 tablespoon lemon zest
- 1 tablespoon lemon juice
- 1 tablespoon unsalted butter
- 1/2 teaspoon sea salt
- 1/2 teaspoon ground black pepper
- 2 teaspoons freshly chopped dill
- 1 teaspoon freshly chopped parsley
- lemon slices for the garnish

Directions:

1. Supply your smoker with wood pellets and follow the start-up procedure. Preheat the grill, with the lid closed, to 325° F.
2. In a small bowl, combine the lemon zest, lemon juice, softened unsalted butter, dill, parsley, sea salt, and ground black pepper.
3. Generously slather the top of the salmon fillet with the mixture and top with a slice of lemon. You may allow marinating for about 10 minutes or so to absorb the mixture.
4. Place the salmon fillets on the hot grill grate, skin-side facing down.
5. Cook the salmon for 20 to 25 minutes, until it reaches an internal temperature of 145 °F and flakes easily, or until the salmon is cooked to your preferred taste.
6. Serve with lemon slices. Enjoy!

Barbecued Scallops

Servings: 4
Cooking Time: 10 Minutes

Ingredients:

- 1 pound large scallops
- 2 tablespoons olive oil
- 1 batch Dill Seafood Rub

Directions:

1. Supply your smoker with wood pellets and follow the start-up procedure. Preheat the grill, with the lid closed, to 375°F.
2. Coat the scallops all over with olive oil and season all sides with the rub.
3. Place the scallops directly on the grill grate and grill for 5 minutes per side. Remove the scallops from the grill and serve immediately.

Teriyaki Smoked Honey Tilapia

Servings: 4
Cooking Time: 120 Minutes

Ingredients:

- 4 tilapia fillets
- 1 cup teriyaki sauce
- 2/3 cup honey
- 1 tbsp sriracha sauce
- Green onions (optional)

Directions:

1. In a large bowl, make the marinade by mixing together the teriyaki sauce, honey,and sriracha. Make sure honey is dissolved and well blended.
2. Place the tilapia fillets in the marinade. Turn the fillets so they are completely coated. Cover with a plastic wrap and marinate in the fridge for about 2 hours.
3. Supply your smoker with wood pellets and follow the start-up procedure. Preheat the grill, with the lid closed, to 275° F.
4. Remove the tilapia fillets from the marinade and transfer them to the grill. Smoke the fillets until they reach an internal temperature of 145°F, about 2 hours.
5. Sprinkle with green onions if desired.

Grilled Fresh Fish

Servings: 2
Cooking Time: 15 Minutes

Ingredients:

- 1 Whole fillet of firm white fish: sea bass, halibut or cod
- Fin & Feather Rub
- 2 Whole lemons

Directions:

1. Supply your smoker with wood pellets and follow the start-up procedure. Preheat the grill, with the lid closed, to 325° F.
2. Season fish with Traeger Fin & Feather Rub and let sit for 30 minutes. Slice lemons in half.
3. Place the fish and the lemons (cut side down) directly on the grill grates. Cook for 10 to 15 minutes until the fish is flaky and is at least 145°F in the thickest part of fish. Be careful not to over cook.
4. Serve with the grilled lemons. Enjoy!

Grilled Oysters With Mignonette

Servings: 2
Cooking Time: 15 Minutes

Ingredients:
- 4 Cup rock salt
- 18 Large oysters
- 4 Tablespoon unsalted butter
- 2 Clove garlic, minced
- kosher salt
- 12 Medium lemon wedges, for serving
- 2 Tablespoon minced shallot
- 1/4 Cup red wine vinegar
- 1/2 Teaspoon freshly ground black pepper

Directions:
1. Choose a shallow serving platter that will hold all of the oysters. Pour the rock salt onto the platter to create a 1/2 inch base. This will steady the oysters for serving.
2. To prepare the oysters, check to ensure they are completely closed. Discard oysters that are not. Wash and lightly scrub the oysters to ensure there is no grit on the surface. This will prevent the grit from entering the oyster once shucked.
3. Using a thick glove or kitchen towel, sturdy the oyster in the hand opposite of the one holding the knife. Using an oyster knife or very sturdy paring knife, locate the "hinge" on each oyster. Place the point of the knife in the hinge, and wiggle the tip of the knife into the oyster until it feels sturdy. Firmly turn the knife to apply a torquing pressure to gently open the oyster.
4. Remove the top shell of the oyster. Using the tip of the knife, loosen the oyster from its shell, leaving the juices intact. Place each loosened oyster on its half shell on a baking sheet.
5. Supply your smoker with wood pellets and follow the start-up procedure. Preheat the grill, with the lid closed, to 450° F.
6. In a small saucepan, melt the butter over medium-low heat. Add the garlic and a generous pinch of salt, and cook until fragrant but not burned, about 1 minute. Remove from the heat. Grill: 450 °F
7. For the Mignonette: Combine the minced shallot, red wine vinegar and 1/2 teaspoon freshly ground black pepper. Set aside.
8. Spoon 1 teaspoon of the garlic butter sauce onto each oyster in its half shell. Carefully place each oyster directly on the grill grates, ensuring they don't slip. Close the lid and allow them to cook for 3 to 4 minutes, until the edges of the oysters have pulled away from the shell. Remove carefully with tongs to keep the juices and butter in the shells. Place directly on the rock salt to balance them. Serve immediately with the mignonette and lemon wedges to squeeze onto the oysters. Enjoy!

Garlic Blackened Catfish

Servings: 4
Cooking Time: 10 Minutes

Ingredients:
- ½ Cup Cajun Seasoning
- ¼ Tsp Cayenne Pepper
- 1 Tsp Granulated Garlic
- 1 Tsp Ground Thyme
- 1 Tsp Onion Powder
- 1 Tsp Ground Oregano
- 1 Tsp Pepper
- 4 (5-Oz.) Skinless Catfish Fillets
- 1 Tbsp Smoked Paprika
- 1 Stick Unsalted Butter

Directions:
1. In a small bowl, combine the Cajun seasoning, smoked paprika, onion powder, granulated garlic, ground oregano, ground thyme, pepper and cayenne pepper.
2. Sprinkle fish with salt and let rest for 20 minutes.

3. Supply your smoker with wood pellets and follow the start-up procedure. Preheat the grill, with the lid closed, to 450° F. If you're using a gas or charcoal grill, set it up for medium-high heat. Place cast iron skillet on the grill and let it preheat.

4. While grill is preheating, sprinkle catfish fillets with seasoning mixture, pressing gently to adhere. Add half the butter to preheated cast iron skillet and swirl to coat, add more butter if needed. Place fillets in hot skillet and cook 3-5 minutes or until a dark crust has been formed. Flip and cook an additional 3-5 minutes or until the fish flakes apart when pressed gently with your finger.

5. Remove fish from grill and sprinkle evenly with fresh parsley. Serve with lemon wedges and enjoy!

Wood-fired Halibut

Servings: 4
Cooking Time: 20 Minutes

Ingredients:
- 1 pound halibut fillet
- 1 batch Dill Seafood Rub

Directions:
1. Supply your smoker with wood pellets and follow the start-up procedure. Preheat the grill, with the lid closed, to 325°F.

2. Sprinkle the halibut fillet on all sides with the rub. Using your hands, work the rub into the meat.

3. Place the halibut directly on the grill grate and grill until its internal temperature reaches 145°F. Remove the halibut from the grill and serve immediately.

Smoked Fish Chowder

Servings: 4
Cooking Time: 60 Minutes

Ingredients:
- 12 Ounce (1-1/2 to 2 lb) skin-on salmon fillet, preferably wild-caught
- Fin & Feather Rub
- 2 Corn Husks
- 3 Slices Bacon, sliced
- 4 Can Cream of Potato Soup, Condensed
- 3 Cup whole milk
- 8 Ounce cream cheese
- 3 green onions, thinly sliced
- 2 Teaspoon hot sauce

Directions:
1. Supply your smoker with wood pellets and follow the start-up procedure. Preheat the grill, with the lid closed, to 180° F.

2. Sprinkle Traeger Fin & Feather rub as needed on salmon. Arrange the salmon skin-side down on the grill grate. Smoke for 30 minutes. Grill: 180 ℉

3. Increase the grill temperature to 350℉. Grill: 350 ℉

4. Cook the salmon for 30 minutes, or until the fish flakes easily with a fork. (The exact time will depend on the thickness of the fillet.) There is no need to turn the fish. Using a large thin spatula, transfer the salmon to a wire rack to cool. Remove the skin. (The salmon can be made a day ahead, wrapped in plastic wrap and refrigerated.) Break into flakes and set aside.

5. Arrange the corn and bacon strips on the grill grate. (The salmon will be roasting while you do this.) Roast the corn and the bacon until the corn is cooked through and browned in spots, turning as needed, and the bacon is crisp, about 15 minutes.

6. In the meantime, bring the cream of potato soup and the milk to a simmer over medium heat in a large saucepan or Dutch oven on the stovetop. Gradually stir in the cream cheese and whisk to blend. Chop the bacon into bits and slice the corn off the cobs using long strokes of a chef's knife.

7. Add to the soup along with the green onions. Stir in the salmon. Heat gently for 5 to 10 minutes. Add the hot sauce to taste. If the chowder is too thick, add more milk. Serve at once. Enjoy!

Traeger Baked Rainbow Trout

Servings: 2
Cooking Time: 20 Minutes

Ingredients:
- 2 Tablespoon olive oil, divided
- 2 Whole rainbow trout, gutted and cleaned, heads and tails still on
- 1/2 Teaspoon fresh dill

- 1/2 Teaspoon fresh thyme
- 1 Teaspoon Jacobsen Salt Co. Pure Kosher Sea Salt
- 1/2 Large onion, sliced
- 1 Large lemon, thinly sliced
- 1 Teaspoon freshly ground black pepper

Directions:

1. Supply your smoker with wood pellets and follow the start-up procedure. Preheat the grill, with the lid closed, to 400° F.

2. Grease a 9x13 inch baking dish with 1 tablespoon olive oil.

3. Place trout in the prepared baking dish and coat fish with remaining olive oil. Season the inside and outside of fish with dill, thyme and salt. Stuff each fish with onion and lemon slices then grind pepper over the top. Place 1 lemon slice on each fish.

4. Bake in the Traeger for 10 minutes. Add 2 tablespoons hot water to the baking dish. Continue baking until fish flakes easily with a fork, about 10 more minutes. Enjoy! Grill: 400 °F

PORK RECIPES

Pickle Brined Grilled Pork Chops

Servings: 4
Cooking Time: 60 Minutes

Ingredients:
- 4 pork chops
- 3 Cup Dill Pickle Brine, jar
- coarse ground black pepper, divided

Directions:
1. Put the pork chops and pickle brine in a resealable plastic bag. Refrigerate for at least 4 hours. Drain well and pat dry with paper towels.
2. Season generously with black pepper.
3. Supply your smoker with wood pellets and follow the start-up procedure. Preheat the grill, with the lid closed, to 300° F.
4. Put the chops directly on the grill grate and grill, turning once, for about 1 hour, or until the internal temperature of the chop is at least 145°F. Grill: 300 °F Probe: 145 °F
5. Let rest for 5 minutes before serving. Enjoy!

Simple Smoked Baby Backs

Servings: 4-8
Cooking Time: 360 Minutes

Ingredients:
- 2 (2- or 3-pound) racks baby back ribs
- 2 tablespoons yellow mustard
- 1 batch Pork Rub

Directions:
1. Supply your smoker with wood pellets and follow the start-up procedure. Preheat the grill, with the lid closed, to 225°F.
2. Remove the membrane from the backside of the ribs. This can be done by cutting just through the membrane in an X pattern and working a paper towel between the membrane and the ribs to pull it off.
3. Coat the ribs on both sides with mustard and season them with the rub. Using your hands, work the rub into the meat.

4. Place the ribs directly on the grill grate and smoke until their internal temperature reaches between 190°F and 200°F.
5. Remove the racks from the grill and cut into individual ribs. Serve immediately.

Smoked Baby Back Ribs

Servings: 4
Cooking Time: 180 Minutes

Ingredients:
- 3 Rack baby back ribs
- kosher salt
- cracked black pepper

Directions:
1. Peel membrane from back side of the ribs and season both sides with salt and pepper.
2. Supply your smoker with wood pellets and follow the start-up procedure. Preheat the grill, with the lid closed, to 225° F.
3. Cook meat side up for two hours. Flip ribs so the meat side is down and cook for an additional hour. Enjoy! Grill: 225 °F

Honey Pork Belly Burnt Ends

Servings: 4
Cooking Time: 270 Minutes

Ingredients:
- 2/3 Cup Bbq Sauce
- 2 Tbsp Butter, Melted
- 2 Tbsp Honey
- 2 Tbsp Olive Oil
- Blackened Sriracha Rub
- 3 Lbs Pork Belly, Skin Removed

Directions:
1. Supply your smoker with wood pellets and follow the start-up procedure. Preheat the grill, with the lid open, to 225° F. If using a gas or charcoal grill, set it up for low, indirect heat.
2. Cut pork belly into 2-inch cubes and place into a large mixing bowl.

3. Drizzle olive oil over pork belly, then generously season with Blackened Sriracha.

4. Transfer seasoned pork belly to a wire rack and place on the grill grate. Cook for 3 hours.

5. Remove the pork belly from the wire rack and transfer into a foil-lined aluminum pan or disposable foil pan.

6. Whisk together BBQ sauce, melted butter, and honey, then pour mixture over pork.

7. Toss to coat, then cover the pan with aluminum foil and return to the grill rack.

8. Cook for another 1 to 1 ½ hours, until the internal temperature reaches 200° F.

9. Remove the foil, transfer pork belly to a cast iron skillet and place in the center of the grill.

10. Open the sear slide and continue cooking for another 5 to 7 minutes, turning halfway, to crisp up the pork.

11. Remove pork belly from the grill, and serve warm.

Smoky Pork Tenderloin

Servings: 4
Cooking Time: 20 Minutes

Ingredients:
- 2 Pork Tenderloins (3-5 Pounds Total), Trimmed of Excess Fat or Silver Skin
- 1 Tablespoon Olive Oil
- 1-2 Tablespoons Fresh Lime Juice
- 1/4 Cup Light Brown Sugar
- 2 Teaspoons Smoked Paprika
- 1 Teaspoon Onion Powder
- 1 Teaspoon Garlic Powder
- 1 Teaspoon Coarse, Kosher Salt
- Pinch of Coarsely Ground Black Pepper

Directions:
1. Stir together the olive oil, lime juice, brown sugar, paprika, onion powder, garlic powder, salt, and pepper in a small bowl.

2. Rub the mixture over the pork and place the meat in a shallow dish. You can grill right away, but for more flavor, cover the dish and refrigerate up to 24 hours.

3. Supply your smoker with wood pellets and follow the start-up procedure. Preheat the grill, with the lid closed, to 375° F.

4. Grill the pork tenderloin for 10 minutes, flip and continue to cook until internal temperature at the thickest part of the meat registers 145 degrees F on an instant-read thermometer, about 8-10 minutes.

5. Remove the pork from the grill and cover with aluminum foil for 10-15 minutes before slicing and serving.

Smoked Traeger Pulled Pork

Servings: 8
Cooking Time: 540 Minutes

Ingredients:
- 1 (6-9 lb) bone-in pork shoulder
- Pork & Poultry Rub
- 2 Cup apple cider
- 'Que BBQ Sauce

Directions:
1. Supply your smoker with wood pellets and follow the start-up procedure. Preheat the grill, with the lid closed, to 250° F.

2. While the Traeger comes to temperature, trim excess fat off pork butt.

3. Generously season with Traeger Pork & Poultry Rub on all sides and let sit for 20 minutes.

4. Place the pork butt fat side up directly on the grill grate and cook until the internal temperature reaches 160°F, about 3 to 5 hours. Grill: 250 °F Probe: 160 °F

5. Remove the pork butt from the grill.

6. On a large baking sheet, stack 4 large pieces of aluminum foil on top of each other, ensuring they are wide enough to wrap the pork butt entirely on all sides. If not, overlap the foil pieces to create a wider base. Place the pork butt in the center on the foil, then bring up the sides of the foil a little bit before pouring the apple cider on top of the pork butt. Wrap the foil tightly around the pork, ensuring the cider does not escape.

7. Place the foil-wrapped pork butt back on the grill fat side up and cook until the internal temperature reaches 204°F, in the thickest part of the meat, about 3 to 4

hours longer depending on the size of the pork butt. Grill: 250 °F Probe: 204 °F

8. Remove from the grill. Allow the pork to rest for 45 minutes in the foil packet.

9. Remove the pork from the foil and pour off any excess liquid into a fat separator.

10. Place the pork in a large dish and shred the meat, removing and discarding the bone and any excess fat. Add separated liquid back into pork and season to taste with additional Traeger Big Game Rub. Optionally, add Traeger 'Que BBQ Sauce or your favorite BBQ sauce to taste.

Spicy Ribs

Servings: 4
Cooking Time: 300 Minutes

Ingredients:
- 2 Finely Minced Chipotle In Adobo
- 1 Cup (Any Kind) Barbecue Sauce
- 1/2 Cup Brown Sugar
- 1/4 Cup Honey
- 1/4 Cup Olive Oil
- 1 Rack St. Louis-Style Rib(S)
- 3 Tablespoons Sweet Heat Rub

Directions:
1. Remove the ribs from their packaging, drain, and pat dry. Using a paper towel, grip the membrane on the back of the ribs and pull off. Discard the membrane and paper towel.

2. In a small mixing bowl, combine the brown sugar, olive oil, honey, BBQ sauce, and chiles in adobo. Using a basting brush, brush the front and back of the ribs generously with the BBQ mixture. Save the basting brush for later along with half of the sauce.

3. Generously season the ribs with Sweet Heat rub, making sure to focus especially on the front of the ribs.

4. Supply your smoker with wood pellets and follow the start-up procedure. Preheat the grill, with the lid open, to 225° F. If you're using a gas or charcoal grill, set it up for low heat. Place the ribs on the grill and smoke at 225°F for 4-6 hours making sure to baste in the sauce every 2 hours.

5. Remove from the grill and serve with additional barbecue sauce.

Competition Style Bbq Pork Ribs

Servings: 6
Cooking Time: 300 Minutes

Ingredients:
- 2 Rack St. Louis-style ribs
- 1 Cup Pork & Poultry Rub
- 1/8 Cup brown sugar
- 4 Tablespoon butter
- 4 Tablespoon agave
- 1 Bottle Sweet & Heat BBQ Sauce

Directions:
1. Supply your smoker with wood pellets and follow the start-up procedure. Preheat the grill, with the lid closed, to 225° F.

2. Remove membrane from back of ribs. Season with Traeger Pork & Poultry Rub on all sides. Let ribs rest for 15 to 20 minutes.

3. Place ribs on the grill, bone-side down and cook for 3 hours. While ribs are cooking, prepare the brown sugar wrap. Spread (approximately the same size as the rack of ribs) half the brown sugar, half the butter and half the agave on top of a double layer of aluminum foil. Repeat for second rack. Grill: 225 °F

4. After 3 hours, place one rack of ribs meat side down in the brown sugar, butter and agave, and wrap. Repeat with second rack. Turn grill up to 250°F and place wrapped ribs, meat side down in grill. Grill: 250 °F

5. Cook for another 1-1/2 hours and check the internal temperature. Desired temperature is 204°F to 205°F. If not at temperature, cook for an additional 30 minutes until temperature is reached. Grill: 250 °F Probe: 204 °F

6. Remove ribs from the grill and foil packet. Place unwrapped ribs back in the grill for an additional 10 minutes. Remove from grill and sauce the meat and bone side with Traeger Sweet & Heat BBQ Sauce and cook for another 10 minutes. Slice ribs and serve. Enjoy!

Smoked Bacon Roses

Servings: 2
Cooking Time: 60 Minutes

Ingredients:

- 1 Pack Bacon, Thick Cut
- 1 Dozen Roses, Fake

Directions:

1. Supply your smoker with wood pellets and follow the start-up procedure. Preheat the grill, with the lid open, to 225° F.
2. Roll each piece of bacon tightly, starting on the thicker side of the strip. Take a toothpick and skewer the middle of the bottom of the bacon roll to keep the bacon from unraveling. With a second toothpick, skewer the bacon roll so that the two toothpicks form an "X" at the bottom of the roll of bacon. Do this to every piece of bacon.
3. Place the bacon rolls directly on the grates of your preheated Grill and smoke for an hour, checking on them every 20 minutes.
4. While the bacon is smoking, rip the petals of the fake roses off of the steams.
5. Once the bacon is fully cooked, remove the toothpicks and pierce the bacon in the head of the steam (where the fake flowers once were). If the bacon isn't staying, you can break a toothpick in half and stick it in the tip of the steam, press firmly and try piercing the bacon again.
6. Place in a nice vase with some babies breath and gift to your Valentine.

Pulled Pork Sliders Hawaiian Rolls

Servings: 6 - 8
Cooking Time: 5 Minutes

Ingredients:

- ½ Cup Apple Cider Vinegar
- 1 Package Of Cabbage
- 2 Tbsp Minced Cilantro
- 1/3 Cup Green Onions, Diced
- 1 Tbsp Mango Magic
- 1 ½ Cup Mayonnaise
- 1 Cup Pineapple, Diced

- 1 Lbs Pulled Pork
- 8 Hawaiian Rolls

Directions:

1. In a large bowl mix together all of the coleslaw ingredients and let set in refrigerator for at least 2 hours.
2. Reheat the pulled pork in a microwave or grill.
3. Serve over the pulled pork on the Hawaiian rolls.

Smoked Pork Tomato Tamales

Servings: 6-8
Cooking Time: 60 Minutes

Ingredients:

- 1 Boneless, Netted Pork Roast
- 1 Cup, Fresh Cilantro, Chopped
- 3 Cloves Garlic, Peeled
- 20 Dried Cornhusks
- 1 Tbsp Lime Juice
- ¼ Cup Olive Oil
- 1 Onion, Quartered
- 4 - 6 Cups Prepared Masa Harina Tamale Dough
- 3 – 4 Serrano Peppers, Deseeded
- 1 Tbsp Sweet Heat Rub
- 1 Lb. Tomatillos, Husked And Washed

Directions:

1. Began by soaking the corn husks in a pan filled with water. Soak for 2 – 4 hours, or if needed, overnight.
2. Unwrap the tomatillos from their shell and place all of them into a grill basket followed by a few Serranos, deseeded, garlic cloves and 1 onion cut into quarters.
3. Supply your smoker with wood pellets and follow the start-up procedure. Preheat the grill, with the lid open, to 400° F. If you're using a gas or charcoal grill, set it up for medium low heat, and use smoke chips to fill your grill with smoke for 15 minutes. Place the grill basket filled with your vegetables and roast them over an open flame on your smoker until vegetables have become charred.
4. Place tomatillos, peppers, garlic and onions in a bowl, cover with plastic wrap, and let stand until cool enough to handle, 10 to 15 minutes.

5. Season the pork roast generously with Sweet Heat Rub and grill at 350°F for 1 hour until the roast has a nice crust on the outside.

6. While the pork roast is cooking, add a handful of cilantro, charred vegetables, 1 tbsp of Sweet Heat Rub, 1 tbsp lime juice, and ¼ cup of olive oil to a food processor. Pulse in food processor until mixture is consistent. Set aside

7. After the pork roast has been grilled for an hour, turn heat down to 275°F. Put roast in pan with about a cup of water, cover with aluminum foil and cook for another 4 hours or until the roast can be shredded. Pour chile verde sauce over shredded pork and toss to combine.

8. To being assembling tamales, place a corn husk on a work surface. Place 2-3 tablespoons of tamale dough on larger end of husk and spread into a rectangle, about ¼" thick, leaving a small border along the edge. Place large tablespoon of chili and pork filling on top of dough. Fold over sides of husk so dough surrounds filling, then fold bottom of husk up and secure closed by tying a thin strip of husk around tamale.

9. To cook tamales, place them in a large metal colander over a large stockpot filled with water. Cover and let steam for 1 hour. After the tamales have been steamed, take them off and grill them at 350°F for about 10-20 minutes until corn husks have charred marks.

Pineapple-pepper Pork Kebabs

Servings: 12-15
Cooking Time: 240 Minutes

Ingredients:
- 1 (20-ounce) bottle hoisin sauce
- ½ cup Sriracha
- ¼ cup honey
- ¼ cup apple cider vinegar
- 2 tablespoons canola oil
- 2 teaspoons minced garlic
- 2 teaspoons onion powder
- 1 teaspoon ground ginger
- 1 teaspoon salt
- 1 teaspoon freshly ground black pepper

- 2 pounds thick-cut pork chops or pork loin, cut into 2-inch cubes
- 10 ounces fresh pineapple, cut into chunks
- 1 red onion, cut into wedges
- 1 bag mini sweet peppers, tops removed and seeded
- 12 metal or wooden skewers (soaked in water for 30 minutes if wooden)

Directions:
1. In a small bowl, stir together the hoisin, Sriracha, honey, vinegar, oil, minced garlic, onion powder, ginger, salt, and black pepper to create the marinade. Reserve ¼ cup for basting.
2. Toss the pork cubes, pineapple chunks, onion wedges, and mini peppers in the remaining marinade. Cover and refrigerate for at least 1 hour or up to 4 hours.
3. Supply your smoker with wood pellets and follow the start-up procedure. Preheat, with the lid closed, to 450°F.
4. Remove the pork, pineapple, and veggies from the marinade; do not rinse. Discard the marinade.
5. Use the double-skewer technique to assemble the kebabs (see Tip below). Thread each of 6 skewers with a piece of pork, a piece of pineapple, a piece of onion, and a sweet mini pepper, making sure that the skewer goes through the left side of the ingredients. Repeat the threading on each skewer two more times. Double-skewer the kebabs by sticking another 6 skewers through the right side of the ingredients.
6. Place the kebabs directly on the grill, close the lid, and smoke for 10 to 12 minutes, turning once. They are done when a meat thermometer inserted in the pork reads 160°F.

Traeger Pulled Pork Sandwiches

Servings: 8
Cooking Time: 660 Minutes

Ingredients:
- 1 (5-7 lb) bone-in pork shoulder
- Pork & Poultry Rub
- 2 Cup apple juice, in food-grade spray bottle
- BBQ Sauce
- 10 hamburger buns

- coleslaw, for serving

Directions:

1. Generously season pork roast on all sides with Traeger Pork & Poultry rub.

2. Supply your smoker with wood pellets and follow the start-up procedure. Preheat the grill, with the lid closed, to 225° F.

3. Put the roast on the grill grate, fat-side up and smoke for 3 hours. Spray the roast with apple juice every hour after the first hour. Grill: 225 °F

4. After 3 hours, transfer pork to a disposable aluminum foil pan large enough to hold the roast. Increase the grill temperature to 250°F, and continue to cook for 6 to 8 additional hours, or until an instant-read meat thermometer inserted in the thickest part, but not touching bone, registers 203°F. If the pork starts to brown too much, cover it loosely with aluminum foil. Grill: 250 °F Probe: 203 °F

5. Carefully transfer the pork roast to a cutting board and let it rest for 20 minutes. Pour the juices from the bottom of the pan into a gravy separator. Discard any fat that has floated to the top.

6. With your hands (preferably protected from the heat with lined, heavy-duty rubber gloves) pull the pork into chunks. Discard the bone and any lumps of fat, including the cap. Pull each chunk into shreds and transfer to a large mixing bowl.

7. Season with additional rub and moisten with the reserved pork juice. Add your favorite Traeger BBQ sauce to the pulled pork and mix well.

8. Pile the pork mixture on the hamburger buns and serve with coleslaw. Enjoy!

St Louis Style Bbq Ribs With Texas Spicy Bbq Sauce

Servings: 8
Cooking Time: 300 Minutes

Ingredients:

- 3 Rack St. Louis-style ribs, membrane removed
- 4 Tablespoon Rub
- 6 Tablespoon butter
- 1 1/2 Cup brown sugar

- 1 1/2 Cup agave
- 1 1/2 Cup Texas Spicy BBQ Sauce

Directions:

1. Supply your smoker with wood pellets and follow the start-up procedure. Preheat the grill, with the lid closed, to 250° F.

2. Season ribs with Traeger rub and place directly on grill grate rib side down or in a Traeger rib rack with the bone resting on the rack. Cook for 3 hours. Grill: 250 °F

3. Stack 2 pieces of tin foil on the table large enough to cover one rack of ribs. In the center of the foil place 3 tablespoons butter, 1/2 cup brown sugar, and 1/2 cup agave. Place the rib rack meat side down on top of the brown sugar mixture and wrap tightly. Repeat with remaining 2 racks.

4. Place all ribs directly on the grill grate meat side down and cook an additional 1-1/2 to 2 hours or until internal temperature reaches 203°F. Grill: 250 °F Probe: 203 °F

5. Remove ribs from the grill and cover each rack with 1/2 cup Texas Spicy BBQ sauce.

6. Rewrap and return to grill an additional 10 minutes allowing sauce to thicken. Grill: 250 °F

7. Remove ribs from the grill, slice and enjoy!

Hanging St. Louis-style Grilled Ribs

Servings: 4
Cooking Time: 270 Minutes

Ingredients:

- 1 1/3 Cup Apple Juice
- 1 2/3 Cup BBQ Sauce, Divided
- Pulled Pork Rub
- 4 Half Racks Spare Ribs, St. Louis Style

Directions:

1. Supply your smoker with wood pellets and follow the start-up procedure. Preheat the grill, with the lid open, to 250° F. If using a gas or charcoal grill, set it up for low, indirect heat.

2. Using a sharp knife, remove the back membrane from the rib racks and pat dry with paper towel. Cut rib racks in half, then season generously with Pulled Pork Rub.

3. Insert a hanging hook under the top rib, then transfer racks to the smoking cabinet. Smoke for 2 ½ hours.

4. Remove ribs from the smoking cabinet and set on heavy duty foil. Mix together ⅔ cup BBQ sauce and ⅓ cup apple juice, then brush thinned BBQ sauce on both sides of ribs. Pour ¼ cup of apple juice around each of the ribs. Fold over foil, then transfer to the grill, meat side down. Increase temperature to 300° F and continue cooking for an additional 2 hours.

5. Remove ribs from the grill, baste with BBQ, then return to the grill and cook for another 10 to 15 minutes. Allow to rest for 15 minutes, then slice and serve hot.

Kodiak Cakes Candied Bacon Crumble Brownies

Servings: 6
Cooking Time: 45 Minutes

Ingredients:
- 1 Box Big Bear Brownie Mix, Kodiak Cakes
- 2 eggs
- 1 Stick butter, melted
- 2 Tablespoon coconut oil
- 2 Tablespoon water
- 2 Cup cooked bacon
- 1/2 Cup Almonds, chopped
- 1/2 Cup sugar

Directions:
1. Supply your smoker with wood pellets and follow the start-up procedure. Preheat the grill, with the lid closed, to 300° F.
2. Spray an 8" baking pan with non-stick spray.
3. Empty Kodiak Cake brownie mix into a medium-size mixing bowl. Add eggs, melted butter, coconut oil, and water. Gently mix, being careful not to overmix. Pour into prepared pan.
4. Place brownies in center of grill grate; bake for 45 minutes. Grill: 300 ˚F
5. While the brownies are baking, begin assembling bacon crumble. Add honey or sugar to a medium-size saucepan, over high heat. Add bacon and almonds. Stir

for 2-3 minutes, or until sugar has dissolved. Remove from heat and let cool.

6. Remove brownies from grill and cool completely. Sprinkle candied bacon crumble over the top of brownies. Enjoy!

Orange & Maple Baked Ham

Servings: 2
Cooking Time: 120 Minutes

Ingredients:
- 2/3 Cup orange juice
- 1/3 Cup maple syrup
- 1/3 Cup Marmalade, Orange
- 1/8 Cup Dijon mustard
- 1 1/3 Tablespoon apple cider vinegar
- 1/2 Teaspoon ground cinnamon
- 1/8 Teaspoon ground cloves
- 2/3 ham

Directions:
1. Supply your smoker with wood pellets and follow the start-up procedure. Preheat the grill, with the lid closed, to 325° F.
2. Meanwhile, make the glaze: In a small saucepan, combine the orange juice, the maple syrup, marmalade, mustard, vinegar, cinnamon, and cloves.
3. Warm over low heat, whisking to combine the ingredients. Remove from the heat and reserve.
4. Place ham in large roasting pan lined with aluminum foil. Place pan on grill and cook for 1.5 hours. Grill: 325 ˚F
5. Open grill and glaze ham with reserved mixture. Continue cooking for another 30 minutes or until a thermometer is inserted into the thickest part of the meat and reaches an internal temperatures of 135 degrees F. Grill: 325 ˚F Probe: 135 ˚F
6. Remove ham from grill and allow to rest for 20 minutes before serving.
7. Warm remaining sauce and serve with ham if desired. Enjoy!

Bacon Wrapped Pickles

Servings: 6
Cooking Time: 60 Minutes

Ingredients:

- 13 Strips Bacon
- 3 Bratwursts, Raw
- 1/2 Cup Colby Jack Cheese, Shredded
- 4 Oz Cream Cheese
- 13 Large Dill Pickles, Spears
- Hickory Bacon Rub
- 2 Scallion, Sliced Thin
- 1/4 Cup Sour Cream

Directions:

1. Supply your smoker with wood pellets and follow the start-up procedure. Preheat the grill, with the lid open, to 375° F.
2. Preheat griddle to medium- low flame.
3. In a mixing bowl combine cream cheese, sour cream, and scallions.
4. Use a hand mixer to blend well, then fold in grated cheddar-jack. Set aside.
5. Cook bratwurst on the griddle. Use a metal spatula to chop up sausage into smaller bits and cook until browned.
6. Remove from the griddle and set aside on a sheet tray to cool.
7. Place pickles on a sheet tray. Cut in half, then remove seeds with a small measuring spoon.
8. Stuff one half of each pickle with cream cheese mixture and top with crumbled bratwurst.
9. Top with the other pickle half, then wrap in bacon.
10. Season bacon-wrapped pickles with Hickory Bacon Rub, place in cast iron skillet, then transfer to grill.
11. Grill pickles for 45 to 55 minutes, until bacon starts to crisp on top. Remove from grill. Serve warm.

Bbq Pork Belly

Servings: 6
Cooking Time: 180 Minutes

Ingredients:

- 1 (3 lb) pork belly, skin removed
- 4 Tablespoon salt

- 1/2 Teaspoon black pepper
- Pork & Poultry Rub

Directions:

1. Supply your smoker with wood pellets and follow the start-up procedure. Preheat the grill, with the lid closed, to 275° F.
2. Meanwhile, season pork belly on both sides with salt, pepper and Traeger Pork & Poultry Rub. Place pork belly directly on the grill grate and cook for 3 to 3-1/2 hours or until the internal temperature reaches 200°F. Grill: 275 °F Probe: 200 °F
3. Remove from grill and let rest 10 to 15 minutes before slicing.
4. Serve in tacos, mac and cheese, nachos or your favorite dish. Enjoy!

Pulled Pork Stew

Servings: 4
Cooking Time: 120 Minutes

Ingredients:

- 16 Ounce salsa verde
- 15 Ounce black beans, drained and rinsed
- 15 Ounce fire roasted red peppers, drained and rinsed
- 1 Pound pulled pork
- 1 Teaspoon ground cumin
- 2 Cup chicken stock
- salt and pepper
- Avocado, Sliced

Directions:

1. Supply your smoker with wood pellets and follow the start-up procedure. Preheat the grill, with the lid closed, to 375° F.
2. Stir in salsa verde, black beans, fire-roasted tomatoes, shredded pork, cumin and chicken broth. Season with salt and pepper to taste.
3. Cook on Traeger for 1 hour stirring every 20 minutes. After 1 hour, cover Dutch oven with lid and cook an additional hour.
4. Top stew with fresh herbs, avocado and sour cream. Serve hot, enjoy!

Spiced Orange Ribs

Servings: 4
Cooking Time: 180 Minutes

Ingredients:

- 1 Tablespoon Adobo Sauce
- 2 (2 1⁄2-Pound) Racks Baby Back Rib
- 1⁄3 Cup Firmly Packed Light Brown Sugar
- 1 Tablespoon Chili Powder
- 5 In Adobo Sauce Chipotle Peppers
- 1⁄3 Cup Leaves Cilantro, Fresh
- 1 Teaspoon Ground Cumin
- 1⁄4 Cup Honey
- 1⁄4 Cup Ketchup
- 2 Tablespoons Lime Juice
- 1 Cup Orange Juice, Fresh
- 5 Tablespoons Sweet Heat Rub

Directions:

1. First, make the barbecue sauce. Into the bowl of a blender, add ¾ cup of orange juice, cilantro, honey, ketchup, lime juice, 2 chipotles in adobo, adobo sauce, and 1 tablespoon of the Sweet Heat Rub. Place the lid on the blender and blend until completely smooth. Pour into a bowl, reserve ½ cup and set aside.

2. Prepare the ribs. Using the paper towels, pull the membrane off of the back of the ribs and discard. In the bowl of a blender, add the orange juice, brown sugar, chipotle peppers, chili powder, ground cumin, and Sweet Heat. Place the lid on the blender and blend until smooth. Pour this mixture over the ribs and massage into the meat. Place the ribs in the refrigerator and marinade for 8 hours.

3. Supply your smoker with wood pellets and follow the start-up procedure. Preheat the grill, with the lid open, to 275° F. Place the ribs, meat side up, and grill for 1 ½ hours. Baste the ribs with the reserved barbecue sauce, then BBQ for another 1 ½ hours, or until the ribs are extremely tender. Remove the ribs from the grill and serve with barbecue sauce.

Smoked Porchetta

Servings: 6
Cooking Time: 360 Minutes

Ingredients:

- 1 Tbs Ancho Chili Powder
- 1/2 Cup Brown Sugar
- 3 Tbs Grilling Seasoning
- 1 Tbs Chopped Italian Parsley
- 1/2 Cup Maple Syrup
- 1 Tsp Dry Oregano
- 1 Tbs Chopped Oregano, Leaves
- 1/2 Pork, Belly (Skinless)
- 1 Whole Pork, Tenderloins
- 6 Slices Prosciutto, Sliced
- 1 Tbs Chopped Rosemary, Fresh
- 1 Tbs Chopped Sage, Leaves
- 1/2 Cup Sugar, Cure

Directions:

1. Sprinkle Sugar Cure on each side and rub in. (You can cure pork belly without using Sodium Nitrite (in the cure mix) but it is much safer if you use it, so I definitely recommend it).

2. In a small bowl, mix brown sugar, maple syrup, ancho chili powder and oregano, and whisk. Slather on both sides of each pork belly piece.

3. Place pork bag (if you can find a 2 gallon or larger one) or container and refrigerate Rotate and flip each 24 hours.

4. After 3 days remove pork belly and rinse each piece thoroughly.

5. If you do not rinse well the porchetta (or bacon) will be too salty due to the sugar cure.

6. Lay pork belly skin side down on a large cutting board.

7. Lightly score the meat side with diamond cuts to allow the seasoning to penetrate.

8. Lightly sprinkle with grilling seasoning, then coat well with the herb mix.

9. Lay out the prosciutto, then lay the pork tenderloin on the pork belly.

10. Lightly sprinkle tenderloin with seasoning, and wrap the pork belly tightly around it.

11. Use cooking twine to tie up tightly.

12. Season the exterior of the pork belly lightly but evenly with grilling seasoning.

13. Supply your smoker with wood pellets and follow the start-up procedure. Preheat the grill, with the lid open, to 250° F.

14. Smoke for 6 hours, or until internal temperature reaches around 175°F.

15. Remove and allow to rest for 20 minutes. Once it cools, then slice thinly and sear in a hot skillet.

16. Let it cool again for about 10 minutes before serving.

Pulled Pork Taquitos With Sour Cream

Servings: 4
Cooking Time: 300 Minutes

Ingredients:

- ⅓ Cup Apple Cider Vinegar
- ½ Cup, Plus Extra For Dipping Bbq Sauce
- 4 Cups Chicken Broth
- 1 Teaspoon Chili Powder
- ⅓ Cup Mustard
- 2 Tbsp Olive Oil
- 6 Tbsp Pulled Pork Rub
- 4 Lb. Pork Shoulder, Bone In
- 1 ½ Cup Sharp Cheddar Cheese, Shredded
- ¼ Cup Sour Cream
- 10 Flour Tortillas

Directions:

1. Supply your smoker with wood pellets and follow the start-up procedure. Preheat the grill, with the lid open, to 400° F. If using a gas or charcoal grill, set the temp to medium heat. In a bowl, combine the chicken broth, mustard, apple cider vinegar, and 1 tablespoon of Pulled Pork Seasoning. Whisk well to combine and set aside.

2. Generously season the pork shoulder with the remaining 3 tablespoons of Pulled Pork Seasoning on all sides of the pork shoulder, then place on the grill and sear on all sides until golden brown, about 10 minutes.

3. Remove the pork shoulder from the grill and place in the disposable aluminum pan. Pour the chicken broth mixture over the pork shoulder. It should come about 1/3 to ½ way up the side of the pork shoulder. Cover the top of the pan tightly with aluminum foil.

4. Reduce the temperature of your grill to 250°F. Place the foil pan on the grill and grill for four to five hours, or until the pork is tender and falling off the bone.

5. Remove the pork from the grill and allow to cool slightly. Place on a cutting board and shred with meat claws, reserving about 2.5 cups. Fire up grill to 425°F.

6. In a mixing bowl, combine sour cream, BBQ sauce, and chili powder. Stir in cheddar cheese and pork until well combined.

7. Lay each tortilla flat on your work surface and scoop about ¼ cup of pork mixture in the center, lengthwise. Roll up tightly and place seam side down on baking sheet. Repeat with all tortillas, then brush tops lightly with olive oil.

8. Transfer baking sheet to grill and cook for 15-20 minutes at 400°F , or until cheese has melted and tortilla edges have turned a golden brown. Serve with extra BBQ sauce for dipping and enjoy!

Baked Sage & Sausage Stuffing

Servings: 4
Cooking Time: 45 Minutes

Ingredients:

- 1 Pound Sage-Flavored Sausage, Such as Bob Evans Or Jimmy Dean
- 1/2 Cup onion, diced
- 1/2 Cup celery, diced
- 14 Ounce (14 oz) package herb seasoned stuffing
- 1/2 Cup dried sweetened cranberries
- 2 Cup low sodium chicken broth
- 6 Tablespoon butter
- butter

Directions:

1. Brown the sausage in a large frying pan, breaking up the sausage with a wooden spoon.

2. Add the onion and celery and cook until softened. Drain any excess fat. Transfer to a large mixing bowl. Add the stuffing mix and cranberries, if using.

3. Warm the chicken broth over medium-low heat; add butter and cook until melted. Toss with the bread/sausage mixture and mix lightly.

4. Butter a 3-qt casserole or baking dish. Do not compress the mixture or it will be dense.

5. Supply your smoker with wood pellets and follow the start-up procedure. Preheat the grill, with the lid closed, to 350° F.

6. Bake the stuffing, covered, for 35 to 45 minutes; uncover during the last 20 minutes of cooking if you prefer a crunchier texture. Grill: 350 °F

7. Remove from grill and serve. Enjoy!

Grilled Pork Tacos Al Pastor

Servings: 8
Cooking Time: 15 Minutes

Ingredients:

- 2 Tsp Annatto Powder
- Cilantro, Chopped
- Corn Tortillas
- 2 Tsp Cumin
- 1 Tsp Granulated Garlic
- 2 Tbsp Guajillo Chili Powder
- Jalapeno Pepper, Minced
- Lime, Wedges
- 1 Tsp Oregano, Dried
- 1/2 Tsp Pepper
- 1/2 Cup Pineapple, Juice
- 1/2 Pineapple, Skinned & Cored
- 2 Lbs Pork Shoulder, Boneless, Sliced Thin
- 1 1/2 Tsp Salt
- 2 Tbsp Tomato Paste
- 2 Tbsp Vegetable Oil
- 1/4 Cup White Vinegar
- Yellow Onion, Chopped

Directions:

1. Prepare marinade: In a mixing bowl, whisk together pineapple juice, vinegar, oil, tomato paste, chili powder, annatto, cumin, granulated garlic, oregano, salt, and pepper. Set aside.

2. Slice pork shoulder into thin slices (around ¼" thick), then place in a resealable plastic bag. Pour marinade over pork, seal bag, and turn to coat. Refrigerate overnight.

3. Supply your smoker with wood pellets and follow the start-up procedure. Preheat the grill, with the lid open, to 450° F. If using a gas or charcoal grill, set it up for high heat.

4. Remove the pork from the marinade and set on the grill. Grill over high heat for 3 to 5 minutes, turning frequently. Transfer to a cutting board to rest for 10 minutes, then slice thin.

5. Grill pineapple for 3 minutes, turning once. Set aside on a cutting board, and chop once cooled.

6. Assemble tacos: tortillas, pork, pineapple, jalapeño, onion, and cilantro. Serve warm with fresh lime wedges.

Stuffed Pork Crown Roast

Servings: 2-4
Cooking Time: 180 Minutes

Ingredients:

- 10 Pound Crown Roast of Pork, 12-14 ribs
- 1 Cup apple juice or cider
- 2 Tablespoon apple cider vinegar
- 2 Tablespoon Dijon mustard
- 1 Tablespoon brown sugar
- 2 Clove garlic, minced
- 2 Tablespoon Thyme or Rosemary, fresh
- 1 Teaspoon salt
- 1 Teaspoon coarse ground black pepper, divided
- 1/2 Cup olive oil
- 8 Cup Your Favorite Stuffing, Prepared According to the Package Directions, or Homemade

Directions:

1. Set the pork on a flat rack in a shallow roasting pan. Cover the end of each bone with a small piece of foil.

2. Make the marinade: Bring the apple cider to a boil over high heat and reduce by half. Remove from the heat, and whisk in the vinegar, mustard, brown sugar, garlic, thyme, and salt and pepper. Slowly whisk in the oil.

3. Using a pastry brush, apply the marinade to the roast, coating all surfaces. Cover it with plastic wrap and allow it to sit until the meat comes to room temperature, about 1 hour.

4. When ready to cook, set grill temperature to High and preheat, lid closed for 15 minutes.

5. Arrange the roasting pan with the pork on the grill grate. Roast for 30 minutes.

6. Reduce the heat to 325°F. Loosely fill the crown with the stuffing, mounding it at the top. Cover the stuffing with foil. (Alternatively, you can bake the stuffing in a separate pan alongside the roast.)

7. Roast the pork for another 1-1/2 hours. Remove the foil from the stuffing and continue to roast until the internal temperature of the meat is 150°F, about 30 minutes to an hour. Make sure the temperature probe doesn't touch bone or you will get a false reading.

8. Remove roast from grill and allow to rest for 15 minutes. Remove the foil covering the bones, but leave the butcher's string on the roast until ready to carve. Transfer to a warm platter.

9. To serve, carve between the bones. Enjoy!

Apple-smoked Pork Tenderloin

Servings: 4-6
Cooking Time: 300 Minutes

Ingredients:
*   2 (1-pound) pork tenderloins
*   1 batch Pork Rub

Directions:
1. Supply your smoker with wood pellets and follow the start-up procedure. Preheat the grill, with the lid closed, to 180°F.

2. Generously season the tenderloins with the rub. Using your hands, work the rub into the meat.

3. Place the tenderloins directly on the grill grate and smoke for 4 or 5 hours, until their internal temperature reaches 145°F.

4. Remove the tenderloins from the grill and let them rest for 5 to 10 minutes before thinly slicing and serving.

Apple & Bourbon Glazed Ham

Servings: 6
Cooking Time: 60 Minutes

Ingredients:
*   1 Large ham
*   1 Cup apple jelly
*   2 Tablespoon Dijon mustard
*   2 Tablespoon bourbon
*   2 Teaspoon fresh lemon juice
*   1/2 Teaspoon ground cloves
*   2 Cup apple juice or cider

Directions:
1. Supply your smoker with wood pellets and follow the start-up procedure. Preheat the grill, with the lid closed, to 325° F.

2. When the grill is hot, place ham directly on the grill grate. Cook for 30 minutes. Grill: 325 °F

3. Meanwhile, in a small saucepan over medium-low heat, melt the apple jelly. Whisk in the apple juice, mustard, bourbon, lemon juice and ground cloves, then remove from the heat and set aside.

4. After 30 minutes, glaze ham with the apple bourbon mixture. Continue cooking for another 30 minutes or until a thermometer that is inserted into the thickest part of the meat reaches an internal temperature of 135°F. Grill: 325 °F Probe: 135 °F

5. Remove ham from grill and allow to rest for 20 minutes before serving. Warm remaining sauce and serve with ham if desired. Enjoy!

Jamaican Jerk Pork Chops

Servings: 4
Cooking Time: 720 Minutes

Ingredients:
*   4 thick pork rib or loin chops, each about 12oz (340g) and 1 inch (2.5cm) thick
*   for the marinade
*   ½ to 1 Scotch bonnet or habanero pepper, destemmed, deseeded, and coarsely chopped, plus more
*   2 scallions, trimmed, white and green parts coarsely chopped
*   1 garlic clove, peeled and coarsely chopped
*   juice of 1 lime
*   2 tbsp vegetable oil
*   2 tbsp distilled water
*   1 tbsp light soy sauce
*   2 tsp coarsely chopped fresh thyme leaves
*   2 tsp peeled and minced fresh ginger
*   2 tsp dark brown sugar or low-carb substitute, plus more
*   1 tsp coarse salt, plus more

- ½ tsp freshly ground black pepper
- ½ tsp ground allspice
- ½ tsp ground nutmeg
- ½ tsp ground cinnamon

Directions:

1. In a blender, make the jerk marinade by combining the ingredients. Blend until fairly smooth. Taste for seasoning, adding more Scotch bonnet, brown sugar, or salt. Place the pork chops in a resealable plastic bag and pour the marinade over them, turning and massaging the bag to thoroughly coat the meat. Refrigerate for 2 to 4 hours.

2. Supply your smoker with wood pellets and follow the start-up procedure. Preheat the grill, with the lid closed, to 425° F.

3. Remove the pork from the marinade and scrape off the excess. (Discard the marinade.) Grill the chops until the internal temperature reaches 145°F (63°C), about 6 to 8 minutes per side.

4. Transfer the chops to a platter. Let rest for 2 minutes before serving.

First-timer's Pulled Pork

Servings: 8
Cooking Time: 540 Minutes

Ingredients:

- 1 bone-in pork shoulder, about 5 to 7lb (2.3 to 3.2kg)
- coarse salt
- freshly ground black pepper
- 1½ cups low-carb beer or sugar-free dark-colored soda
- for the sauce
- 1½ cups apple cider vinegar
- ½ cup distilled water
- 2 tbsp ketchup
- 1½ tbsp granulated brown sugar or low-carb substitute
- 1 tsp coarse salt, plus more
- 1 tsp freshly ground black pepper
- ½ to 1 tsp crushed red pepper flakes

Directions:

1. Supply your smoker with wood pellets and follow the start-up procedure. Preheat the grill, with the lid closed, to 250° F.

2. In a medium saucepan on the stovetop over medium-high, make the vinegar sauce by bringing the ingredients to a boil. Whisk to dissolve the sugar and salt. Let the sauce cool to room temperature and then transfer to a jar with a tight-fitting lid. Set aside.

3. Season the pork shoulder on all sides with salt and pepper. Place the pork on the grate and smoke until the bone releases easily from the meat and the internal temperature reaches 200°F (93°C), about 7 to 9 hours. Wrap the pork tightly in a large piece of heavy-duty aluminum foil and let rest in an insulated cooler for up to 1 hour.

4. Carefully remove the pork from the foil and reserve the juices. Wear heatproof gloves to pull the pork into chunks. Discard the bone and any large lumps of fat. Pull the meat into shreds and transfer to a clean aluminum foil roasting pan. Moisten with some of the reserved juices. Taste, adding more salt and pepper. Serve with the vinegar sauce.

Maple Baby Backs

Servings: 4-6
Cooking Time: 240 Minutes

Ingredients:

- 2 (2- or 3-pound) racks baby back ribs
- 2 tablespoons yellow mustard
- 1 batch Sweet Brown Sugar Rub
- ½ cup plus 2 tablespoons maple syrup, divided
- 2 tablespoons light brown sugar
- 1 cup Pepsi or other non-diet cola
- ¼ cup The Ultimate BBQ Sauce

Directions:

1. Supply your smoker with wood pellets and follow the start-up procedure. Preheat the grill, with the lid closed, to 180°F.

2. Remove the membrane from the backside of the ribs. This can be done by cutting just through the membrane in an X pattern and working a paper towel between the membrane and the ribs to pull it off.

3. Coat the ribs on both sides with mustard and season them with the rub. Using your hands, work the rub into the meat.

4. Place the ribs directly on the grill grate and smoke for 3 hours.

5. Remove the ribs from the grill and place them, bone-side up, on enough aluminum foil to wrap the ribs completely. Drizzle 2 tablespoons of maple syrup over the ribs and sprinkle them with 1 tablespoon of brown sugar. Flip the ribs and repeat the maple syrup and brown sugar application on the meat side.

6. Increase the grill's temperature to 300°F.

7. Fold in three sides of the foil around the ribs and add the cola. Fold in the last side, completely enclosing the ribs and liquid. Return the ribs to the grill and cook for 30 to 45 minutes.

8. Remove the ribs from the grill and unwrap them from the foil.

9. In a small bowl, stir together the barbecue sauce and remaining 6 tablespoons of maple syrup. Use this to baste the ribs. Return the ribs to the grill, without the foil, and cook for 15 minutes to caramelize the sauce.

10. Cut into individual ribs and serve immediately.

Grilled Dr. Pepper Ribs

Servings: 4
Cooking Time: 300 Minutes

Ingredients:
- Aluminum Foil
- 2 Racks Baby Back Ribs
- 1 Cup Bbq Sauce
- 1 Stick Butter, Melted
- 1/2 Cup Dark Brown Sugar
- 12 Oz Dr. Pepper Soda
- 1/4 Cup Sweet Rib Rub
- 1/4 Cup Yellow Mustard

Directions:
1. Supply your smoker with wood pellets and follow the start-up procedure. Preheat the grill, with the lid open, to 225° F. If using a gas or charcoal grill, set it up for low, indirect heat.

2. After the grill comes to temp, place the ribs directly on the grill grates, close the lid, and smoke for 2 hours.

3. In a glass measuring cup, whisk together butter, brown sugar, and 8 ounces of Dr. Pepper.

4. Pour half of the mixture on a foil-lined sheet tray.

5. Place ribs, meat-side down, on top of the mixture, then pour remaining mixture on the bone-side. Tent the sheet tray with foil, then return to the grill for another 2 hours.

6. Remove ribs from liquid and set meat-side up directly on the grill grate.

7. Whisk together BBQ sauce and 4 ounces of Dr. Pepper, then brush half of the sauce all over the ribs.

8. Increase temperature to 275°F and cook an additional 30 to 60 minutes until ribs are tender, and meat pulls away from the bones.

9. Place ribs on a sheet tray, allow to rest for 10 minutes, then slice and serve with remaining BBQ sauce.

Cajun Double-smoked Ham

Servings: 12-15
Cooking Time: 300 Minutes

Ingredients:
- 1 (5- or 6-pound) bone-in smoked ham
- 1 batch Cajun Rub
- 3 tablespoons honey

Directions:
1. Supply your smoker with wood pellets and follow the start-up procedure. Preheat the grill, with the lid closed, to 225°F.

2. Generously season the ham with the rub and place it either in a pan or directly on the grill grate. Smoke it for 1 hour.

3. Drizzle the honey over the ham and continue to smoke it until the ham's internal temperature reaches 145°F.

4. Remove the ham from the grill and let it rest for 5 to 10 minutes, before thinly slicing and serving.

Bacon-draped Injected Pork Loin Roast

Servings: 4
Cooking Time: 180 Minutes

Ingredients:
- 1 Cup apple juice
- 1/4 Cup water
- 1 Teaspoon salt
- 1 Teaspoon Worcestershire sauce
- 3 Pound (3 lb) center-cut pork loin
- Sweet Rub
- 10 Slices bacon

Directions:
1. In a small bowl combine apple juice, water, salt, and Worcestershire; stir to dissolve the salt crystals.Plunge the injector into the sauce and retract the needle to draw up the liquid. Liberally inject the meat.
2. Plunge the injector into the sauce and retract the needle to draw up the liquid. Liberally inject the meat.
3. Season the meat all over with the Traeger Sweet Rub.
4. Supply your smoker with wood pellets and follow the start-up procedure. Preheat the grill, with the lid closed, to 225° F.
5. Drape the loin with the bacon slices. Put the roast directly on the grill grate and smoke for 3 to 4 hours, or until the internal temperature of the meat is at least 145 degrees F on an instant-read thermometer. Grill: 225 °F Probe: 145 °F
6. Transfer the pork to a cutting board and let rest for 10 minutes before carving and serving. Enjoy!

Pulled Pork Corn Tortillas

Servings: 4
Cooking Time: 15 Minutes

Ingredients:
- Cilantro
- Cilantro, Chopped
- 8 Corn Tortillas
- Jalepeno, Sliced
- 1 Lime, Wedges
- 2 Cups Pulled Pork
- Radishes, Sliced
- White Onion, Diced

Directions:
1. Supply your smoker with wood pellets and follow the start-up procedure. Preheat the grill, with the lid open, to 350° F. Grill the corn tortillas until they are softened and have charred spots, about 30 seconds.
2. To assemble the carnitas, add the pulled pork to the tortillas, and top with radishes, diced onion, cilantro, jalapeno and a squeeze of lime juice, if desired. Serve and enjoy!

Classic Pulled Pork

Servings: 8-12
Cooking Time: 1200 Minutes

Ingredients:
- 1 (6- to 8-pound) bone-in pork shoulder
- 2 tablespoons yellow mustard
- 1 batch Pork Rub

Directions:
1. Supply your smoker with wood pellets and follow the start-up procedure. Preheat the grill, with the lid closed, to 225°F.
2. Coat the pork shoulder all over with mustard and season it with the rub. Using your hands, work the rub into the meat.
3. Place the shoulder on the grill grate and smoke until its internal temperature reaches 195°F.
4. Pull the shoulder from the grill and wrap it completely in aluminum foil or butcher paper. Place it in a cooler, cover the cooler, and let it rest for 1 or 2 hours.
5. Remove the pork shoulder from the cooler and unwrap it. Remove the shoulder bone and pull the pork apart using just your fingers. Serve immediately as desired. Leftovers are encouraged.

Pulled Pork Shoulder And Chicken

Servings: 6 - 8
Cooking Time: 300 Minutes

Ingredients:
- 1/3 Cup Apple Cider Vinegar

- 4 Cups Chicken Broth
- 1/3 Cup Ketchup
- 2 Tbsp Pulled Pork Seasoning
- 4 Lbs. Pork Shoulder, Bone In

Directions:

1. Supply your smoker with wood pellets and follow the start-up procedure. Preheat the grill, with the lid open, to 350° F. In a bowl, combine the chicken broth, ketchup, apple cider vinegar, and 1 tablespoon of Pulled Pork Seasoning. Whisk well to combine and set aside.

2. Generously season the pork shoulder with the remaining 3 tablespoons of Pulled Pork Seasoning on all sides of the pork shoulder, then place on the grill and sear on all sides until golden brown, about 10 minutes.

3. Remove the pork shoulder from the grill and place in the disposable aluminum pan. Pour the chicken broth mixture over the pork shoulder. It should come about 1/3 to ½ way up the side of the pork shoulder. Cover the top of the pan tightly with aluminum foil.

4. Reduce the temperature of your grill to 250°F. Place the foil pan on the grill and grill for four to five hours, or until the pork is tender and falling off the bone.

5. Remove the pork from the grill and allow to cool slightly. Drain the liquid from the pan, reserving about a cup, then shred the pork and cover with the reserved liquid. Serve and enjoy!

Baked German Pork Schnitzel With Grilled Lemons

Servings: 2

Cooking Time: 20 Minutes

Ingredients:

- 16 Ounce pork chops
- salt
- black pepper
- 1 Teaspoon garlic powder
- 1 Teaspoon paprika
- 2 eggs
- 1 Cup panko breadcrumbs
- 1/2 Cup flour
- 2 Whole lemon, halved

Directions:

1. Supply your smoker with wood pellets and follow the start-up procedure. Preheat the grill, with the lid closed, to High heat.

2. Place pork chops individually between 2 pieces of plastic wrap. Pound with a meat mallet until they are around 1/4 to 1/8" thick. Season both sides generously with salt and black pepper.

3. Mix the garlic powder and paprika in a bowl. In another bowl whisk the eggs. In a third bowl add the breadcrumbs.

4. Dip pork cutlets one by one into flour shaking off any excess, then into eggs and then into the breadcrumbs. Place breaded pork cutlets onto a lightly oiled wire rack over a baking sheet.

5. Cook for 15 minutes then flip and bake for another 5 minutes. When you open the grill to flip pork, place sliced lemons directly on grill grate flesh side down. Grill: 500 °F

6. Remove from grill and serve immediately with grilled lemons. Enjoy!

Balsamic Brussels Sprouts With Bacon

Servings: 8

Cooking Time: 25 Minutes

Ingredients:

- 6 Strips thick-cut bacon
- 2 Pound Brussels sprouts, trimmed and halved
- 1 Small onion, diced
- 2 Tablespoon olive oil or vegetable oil
- freshly ground black pepper
- salt
- 1/2 Cup chicken stock
- 1 Tablespoon balsamic vinegar

Directions:

1. Supply your smoker with wood pellets and follow the start-up procedure. Preheat the grill, with the lid closed, to 450° F.

2. Place the bacon strips directly on the grill grate and cook for 20 minutes. Grill: 450 °F

3. Line a large baking sheet with foil for easy cleanup. Place the onion and sprouts cut-side down on the baking sheet, drizzle with oil and season with salt and pepper.

4. Place the baking sheet directly on the grill grate next to the bacon and roast until they turn a light golden brown, about 8 to 10 minutes. Grill: 450 °F

5. Add the cooked bacon, pour chicken stock and balsamic vinegar over the sprouts, mix and continue to cook until the liquid has thickened. Remove from heat. Enjoy!

Smoked Pork Spare Ribs

Servings: 8
Cooking Time: 240 Minutes

Ingredients:
- 2 Rack (6 lb) pork spare ribs, trimmed
- 3 Tablespoon Pork & Poultry Rub
- 1 Cup apple juice, cider or beer
- 9 Ounce BBQ Sauce

Directions:
1. Supply your smoker with wood pellets and follow the start-up procedure. Preheat the grill, with the lid closed, to 250° F.

2. If your butcher hasn't done so already, remove the silver-skin on the back of the ribs and trim off any excess fat.

3. Season the ribs on all sides with Traeger Pork & Poultry rub.

4. Arrange the racks of spare ribs on the grill grate, bone-side down and cook for 3 to 4 hours. After the first hour, spray the ribs with apple juice. Continue spraying every hour after that with apple juice. Grill: 250 °F

5. Start checking the temp after 2 hours. The finished internal temperature should be 203°F, about 3 to 4 hours. Grill: 250 °F Probe: 203 °F

6. When the internal temperature registers 203°F, brush the ribs on all sides with Traeger BBQ sauce of your choice. Return ribs to the grill and cook for an additional 30 to 60 minutes to tighten the sauce.

7. To serve, cut each slab in half or into individual ribs and serve with additional BBQ sauce on the side. Enjoy!

Bbq Pulled Pork With Sweet & Heat Bbq Sauce

Servings: 4

Cooking Time: 540 Minutes

Ingredients:
- 10 Pound Bone-In Pork Butt
- 2 Tablespoon Pork & Poultry Rub
- 1 1/2 Cup apple juice
- 4 Tablespoon brown sugar
- 1 Tablespoon salt
- 1 To Taste salt
- 1 To Taste Pork & Poultry Rub
- 1 As Needed Sweet & Heat BBQ Sauce

Directions:
1. Trim pork butt of all excess fat leaving 1/4" of the fat cap attached. Combine 2 Tbsp Pork and Poultry rub, apple juice, brown sugar, and salt in a small bowl stirring until most of the sugar and salt are dissolved. Inject the pork butt every square inch or so with the apple juice mixture. Season the exterior of the pork butt with remaining rub.

2. Supply your smoker with wood pellets and follow the start-up procedure. Preheat the grill, with the lid closed, to 225° F.

3. Place pork butt directly on the grill grate and cook for about 6 hours or until the internal temperature reaches 160°F. Grill: 225 °F Probe: 160 °F

4. Wrap the pork butt in two layers of foil and pour in 1/2 cup of apple juice. Secure tin foil tightly to contain the apple juice. Increase temperature to 275°F and return to grill in a pan large enough to hold the pork butt in case of leaks. Cook an additional 3 hours or until internal temperature reaches 205°F. Grill: 275 °F Probe: 205 °F

5. Remove from the grill and discard the bone. Shred the pork removing any excess fat or tendons. Season with additional Pork and Poultry Rub and salt if needed.

6. Add Sweet & Heat BBQ sauce and serve. Enjoy!

Bacon Wrapped Asparagus

Servings: 4
Cooking Time: 20 Minutes

Ingredients:
- 1 Bunch asparagus
- 1 Tablespoon olive oil
- 1/2 Teaspoon garlic powder

- 1/2 Teaspoon onion powder
- salt and pepper
- 1 Pound Bacon, sliced

Directions:

1. Coat the Asparagus evenly with olive oil, then sprinkle the asparagus evenly with, garlic powder, onion powder, salt and pepper. Individually wrap each asparagus with 1 piece of thin cut bacon.

2. Supply your smoker with wood pellets and follow the start-up procedure. Preheat the grill, with the lid closed, to 450° F.

3. Place the wrapped asparagus on the grill and roast for 15-20 minutes, or until the bacon is crispy. Enjoy!

Smoked Spare Ribs

Servings: 4-8
Cooking Time: 360 Minutes

Ingredients:

- 2 (2- or 3-pound) racks spare ribs
- 2 tablespoons yellow mustard
- 1 batch Sweet Brown Sugar Rub
- ¼ cup The Ultimate BBQ Sauce

Directions:

1. Supply your smoker with wood pellets and follow the start-up procedure. Preheat the grill, with the lid closed, to 225°F.

2. Remove the membrane from the backside of the ribs. This can be done by cutting just through the membrane in an X pattern and working a paper towel between the membrane and the ribs to pull it off.

3. Coat the ribs on both sides with mustard and season with the rub. Using your hands, work the rub into the meat.

4. Place the ribs directly on the grill grate and smoke until their internal temperature reaches between 190°F and 200°F.

5. Baste both sides of the ribs with barbecue sauce.

6. Increase the grill's temperature to 300°F and continue to cook the ribs for 15 minutes more.

7. Remove the racks from the grill, cut them into individual ribs, and serve immediately.

Smoked Rack Of Pork

Servings: 6
Cooking Time: 360 Minutes

Ingredients:

- 4 Bay Leaves
- 2 Jalapeno Peppers
- 1 Six Bone Rack Of Pork
- 1 Cup Salt
- Salt & Freshly Ground Black Pepper
- 2 Tbsp Smokey Apple Chipotle Rub
- 10 Thyme, Fresh Sprigs
- 1 Gallon Water

Directions:

1. To make the rack of pork: Combine the salt, water, bay, thyme and jalapeño in a large stock pot and bring to a boil, let boil for 10 minutes until salt is dissolved.

2. Remove from heat and let cool completely, add pork to the brine and brine overnight. Remove from the brine and rinse. Pat dry and season with Apple Chipotle seasoning and salt and pepper.

3. Supply your smoker with wood pellets and follow the start-up procedure. Preheat the grill, with the lid open, to 140° F. Place the rack of pork on the smoker with a probe inserted and cook for about 5 to 6 hours.

4. Turn the heat up to 450°F and open the heat shield.

5. Sear the pork on all sides, once seared move to a cutting board and tent with foil, rest for 20 minutes then slice in between each bone and serve.

6. To make the pickled fennel: Place the fennel in a bowl. In a small saucepan over medium low heat, add the pickling spice and toast for about 2 minutes or until fragrant.

7. Add the cider vinegar and bring to a boil over high heat. Add the sugar, salt and water and bring to a boil.

8. Cook for 10 minutes over medium high heat to meld the flavors. Strain over the fennel and set aside to cool. Once cool cover and place in the fridge until ready to use.

9. To make the caramelized sweet potato puree: In a large pan add the olive oil over high heat until the oil is shimmering, add the sweet potatoes and cook browning on all sides.

10. Once the sweet potatoes are caramelized add 1 cup of the water and cook until it has evaporated and repeat the process with the remaining water.

11. In a saucepan add the milk and the cream and warm over low heat. Once the sweet potatoes are tender add them to a blender with the milk mixture and blend until smooth but be careful not to over process and turn the potatoes into glue.

12. To make the mustard gravy: Add the olive oil to a large pan over medium high heat, once shimmering, add the shallots and cook until translucent but not browned.

13. Add the bourbon and cooked until almost entirely reduced. Add the heavy cream and the mustard and cook for about 8 to 10 minutes stirring often until the sauce thickens and coats the back of a spoon.

14. Stir in the parsley and season with salt and pepper.

15. To make the fried shallots: Place the shallots in a small bowl and cover them with the milk, let soak in the milk for at least 1 hour.

16. Drain the shallots and transfer them to a large Ziplock bag, add the flour, salt and pepper. Seal the bag and shake well to coat all the shallots in the flour. Remove from the bag shaking off the excess flour.

17. Heat the oil to 350°F in a deep pot. Fry the shallots until golden brown then remove them to a plate lined with paper towels. Season with salt.

18. To put it all together and plate: Spread the puree in a circle in the middle of the plate, place a small handful of the pickled fennel on one side of the puree, Place the pork leaning on the fennel, Spoon over the sauce and top with the fried shallots and the micro arugula.

Bbq Pork Shoulder Steaks

Servings: 4
Cooking Time: 120 Minutes

Ingredients:
- 4 (1 to 1-1/4 inch thick) pork shoulder steaks
- 1/2 Cup mustard
- Pork & Poultry Rub
- 1/2 Cup apple juice
- 1 Cup 'Que BBQ Sauce

Directions:

1. Slather the pork steaks on all sides with the mustard and season with the Traeger Pork & Poultry Rub. (The mustard will help keep the pork moist, but the taste will be unnoticeable in the final product.)

2. Supply your smoker with wood pellets and follow the start-up procedure. Preheat the grill, with the lid closed, to 180° F.

3. Arrange the steaks on the grill grate. Smoke for 1-1/2 hours. Grill: 180 °F

4. Remove the pork steaks to a plate and increase temperature to 225°F. Preheat 5 to 10 minutes. Grill: 225 °F

5. Meanwhile, wrap each steak with aluminum foil, adding in a couple tablespoons of apple juice.

6. Cook the steaks for another hour or so or until they are tender (about 160°F on an instant-read meat thermometer). Grill: 225 °F Probe: 160 °F

7. The last 15 minutes, take the pork steaks out of the foil and put them directly on the grill.

8. Brush each steak on both sides with the Traeger 'Que BBQ Sauce or your favorite barbecue sauce.

9. Let the steaks rest for 3 minutes before serving. Enjoy!

Beer Pork Belly Chili Con Carne

Servings: 4
Cooking Time: 120 Minutes

Ingredients:
- Avocado, Diced
- 2 Bay Leaves
- 1 Lbs Beef Stew Meat
- 12 Oz Beef Stock
- 12 Oz Beer, Bottle
- 15 Oz Black Beans, Rinsed And Drained
- 3 Tbsp Chili Powder
- Cilantro, Chopped
- 1 Tsp Coriander, Ground
- 2 Tsp Cumin, Ground
- 1 Tbsp Flour
- 4 Garlic Cloves, Minced
- 2 Tsp Mexican Oregano, Dried
- 2 Tbsp Olive Oil

- 2 Oz Pancetta, Diced
- Pork Belly, Cut Into 1 Inch Chunks
- 2 Red Onion, Chopped
- Rice, Cooked
- To Taste, Salt & Pepper
- Scallion, Sliced Thin
- 1/4 Cup Tomato Purée

Directions:

1. Supply your smoker with wood pellets and follow the start-up procedure. Preheat the grill, with the lid open, to 425° F. If using a gas or charcoal grill, set it up for medium-high heat. Place Dutch oven on grill and allow to preheat.

2. Heat the olive oil in the Dutch oven, then sauté the pancetta until crisp. Add the onions and sauté for 3 minutes, then add the garlic and sauté 1 minute, until fragrant. Remove mixture with a slotted spoon and set aside.

3. Add the pork belly and beef to the pot to brown, then add the chili powder, cumin, oregano, and coriander. Add the flour and cook for 2 minutes, stirring constantly.

4. Add the beer, beef stock, and tomato purée. Stir well, then return the pancetta mixture to the pot. Add the black beans and bay leaves, then season with salt and pepper.

5. Bring chili to a simmer, then reduce temperature to 325°F and simmer, uncovered, for 2 hours, stirring occasionally, until meat is tender, and sauce has thickened.

6. Remove the chili from the grill, then serve warm with cooked rice, avocado, fresh cilantro, and scallions.

Bbq Brown Sugar Bacon Bites

Servings: 2
Cooking Time: 25 Minutes

Ingredients:
- 1/2 Cup brown sugar
- 1 Tablespoon Fennel, ground
- 2 Teaspoon kosher salt
- 1 Teaspoon ground black pepper
- 1 Pound Pork Belly, diced

Directions:

1. Fold a 12" x 36" piece of aluminum foil in half and crimp the edges so there is a rim. Using a fork, poke holes in the bottom of the foil. This way some of the bacon fat will be rendered out and the bacon bites will crisp.

2. Supply your smoker with wood pellets and follow the start-up procedure. Preheat the grill, with the lid closed, to 350° F.

3. In a large bowl, combine the brown sugar, ground fennel, salt, and black pepper. Stir to combine.

4. Place the diced pork belly into the mixture and toss until well-coated. Transfer the pork pieces to the foil.

5. Place on the grill and bake until the pieces are crispy, glazed, and bubbly, about 20-30 minutes. Enjoy!

Grilled German Sausage With A Smoky Traeger Twist

Servings: 8
Cooking Time: 120 Minutes

Ingredients:
- 2 Tablespoon Jacobsen Salt Co. Pure Kosher Sea Salt
- 1 Teaspoon The Sausage Maker Instacure #1
- 1 Tablespoon ground nutmeg
- 2 Teaspoon ground mace
- 1 Teaspoon ground ginger
- 4 Pound ground pork, 80% lean
- 1 Pound ground veal or ground beef
- 2 Large eggs
- 1 Cup nonfat dry milk powder

Directions:

1. Combine salt, Instacure #1, nutmeg, mace and ginger in a large pitcher or small bowl. Add the milk and eggs. Beat until well combined. Pour the egg mixture over the ground meat and mix gently. Using your hands, mix in the milk powder until evenly distributed.

2. Form the meat into sausage links, roughly 4 to 6 inches in length.

3. Supply your smoker with wood pellets and follow the start-up procedure. Preheat the grill, with the lid closed, to 225° F.

4. Smoke for approximately 2 hours, or until the internal temperature reaches 175°F. Serve immediately or refrigerate until ready to serve. Enjoy! Grill: 225 °F Probe: 175 °F

Bbq Pork Short Ribs

Servings: 4
Cooking Time: 360 Minutes

Ingredients:

- 2 Pork Short Rib Racks With At Least 1 1/2-2" of Meat On Bone
- Pork & Poultry Rub

Directions:

1. Clean and trim short ribs. Season generously on all sides with Traeger Pork and Poultry rub.
2. Supply your smoker with wood pellets and follow the start-up procedure. Preheat the grill, with the lid closed, to 250° F.
3. Place ribs directly on the grill grate and cook for 4-6 hours or until the internal temperature reaches 202-204°F when an instant read thermometer is inserted in the thickest part of meat. Spritz with apple juice every hour if desired. Grill: 250 °F Probe: 202 °F
4. Remove from grill and allow to rest 10 minutes before slicing. Cut into individual ribs and serve with your favorite sides. Enjoy!

Beer Braised Garlic Bbq Pork Butt

Servings: 6-8
Cooking Time: 300 Minutes

Ingredients:

- One 12Oz Bottle Dark Beer
- 1/2 Cup Brown Sugar
- 2 Tablespoons Granulated Garlic
- 4 Tablespoons Honey
- 1 Cup Ketchup
- 1 Tablespoon Olive Oil
- Pulled Pork Rub
- 1 Pork Butt, Boneless
- 2 Tablespoons Worcestershire Sauce
- 4 Tablespoons Yellow Mustard

Directions:

1. Generously season the pork butt with Pulled Pork Rub, making sure to rub the seasoning in on all surfaces of roast. Place the pork onto a roasting rack inside a 9x13 pan.

2. Pour about half a bottle of dark beer into the bottom of the pan and save the remaining amount of beer, you'll need this later.
3. Supply your smoker with wood pellets and follow the start-up procedure. Preheat the grill, with the lid open, to high heat. If you're using a gas or charcoal, set it up for high direct heat. Place the pan in the center of the grill and grill for 30 minutes until the pork roast is dark in color and charred in some spots.
4. Remove the pork from the grill and decrease the temperature of the grill to 325°F. Set aside and began to make the BBQ sauce.
5. In a medium sized bowl, add ketchup, brown sugar, yellow mustard, honey, Worcestershire, granulated garlic, half bottle of dark beer, and finally 1 tbsp of Pulled Pork Rub. Mix together thoroughly.
6. Take the sauce and pour it over the roast, cover with aluminum foil.
7. Cook the roast for 4 - 6 hours or until the meat is falling apart tender and the bone easily comes away from the meat and reaches an internal temperature of 200°F. Remove the pork from the grill and allow it to rest for 10-15 minutes.
8. Shred the pork with meat claws or forks, discarding any fat or gristle. Toss the shredded pork with the barbecue sauce and serve immediately.

Home-cured Picnic Ham With Mustard Caviar

Servings: 8
Cooking Time: 420 Minutes

Ingredients:

- 1 pork shoulder roast, about 5lb (2.3kg) total
- 1 cup distilled water, apple cider, or apple juice, plus more
- Mustard Caviar
- for the brine
- 1 cup kosher salt
- 5 tsp pink curing salt #1
- 1 cup light brown sugar or turbinado sugar or low-carb substitute
- ¼ cup molasses or honey

- 1 gallon (3.8 liters) distilled water, divided, plus more

Directions:

1. Trim any excess fat from the pork shoulder, leaving at least ¼ inch. Use a sharp knife to score the skin of the ham in the classic diamond pattern, making the cuts about 1 inch (2.5cm) apart, but don't penetrate the meat. (If you purchased a shoulder without skin, skip this step.)
2. In a stockpot on the stovetop over medium-high heat, make the brine by combining the salts, brown sugar, molasses, and water. Bring the mixture to a boil. Whisk to dissolve the salts and sugar. Remove the stockpot from the stovetop and let the brine cool to room temperature.
3. Submerge the pork shoulder in the brine. If it floats, place a resealable bag of ice on top. Refrigerate for 3 days.
4. Place the ham in a clean container and cover with cold water. Let the ham soak for 30 minutes. Drain and pat dry with paper towels.
5. Supply your smoker with wood pellets and follow the start-up procedure. Preheat the grill, with the lid closed, to 225° F.
6. Place the ham on the grate and grill until the internal temperature in the thickest part of the meat reaches 160°F (71°C), about 4 to 5 hours. Remove the ham from the grill. Let the ham come to room temperature. Cover and refrigerate for up to 3 days. This helps establish the ham's smokiness.
7. Preheat the grill to 325°F (163°C).
8. Transfer the ham to an aluminum foil roasting pan and add the water to the bottom of the pan. Place the pan on the grate and roast the ham until the skin is nicely browned and the internal temperature reaches 145°F (63°C), about 1½ to 2 hours.
9. Remove the ham from the grill and let rest for 10 minutes. Carve the ham and serve with the mustard caviar.

Smoke-roasted Beer-braised Brats

Servings: 8
Cooking Time: 65 Minutes

Ingredients:

- 8 Wisconsin-style bratwursts
- low-carb beer (enough to cover the brats)
- 2 tbsp unsalted butter
- 2 large sweet onions, peeled and sliced crosswise
- 2 garlic cloves, peeled and smashed with a chef's knife
- 8 brat buns (optional)
- coarse ground mustard or German-style mustard

Directions:

1. Supply your smoker with wood pellets and follow the start-up procedure. Preheat the grill, with the lid closed, to 325° F.
2. Place the brats on the grate at a diagonal to the bars. (Don't pierce the brats or the juices will run out.) Grill until the skin is nicely browned, about 40 to 45 minutes.
3. In a Dutch oven on the stovetop over medium-high heat, bring the beer, butter, onions, and garlic to a boil. Transfer the Dutch oven to the grill.
4. Use tongs to transfer the brats to the Dutch oven and let them steep for at least 20 minutes. The brats will stay at serving temperature—160°F (71°C)—for 1 hour or more.
5. Remove the Dutch oven from the grill and serve the brats on buns (if using) with mustard.

Smoked Ham

Servings: 12-15
Cooking Time: 300 Minutes

Ingredients:

- 1 (10-pound) fresh ham, skin removed
- 2 tablespoons olive oil
- 1 batch Rosemary-Garlic Lamb Seasoning

Directions:

1. Supply your smoker with wood pellets and follow the start-up procedure. Preheat the grill, with the lid closed, to 180°F.
2. Rub the ham all over with olive oil and sprinkle it with the seasoning.
3. Place the ham directly on the grill grate and smoke for 3 hours.

4. Increase the grill's temperature to 375°F and continue to smoke the ham until its internal temperature reaches 170°F.

5. Remove the ham from the grill and let it rest for 10 minutes, before carving and serving.

Unique Carolina Mustard Ribs

Servings: 4
Cooking Time: 300 Minutes

Ingredients:
- 1 Rack St. Louis Style Ribs
- 2 Cups Apple Juice
- 1/4 Cup Cider Vinegar
- 1/4 Cup Dark Brown Sugar
- 1/4 Cup Honey
- 1 Tablespoon Hot Sauce
- 2 Tablespoons Ketchup
- 7 Tablespoon Sweet Rib Rub
- 1 Tablespoon Worcestershire Sauce
- 2 Cups, Prepared Yellow Mustard

Directions:
1. Make the sauce for the ribs. In a large mixing bowl, combine 1 cup of the yellow mustard, cider vinegar, dark brown sugar, honey, ketchup, Worcestershire sauce, hot sauce, and 1 tablespoon of the Sweet Rib Rub. Mix well to combine and set in the refrigerator until ready to use.
2. Make the ribs. Using a paper towel, peel the membrane off of the backs of the rib racks and discard. Generously coat the ribs in a thin coat of mustard, and sprinkle all over with Sweet Rib Rub.
3. Supply your smoker with wood pellets and follow the start-up procedure. Preheat the grill, with the lid closed, to 275° F. If you're using a gas or charcoal grill set it up for low, indirect heat. Place the ribs meaty-side up and grill for 2-3 hours. Once the ribs have grilled for 2-3 hours, fill a spray bottle with 2 cups of apple juice and spray the ribs to keep them moist. Continue to grill the ribs, spraying every 45 minutes, until the meat bends slightly at the ends when lifted and is a deep mahogany color, about another 2-3 hours.
4. Remove the ribs from the grill and brush with mustard sauce, then slice and serve immediately.

Home-cured Hickory-smoked Bacon

Servings: 4
Cooking Time: 180 Minutes

Ingredients:
- 1 pork belly, about 5lb (2.3kg) and 1½ inches (3.75cm) thick, rind removed
- for the cure
- ⅓ cup kosher salt
- ⅓ light brown sugar, turbinado sugar, or maple sugar or low-carb substitute
- 3 tbsp freshly ground black pepper
- 3 bay leaves, crumbled
- 2 tsp pink curing salt #1
- 2 tsp granulated garlic

Directions:
1. Rinse the pork belly under cold running water and pat dry with paper towels. Place in a resealable plastic bag.
2. In a small bowl, make the cure by combining the ingredients, ensuring to especially distribute the pink curing salt. Sprinkle the rub as evenly as possible on the pork belly and use your hands to thoroughly distribute it. (You might want to wear disposable gloves.) Close the bag and refrigerate for 7 days, turning once a day and occasionally massaging the spices into the meat. Some liquid will appear in the bag and the pork belly will start firming up.
3. Rinse the pork under cold running water and pat dry with paper towels. Place the pork belly on a wire rack placed on a rimmed sheet pan. Refrigerate uncovered for 48 hours so it has an opportunity to develop a pellicle—a surface that's very amenable to receiving smoke.
4. Supply your smoker with wood pellets and follow the start-up procedure. Preheat the grill, with the lid closed, to 200° F.
5. Place the sheet pan on the grate and smoke the pork until the internal temperature reaches 150°F (66°C), about 2 to 3 hours.
6. Remove the pan from the grill and let the bacon cool. Cover and refrigerate until it's firmed up again. Slice while cold and either grill or fry the first slices of the batch. Wrap the bacon in plastic wrap. Refrigerate for up to 1 week or freeze for up to 3 months.

Apple-smoked Bacon

Servings: 4-6
Cooking Time: 30 Minutes

Ingredients:
- 1 (1-pound) package thick-sliced bacon

Directions:
1. Supply your smoker with wood pellets and follow the start-up procedure. Preheat the grill, with the lid closed, to 275°F.
2. Supply your smoker with wood pellets and follow the start-up procedure. Preheat the grill, with the lid closed, to 275°F.

Baked Honey Glazed Ham

Servings: 8
Cooking Time: 120 Minutes

Ingredients:
- 1 (6-8 lb) Snake River Farms Kurobuta Half Bone-In Ham
- 20 whole cloves
- 1 Stick butter, softened
- 1/4 Cup dark corn syrup
- 1 Cup honey, room temperature

Directions:
1. Supply your smoker with wood pellets and follow the start-up procedure. Preheat the grill, with the lid closed, to 325° F.
2. Score ham. Smear the entire ham with softened butter and stud with the whole cloves and place ham in foil-lined pan.
3. Combine the dark corn syrup and honey. Warm to combine if needed. Pour 3/4 of the glaze over ham, and bake for 1-1/2 to 2 hours on the grill or until the ham reaches 140°F. Grill: 325 °F Probe: 140 °F
4. Baste ham every 20 minutes with remaining honey glaze. Grill: 325 °F Probe: 140 °F
5. Remove from grill and let rest a few minutes.
6. Slice and serve. Enjoy!

Whiskey- & Cider-brined Pork Shoulder

Servings: 8
Cooking Time: 540 Minutes

Ingredients:
- 1 bone-in pork shoulder, about 5 to 7lb (2.3 to 3.2kg)
- fresh coarsely ground black pepper
- granulated garlic
- 1 cup apple juice or apple cider
- low-carb barbecue sauce, warmed
- hamburger buns (optional)
- for the brine
- 1 gallon (3.8 liters) cold distilled water
- 1 cup coarse salt
- 1¼ cup whiskey, divided
- ½ cup light brown sugar or low-carb substitute

Directions:
1. In a large saucepot on the stovetop over medium-high heat, make the brine by bringing the water, salt, 1 cup of whiskey, and brown sugar to a boil. Stir with a long-handled wooden spoon until the salt and sugar dissolve. Let the brine cool to room temperature. Cover and cool completely in the refrigerator.
2. Submerge the pork in the brine. If it floats, place a resealable bag of ice on top. Refrigerate for 24 hours.
3. Supply your smoker with wood pellets and follow the start-up procedure. Preheat the grill, with the lid closed, to 250° F.
4. Remove the pork shoulder from the brine and pat dry with paper towels. (Discard the brine.) Season the pork with pepper and granulated garlic. Place the pork on the grate and smoke until the internal temperature reaches 165°F (74°C), about 5 hours.
5. Transfer the pork to an aluminum foil roasting pan and add the apple juice and the remaining ¼ cup of whiskey. Cover tightly with aluminum foil. Place the pan on the grate and cook the pork until the bone releases easily from the meat and the internal temperature reaches 200°F (93°C), about 3 hours more. (Be careful when lifting a corner of the foil to check on the roast because steam will escape.)

6. Remove the pan from the grill and let the pork rest for 20 minutes. Reserve the juices.

7. Wearing heatproof gloves, pull the pork into chunks. Discard the bone or any large lumps of fat. Pull the meat into shreds and transfer to a clean aluminum foil roasting pan. Moisten with the barbecue sauce or serve the sauce on the side. Stir in some of the drippings—not too much because you don't want the pork to be swimming in its juices. Serve on buns (if using).

Pig On A Stick With Buffalo Glaze

Servings: 12
Cooking Time: 75 Minutes

Ingredients:

- 4lb (1.8kg) pork shanks, each about 4 to 6oz (110 to 170g), trimmed and thawed if frozen
- 1½ cups sugar-free dark-colored soda, sugar-free root beer, or no-sugar-added apple juice
- for the brine (optional)
- 1 gallon (3.8 liters) distilled water
- ¾ cup kosher salt
- 5 tsp pink curing salt #1
- for the glaze (optional)
- ½ cup unsalted butter
- 1 cup hot sauce
- 2 tsp granulated garlic
- 1 tsp Worcestershire sauce

Directions:

1. In a stockpot on the stovetop over medium-high heat, make the brine by combining the ingredients and bringing the mixture to a boil. Stir until the salts dissolve. Remove the pot from the stovetop and let the brine cool to room temperature.

2. Add the pork shanks to the brine. Cover and refrigerate for 2 days.

3. Supply your smoker with wood pellets and follow the start-up procedure. Preheat the grill, with the lid closed, to 180° F.

4. Drain the pork shanks and discard the brine. (If you didn't brine the pork shanks, season them on all sides with your favorite barbecue rub.) Place the pork on the grate and smoke for 3 hours. Transfer the shanks to an aluminum roasting pan.

5. Raise the temperature to 275°F (135°C).

6. Add the soda to the pan and cover tightly with aluminum foil. Place the pan on the grate and braise the meat until it's tender but still attached to the bone, about 2 to 3 hours. Be careful when removing the foil because steam will escape. Remove the pan from the grill and set aside.

7. Raise the temperature to 325°F (163°C).

8. In a saucepan on the stovetop over medium heat, make the buffalo glaze by melting the butter. Stir in the remaining ingredients. Let the sauce simmer for 5 minutes to allow the flavors to blend.

9. Dip the pork shanks into the glaze and then transfer them to an aluminum foil roasting pan. Cover tightly with aluminum foil. Place the pan on the grate and cook the shanks until hot, about 30 minutes.

10. Remove the pan from the grill. Serve the pork with plenty of napkins.

Barbecued Tenderloin

Servings: 4-6
Cooking Time: 30 Minutes

Ingredients:
- 2 (1-pound) pork tenderloins
- 1 batch Sweet and Spicy Cinnamon Rub

Directions:

1. Supply your smoker with wood pellets and follow the start-up procedure. Preheat the grill, with the lid closed, to 350°F.

2. Generously season the tenderloins with the rub. Using your hands, work the rub into the meat.

3. Place the tenderloins directly on the grill grate and smoke until their internal temperature reaches 145°F.

4. Remove the tenderloins from the grill and let them rest for 5 to 10 minutes, before thinly slicing and serving.

Egg Bacon French Toast Panini

Servings: 2
Cooking Time: 10 Minutes

Ingredients:

- 6 Bacon Slices
- 1 Tbsp Black Pepper
- 4 Brioche Sandwich Slices, Day Old
- 2 Tbsp Butter
- 1 Tbsp Cinnamon-Sugar
- 6 Eggs
- 1 Tbsp Heavy Cream
- 1 Tbsp Maple Syrup
- 1 Tbsp Salt

Directions:

1. Supply your smoker with wood pellets and follow the start-up procedure. Preheat the grill, with the lid open, to 375° F. If using a gas or charcoal grill, set heat to medium heat. For all other grills, preheat cast iron skillet on grill grates.
2. Place butter on griddle and spread to coat surface.
3. In a pie plate, whisk together 2 eggs, heavy cream, and maple syrup.
4. Soak both sides of bread slices in egg mixture and transfer to griddle. Cook for 2 minutes, flipping halfway until egg mixture is cooked and golden. Set aside.
5. Lay bacon on the griddle, and cook 3 minutes per side, until golden.
6. Transfer to lower right-hand corner of griddle to keep warm.
7. Crack 4 eggs on top of rendered bacon fat. Season with salt and pepper. Cook 1 minute per side, or to desired doneness.
8. Lay eggs on top of French toast, add bacon, then place the other slice of French Toast on top.
9. Transfer back to griddle for another minute to warm, sprinkle with extra cinnamon-sugar, then slice in half and serve hot.

Pork Tenderloin With Bourbon Peaches

Servings: 6
Cooking Time: 27 Minutes

Ingredients:

- 2 pork tenderloins, about 2lb (1kg) total, trimmed of silver skin and excess fat
- extra virgin olive oil
- for the rub
- 3 tbsp coarse salt
- 3 tbsp freshly ground black pepper
- 3 tbsp smoked or regular paprika
- 3 tbsp granulated light brown sugar or low-carb substitute
- 2 tbsp instant coffee
- 1 tbsp granulated garlic
- 2 tsp ground cumin
- 1 tsp chili powder
- for the peaches
- 4 freestone peaches, about 1lb (450g) total, peeled, pitted, and sliced
- 1 tbsp freshly squeezed lemon juice
- ¼ cup unsalted butter
- 4 tbsp granulated light brown sugar or low-carb substitute
- 2 tbsp bourbon
- ½ tsp ground cinnamon
- ½ tsp pure vanilla extract
- pinch of coarse salt

Directions:

1. Supply your smoker with wood pellets and follow the start-up procedure. Preheat the grill, with the lid closed, to 400° F.
2. In a small bowl, make the rub by combining the ingredients. Coat the tenderloins in olive oil and season with the rub.
3. Place the peaches and lemon juice in a medium bowl, turning the peaches gently to coat. Measure the other ingredients and then take them and the peaches grill side.
4. Place 1 tablespoon of olive oil in the hot skillet and add the tenderloins. Quickly sear the pork, about 2 to 3 minute per side, turning as needed with tongs. When they're nicely browned, transfer the tenderloins to the grate. Cook until the internal temperature in the thickest part of the meat reaches 145°F (63°C), about 8 minutes. For moist meat, don't cook the tenderloins beyond 155°F (68°C).

5. Transfer the pork to a cutting board and tent with aluminum foil.

6. Replace the cast iron skillet with a clean one and close the grill lid to let it heat. Once hot, make the bourbon peaches by melting the butter. Add the brown sugar, bourbon, cinnamon, vanilla, and salt. Cook the mixture until it bubbles, about 5 to 8 minutes. Add the peaches and cook for 5 to 8 minutes more, turning the peaches carefully with a spoon to coat. Carefully transfer the skillet to a trivet or another heatproof surface.

7. Slice the pork on a diagonal into ½-inch (1.25cm) slices. Shingle the slices on a platter. Spoon the peaches around the pork or serve separately.

Leftover Pulled Pork With Eggs

Servings: 4

Cooking Time: 20 Minutes

Ingredients:
- 1 Teaspoon Coarse Black Pepper
- 4 Eggs
- 1 Green Bell Pepper, Diced
- 1 Teaspoon Kosher Salt
- 3 Tablespoons Olive Oil
- 1 Small Onion, Diced
- 1 Tablespoon Hickory Bacon Seasoning
- 2 Cups Of Leftover Pulled Pork
- 1 Red Bell Peppers, Diced
- 1 ½ Pounds Red Potatoes, Diced

Directions:

1. Supply your smoker with wood pellets and follow the start-up procedure. Preheat the grill, with the lid open, to 350° F.

2. In a large bowl, toss the potatoes with 2 tablespoons of olive oil and Hickory Bacon seasoning. You want to get the potatoes coated well and evenly with the oil and seasoning.

3. Add the potatoes to the skillet and cook on the grill for 12-15 minutes or until they're cooked all the way through and browned. Remove from the pan and set aside.

4. Add 1 more tablespoon of olive to the pan and cook the peppers and onion for 2-3 minutes or until soft. Remove from the pan and set aside.

5. Add the pork to the pan and cook until warmed through. Because the pork is already cooked this should only be 1-2 minutes so the meat stays moist.

6. Add the potatoes, peppers and onions back to the pan, then give everything in the skillet a quick mix, so the hash is evenly blended.

7. Crack the 4 eggs on top of the hash. Try to space them evenly around. Sprinkle the teaspoons of salt and pepper on top of the eggs, then place the lid on top of the pan and allow the eggs to cook for 5-6 minutes, or until the whites are firm and the yolks are still runny.

8. Remove from the grill and serve immediately.

Bbq Rib Sandwich

Servings: 2

Cooking Time: 180 Minutes

Ingredients:
- 3 Rack baby back pork ribs
- cracked black pepper
- kosher salt
- 1 Cup 'Que BBQ Sauce
- 4 hoagie rolls
- 1 Jar Pickles
- 1 yellow onion, thinly sliced

Directions:

1. Peel membrane from back side of the ribs. Lightly season with cracked black pepper and salt.

2. Supply your smoker with wood pellets and follow the start-up procedure. Preheat the grill, with the lid closed, to 225° F.

3. Cook meaty side up for two hours, then flip the ribs to meaty side down and cook for one more hour. Grill: 225 °F

4. Remove ribs from grill and flip over so they are laying bone side up on a cutting board. Using a sharp knife, cut down the center of each bone and remove bones using your fingers.

5. Flip ribs back over and brush with half of the Traeger 'Que BBQ Sauce. Place back on the grill for 5-

10 minutes to set the sauce. Remove from the grill and set aside.

6. Cut rib racks to match the length of the hoagie rolls. Split the hoagie rolls in half and place ribs on the bottom bun.

7. Top with pickles, onions, more BBQ sauce and top bun. Enjoy!

Hawaiian Pulled Pig

Servings: 4
Cooking Time: 300 Minutes

Ingredients:

- 7 Pound bone-in pork shoulder
- 3 Tablespoon Jacobsen Salt Co. Pure Kosher Sea Salt
- ground black pepper
- 2 Whole Banana Leaves

Directions:

1. Season the pork shoulder with Jacobsen Salt and pepper.

2. Place a banana leaf on your work surface. Lay the pork shoulder in the center of it, and draw up the ends as if you were wrapping a gift. Lay the second banana leaf at right angles to the first and draw up the ends to enclose the meat. Wrap the entire package tightly in aluminum foil. Refrigerate overnight.

3. Supply your smoker with wood pellets and follow the start-up procedure. Preheat the grill, with the lid closed, to 300° F.

4. Place the wrapped pork directly on the grill grate and cook until the pork is falling-apart-tender, 5 to 6 hours, or until it has reached an internal temperature of 190 degrees F. Grill: 300 °F Probe: 190 °F

5. Transfer the pork to a cutting board and let rest, still wrapped, for 20 minutes. Carefully unwrap the pork and save any juices that accumulated in the foil.

6. Tear the pork into chunks and shreds, discarding any lumps of fat or bone. Enjoy!

Maple Syrup Bacon Wrapped Tenderloin

Servings: 5

Cooking Time: 30 Minutes

Ingredients:

- 1 Package Bacon, Thick Cut
- 1/4 Cup Maple Syrup
- 2 Tbsp Olive Oil
- 3 Tbsp Competition Smoked Rub
- 1 Trimmed With Silver Skin Removed Pork, Tenderloin

Directions:

1. Lay the strips of bacon out flat, with each strip slightly overlapping the other.

2. Sprinkle the pork tenderloin with 1 tablespoon of the Competition Smoked Rub and lay in the center.

3. Wrap with bacon over the tenderloin and tuck in the ends.

4. In a small bowl, mix the olive oil, maple syrup and remaining seasoning together and brush onto the wrapped tenderloin.

5. Supply your smoker with wood pellets and follow the start-up procedure. Preheat the grill, with the lid open, to 350° F.

6. When the grill is ready, place your tenderloin on the grill and cook, turning, for 15 minutes.

7. Increase the grill temperature to 400°F and grill for another 15 minutes or until the internal temperature is 145°F. Serve and enjoy!

Hot & Fast Smoked Baby Back Ribs

Servings: 6
Cooking Time: 180 Minutes

Ingredients:

- 3 Rack baby back ribs
- Pork & Poultry Rub
- 2 Cup apple juice

Directions:

1. Supply your smoker with wood pellets and follow the start-up procedure. Preheat the grill, with the lid closed, to 300° F.

2. Pull membrane from back of the ribs and trim any excess fat.

3. Season front and back of ribs with the Traeger Pork & Poultry Rub. Let rest on counter for 10 minutes. Grill: 300 °F

4. Place ribs directly on the grill and cook for 30 minutes. Grill: 300 °F

5. While ribs cook, put apple juice in a spray bottle. Spray ribs with apple juice after the first 30 minutes of cooking and every 30 minutes after, about 2-1/2 hours. Grill: 300 °F Probe: 202 °F

6. Check the internal temperature of the ribs. The desired temperature is 202°F. If the desired temperature has not been reached, check every 20 minutes until it comes to temperature. Grill: 300 °F Probe: 202 °F

7. Remove ribs from grill and let rest 10 minutes before slicing and serving. Enjoy!

Traeger Cajun Broil

Servings: 8
Cooking Time: 60 Minutes

Ingredients:

- 2 Tablespoon olive oil
- 2 Pound red potatoes
- Old Bay Seasoning
- 6 Corn Ears, each cut into thirds
- 2 Pound smoked kielbasa sausage
- 3 Pound large shrimp with tails, deveined
- 2 Tablespoon butter

Directions:

1. Supply your smoker with wood pellets and follow the start-up procedure. Preheat the grill, with the lid closed, to 450° F.

2. Drizzle potatoes with half of the olive oil and lightly season with Old Bay seasoning. Place directly on the grill grate. Roast 20 minutes or until tender. Grill: 450 °F

3. Drizzle corn with remaining olive oil and lightly season with Old Bay seasoning. Place corn and kielbasa directly on the grill grate next to the potatoes. Roast 15 minutes. Grill: 450 °F

4. Season shrimp with Old Bay seasoning. Place shrimp directly on grill grate next to the rest of the items and cook for 10 minutes, or until bright pink and cooked through. Grill: 450 °F

5. Remove everything from the grill and transfer to a large bowl. Add butter and season with more Old Bay seasoning to taste. Toss to coat and serve immediately. Enjoy!

Grilled Lasagna With Cold-smoked Mozzarella

Servings: 8-12
Cooking Time: 70 Minutes

Ingredients:

- 15 Oz. Ricotta Cheese
- 3 Cups Cold-Smoked Mozzarella, Grated Divided
- 2 Eggs
- 6 Garlic Cloves, Chopped
- 1 Tsp Garlic Powder
- 1 Cup Grated Parmesan Cheese, Divided
- 1 Lb. Italian Sausage
- 1 Tbsp Italian Seasoning
- 1 Pkg. "No-Bake" Lasagna Noodles
- 48 Oz. Marinara Sauce
- 1 Lb. Mozzarella Block
- 1 Tbsp Olive Oil
- 1 Tbsp Chopped Oregano
- ¼ Cup Italian Parsley, Chopped
- 1 Yellow Onion, Chopped

Directions:

1. In a glass bowl, mix together the eggs, Italian seasoning, garlic powder, ricotta cheese, ½ cup parmesan cheese, and 1 cup of smoked mozzarella, and 2 tablespoons of parsley. Cover and refrigerate for 1 hour.

2. Supply your smoker with wood pellets and follow the start-up procedure. Preheat the grill, with the lid open, to 400° F. If using a gas or charcoal grill, set it up for medium-high heat. Place a cast iron skillet on the grill grates and allow to preheat.

3. Heat olive oil in skillet, then add Italian sausage and cook for 5 minutes, then add in onion and garlic, and cook an additional 3 minutes. Remove from heat and stir in 1 tablespoon of parsley and dried oregano. Set aside and reduce grill temperature to 350° F.

4. To assemble, begin by covering the bottom of a 9x13 pan with 1 cup of sauce. For the first layer, place a single

layer of uncooked noodles over the sauce, followed by ⅓ of the ricotta cheese mixture, half of the Italian sausage, 1 cup of mozzarella cheese, and 1 cup of sauce. Repeat for layer two with a single layer of uncooked lasagna noodles, ⅓ of the ricotta cheese mixture, and 1 ½ cups of sauce. Repeat for layer three with a layer of uncooked lasagna noodles, remaining ricotta mixture, remaining Italian sausage, 1 cup of sauce. For the final layer, add a layer of uncooked lasagna noodles, remaining sauce, and remaining 1 cup mozzarella plus ½ cup parmesan.

5. Transfer lasagna to grill and cook, covered with foil, for 35 minutes. Remove foil and continue cooking for 10 minutes, sprinkle with additional parmesan and parsley, if desired. Remove from grill and let stand 15 minutes before serving.

Roasted Bacon Weave Holiday Ham

Servings: 6
Cooking Time: 180 Minutes

Ingredients:
- 1 1/2 Pound Bacon, sliced
- 1 Large Ham, Bone-In
- whole cloves
- 1 1/2 Cup pineapple juice
- 2 Cup ginger beer
- 1/4 Cup brown sugar
- 2 Tablespoon mustard

Directions:
1. Create a bacon weave on parchment paper.
2. Put the ham in a disposable roasting pan. Gently transfer the bacon weave to the top of the ham and stud the bacon with the cloves (if desired).
3. Pour 1 cup of pineapple juice and 1 cup of ginger beer/ale into the bottom of the roasting pan.
4. Supply your smoker with wood pellets and follow the start-up procedure. Preheat the grill, with the lid closed, to 300° F.
5. Cover the roasting pan with foil and put on the Traeger. Cook the ham until it reaches 145°F (somewhere between 2 to 3 hours). Grill: 300 °F Probe: 145 °F

6. Meanwhile mix together the glaze. Combine the remaining 1/2 cup of pineapple juice, 1 cup ginger beer/ale, brown sugar and mustard in a saucepan on the stovetop. Cook until it thickens slightly, then brush on the ham.
7. Put the uncovered ham back on Traeger and cook until the temperature reaches 160°F. Grill: 300 °F Probe: 160 °F
8. Let the ham rest 5 minutes before slicing and serving. Reserve the juices to pour over the ham. Enjoy!

Double-decker Pulled Pork Nachos With Smoked Cheese

Servings: 4
Cooking Time: 55 Minutes

Ingredients:
- 8 Ounce pepper jack cheese
- 8 Ounce Cheese, sharp cheddar
- tortilla chips
- 2 Cup leftover pulled pork
- black olives
- jalapeño, diced
- cilantro

Directions:
1. Supply your smoker with wood pellets and follow the start-up procedure. Preheat the grill, with the lid closed, to 165° F.
2. Place the cheese (frozen) on a rack on top of a tray filled with ice. You may want to cut the cheese into smaller portions, maybe 2 or 3 chunks per block, to help it smoke more quickly.
3. Smoke the cheeses for 45 to 60 minutes; allow to cool. Shred the cheeses (about 1 cup of each), and set aside. Grill: 165 °F
4. Turn the heat on the Traeger up to 350 degrees and preheat, lid closed, for 10 to 15 minutes. Grill: 350 °F
5. Lay out your tortilla chips on large baking sheet and top evenly with the shredded, smoked cheeses. Place the baking sheet on the Traeger grill grate and cook for about 10 minutes, or until the cheese is melted and bubbly. Grill: 350 °F

6. Remove the pan from the Traeger and start to assemble the double-decker nachos. Assemble the nachos with a layer of cheesy chips on the bottom, some pulled pork, and more cheesy chips on top. Finish it off with your favorite nacho toppings. Serve warm.

Cocoa-crusted Pork Tenderloin

Servings: 4
Cooking Time: 25 Minutes

Ingredients:

- 1 pork tenderloin
- 1/2 Teaspoon Fennel, ground
- 2 Teaspoon unsweetened cocoa powder
- 1 Teaspoon smoked paprika
- 1/2 Teaspoon kosher salt
- 1/2 Teaspoon black pepper
- 1 Tablespoon extra-virgin olive oil
- 3 green onions, thinly sliced

Directions:

1. With a paring knife, remove the silver skin and connective tissue from the loin. In a small mixing bowl, combine the remaining ingredients, making paste. Rub the paste on the pork loin, and refrigerate for 30 minutes.
2. Supply your smoker with wood pellets and follow the start-up procedure. Preheat the grill, with the lid closed, to 450° F.
3. Place the loin on the front of the grill and sear it on all sides. After it has been seared, reduce the temperature to 350°F and move the pork to the center of the grill. Grill: 350 °F
4. Continue to cook for 10- 15 minutes, or until it has reached an internal meat temp of 145°F for medium to medium well. Probe: 145 °F
5. Once it has cooked, remove it from the grill and let rest for at least 8 to 10 minutes before slicing. Garnish with green onions. Enjoy!

Delicious Smoked Bone-in Pork Chops

Servings: 4
Cooking Time: 90 Minutes

Ingredients:

- 1/2 Cup Apple Cider Vinegar
- 4 Pork Butt Roast, Bone-In
- 2 Tbsp Salt
- 1 Tbsp Sugar
- 4 Tablespoons Tennessee Apple Butter Seasoning
- 1/4 Cup Vinegar, Red Wine
- 1/4 Cup Water

Directions:

1. Supply your smoker with wood pellets and follow the start-up procedure. Preheat the grill, with the lid closed, to 250° F.
2. In a large mixing bowl, combine the sugar, red wine vinegar, salt, 2 tablespoons of Tennessee Apple Butter and water to create a brine for the pork chops. Whisk the brine well until the sugar, salt and Tennessee Apple Butter have dissolved.
3. Generously rub the pork chops on all sides with olive oil and season on all sides with the Tennessee Apple Butter. Make sure the meat is coated on all sides.
4. Place the pork chops in the smoker, insert a temperature probe into the thickest part of one of the pork chops, and smoke until the internal temperature reaches 145°F, or about 1 hour 30 minutes. The pork chops should have developed a good color and be juicy, but no longer be pink in the center.
5. Remove the pork chops from the smoker and allow them to rest for 5-10 minutes under tented aluminum foil, then slice along the grain and serve.

Smoked Apple Pork Belly

Servings: 12
Cooking Time: 370 Minutes

Ingredients:

- 4 Pounds Slab Pork Belly (Uncured)
- 2 Cups Apple Juice (Divided Use)
- ½ Cup BBQ Sauce
- ¼ Cup Signature Sweet Rub

Directions:

1. Supply your smoker with wood pellets and follow the start-up procedure. Preheat the grill, with the lid closed, to 250° F.

2. Score the top layer of fat on the pork belly in 1 inch squares. Don't cut too deep, just barely into the muscle. Season liberally with the Sweet Rub on all sides.

3. Place the seasoned pork belly on the grill and smoke until the internal temperature reaches 165 degrees F (about 6 hours). Spritz with the apple juice every hour while it is cooking.

4. Once the belly reaches 165 degrees F, remove from the grill and wrap in heavy duty tinfoil with 1/2 cup of the apple juice. Seal the edges of the foil completely and return to the grill until the internal temperature reaches 200 degrees F.

5. Carefully remove the belly from the foil and drizzle with the apple juices from the foil. Return the pork belly to the grill and brush with BBQ sauce. Cook on the grill for 10 more minutes.

6. Remove the finished pork belly from the grill and let it rest for 10-15 more minutes before serving.

Bacon Stuffed Onion Rings

Servings: 6
Cooking Time: 120 Minutes

Ingredients:
- 1 Pack Bacon
- 2 White Onions

Directions:
1. Supply your smoker with wood pellets and follow the start-up procedure. Preheat the grill, with the lid open, to 250° F.
2. Peel each onion and cut into thirds, separating the onion slices into rings. Using two slices of bacon, wrap around the onion ring until the ring is fully covered, securing in place with a toothpick. Continue until all the bacon is used up.
3. Place the onion rings on the and smoke until the bacon is cooked, about 120 minutes.

Grilled Ham & Egg Cups

Servings: 6
Cooking Time: 25 Minutes

Ingredients:
- 12 Pieces ham

- 12 eggs
- Cup Cream, whipping
- salt and pepper
- 1 Cup shredded cheddar cheese
- chives, chopped

Directions:
1. Supply your smoker with wood pellets and follow the start-up procedure. Preheat the grill, with the lid closed, to 350° F.
2. Spray the wells of a muffin tin with cooking spray. Cut the ham to be sized just a little bigger than each muffin well.
3. Arrange the ham slices directly on the grill grate and cook for 5 to 10 minutes per side, or until nice grill marks appear. Leave the grill on.
4. Whisk together eggs and heavy whipping cream. Season mixture with salt and pepper.
5. Bake for 12 to 15 minutes, or until the eggs are cooked to your liking. Top with cheese the last few minutes of cooking, if desired.
6. Carefully remove the ham and egg cups and serve immediately with some fresh chopped chives or cilantro. Enjoy!

Baby Back Ribs With Mustard Slather

Servings: 4
Cooking Time: 120 Minutes

Ingredients:
- 2 racks of baby back ribs, each about 2lb (1kg)
- all-purpose barbecue rub
- low-carb barbecue sauce (optional)
- for the mustard
- ½ cup yellow or brown mustard
- 2 tbsp dill pickle juice or apple cider vinegar

Directions:
1. Supply your smoker with wood pellets and follow the start-up procedure. Preheat the grill, with the lid closed, to 325° F.
2. Remove the thick membrane on the bone side of the ribs. Don't remove the thin membrane on top of the bones because it holds them together. Trim off any odd

bits of meat or excess fat. Place the ribs on a rimmed sheet pan.

3. In a small bowl, make the mustard slather by combining the mustard and pickle juice. Brush the ribs on both sides with the mixture and then season with the barbecue rub.

4. Place the ribs on the grate and smoke until the ribs are tender, about 1½ to 2 hours. (A toothpick inserted between bones should go in with little resistance. The meat will also have pulled back from the bone about ½ inch [1.25cm].) Brush the ribs with barbecue sauce (if using) during the last 10 minutes of smoking. Place the ribs meat side down on the grate for 5 minutes. Turn and grill for 5 minutes more. This sets the sauce.

5. Transfer the ribs to a cutting board. Use a sharp knife to cut the slabs in half or into individual ribs. Serve immediately with more barbecue sauce.

Bbq Pork Chops

Servings: 4
Cooking Time: 30 Minutes

Ingredients:
- 4 8-To-10-Ounce Bone-In Pork Loin Chops, Trimmed Of Excess Fat
- 1/2 Cup Brown Sugar
- 2 Garlic Clove, Minced
- 2 Tbsp Honey
- 1 Cup Ketchup
- 1/4 Cup Molasses
- Sweet Rib Rub Seasoning
- 2 Tbsp Worcestershire Sauce

Directions:
1. First, place pork chops onto sheet pan lined with butcher paper. Season generously with Sweet Rib Rub, making sure to coat all sides of the chops. Set aside while you make the glaze.

2. In a medium sized mixing bowl, combine the ketchup, brown sugar, molasses, honey, garlic, Worcestershire, and 1 tbsp Sweet Rib Rub. Mix well, add 1 shot of bourbon, mix again until sauce becomes smooth. Transfer sauce into an oven proof sauce pan.

3. Supply your smoker with wood pellets and follow the start-up procedure. Preheat the grill, with the lid open, to 375° F. If you're using a gas or charcoal grill, set it up for medium direct heat.

4. Grill the pork chops for 10-15 minutes per side. Place the saucepan on the grill and allow the sauce to come to a boil. Glaze the chops on both sides and let the glaze caramelize onto the chops.

5. Grill the pork chops until they are lightly charred and reach an internal temperature of 145°F - 165°F. Remove the pork chops from the grill and allow them to rest for 5 minutes.

6. Once the pork chops have finished resting, glaze them again if you choose to. Serve immediately.

Traeger Roasted Easter Ham

Servings: 8
Cooking Time: 60 Minutes

Ingredients:
- 1 (6-7 lb) bone-in ham
- 1 Cup Sweet & Heat BBQ Sauce
- 2 Cup brown sugar
- 1/2 Cup pineapple juice

Directions:
1. Supply your smoker with wood pellets and follow the start-up procedure. Preheat the grill, with the lid closed, to 225° F.

2. Place ham in grill and cook for 60 minutes. Grill: 225 °F

3. While the ham is cooking, mix together the Traeger Sweet & Heat BBQ Sauce, brown sugar and pineapple juice.

4. Glaze ham with the sauce every 10 minutes during the last 30 minutes. Remove ham from grill and serve. Enjoy!

Bbq Bacon-wrapped Water Chestnuts

Servings: 6
Cooking Time: 35 Minutes

Ingredients:
- 1 Pound bacon
- 2 Can Water Chestnuts

- 1/3 Cup brown sugar
- 1/3 Cup mayonnaise
- 1/3 Cup Texas Spicy BBQ Sauce

Directions:

1. Supply your smoker with wood pellets and follow the start-up procedure. Preheat the grill, with the lid closed, to 350° F.

2. Line a rimmed baking sheet with aluminum foil. Cut each piece of bacon into thirds or halves. Wrap each water chestnut with a piece of bacon large enough to encircle it and secure the bacon with a toothpick.

3. Arrange the bacon-wrapped chestnuts in a single layer on the prepared baking sheet. Bake for 20 minutes. Leave the grill on. Grill: 350 ˚F

4. Meanwhile, whisk the mayonnaise, brown sugar, and Traeger Spicy Barbecue Sauce in a mixing bowl. Pour the sauce over the chestnuts and return to the grill to bake for 10 to 15 minutes more. Transfer to a platter for serving. Enjoy!

Bbq Pulled Pork Grilled Cheese Sandwich

Servings: 8

Cooking Time: 540 Minutes

Ingredients:

- 1 Pork Butt, bone-in, 8-10 lbs.
- 2 Tablespoon Pork & Poultry Rub
- 1 1/2 Cup apple juice
- 4 Tablespoon brown sugar
- 1 Tablespoon salt
- Sweet & Heat BBQ Sauce
- 16 Pieces White Bread
- cheddar cheese
- butter, softened

Directions:

1. Trim pork butt of all excess fat leaving 1/4-inch of the fat cap attached.

2. Combine 2 Tbsp Traeger Pork & Poultry Rub, apple juice, brown sugar and salt in a small bowl stirring until most of the sugar and salt are dissolved.

3. Inject the pork butt every square inch or so with the apple juice mixture. Season the exterior of the pork butt with remaining rub.

4. Supply your smoker with wood pellets and follow the start-up procedure. Preheat the grill, with the lid closed, to 250° F.

5. Place pork butt directly on the grill grate and cook for about 6 hours or until the internal temperature reaches 160 degrees F. Remove pork butt from grill and wrap in two layers of foil. Pour in 1/2 cup of apple juice. Secure tin foil tightly to contain the apple juice. Grill: 250 ˚F Probe: 160 ˚F

6. Increase temperature to 275 degrees F and return to grill in a pan large enough to hold the pork butt in case of leaks. Cook an additional 3 hours or until internal temperature reaches 205 degrees F. Grill: 275 ˚F Probe: 205 ˚F

7. Remove from the grill and discard the bone. Shred the pork removing any excess fat or tendons. Season with additional Traeger Pork & Poultry Rub and salt if needed. Add Traeger Sweet & Heat BBQ Sauce and mix to combine. Set pork aside.

8. For the grilled cheese sandwiches: Butter two pieces of bread and place one in a pan warmed over medium heat, butter side down. Place a slice of cheddar cheese on top of the bread and top with pulled pork. Place another slice of cheese on top of pork and finish with the other slice of bread, butter side up.

9. Cook on first side 5-7 minutes until bread is lightly browned. Flip and cook for another 5-7 minutes. Remove from heat and slice in half. Enjoy!

BEEF LAMB AND GAME RECIPES

Smoked Beef Back Ribs

Servings: 6
Cooking Time: 480 Minutes

Ingredients:
- 2 Rack beef back ribs
- 1/2 Cup Beef Rub

Directions:
1. If your butcher has not already done so, remove the thin papery membrane from the bone-side of the ribs by working the tip of a butter knife underneath the membrane over a middle bone. Use paper towels to get a firm grip, then tear the membrane off.
2. Season both sides of ribs with Traeger Beef Rub.
3. Supply your smoker with wood pellets and follow the start-up procedure. Preheat the grill, with the lid closed, to 225° F.
4. Arrange the ribs on the grill grate, bone side down. Cook for 8-10 hours, or until internal temperature reaches 205℉. Grill: 225 ℉ Probe: 205 ℉
5. Remove ribs from grill and let rest, lightly covered for 20 minutes before slicing and serving. Enjoy!

Smoked Texas Bbq Brisket

Servings: 8
Cooking Time: 600 Minutes

Ingredients:
- 1 (14-18 lb) whole packer brisket
- Meat Church Holy Cow BBQ Rub
- Meat Church Holy Gospel BBQ Rub

Directions:
1. Trim any hard fat from all sides of the brisket, being careful not to dig too deep into the meat. Trim the sides of any excess or loose fat. Trim the fat side of the brisket to 1/4 inch thick.
2. Season all sides evenly with Meat Church Holy Cow Rub. Optionally add a light layer of Meat Church Holy Gospel Rub. Let the brisket sit in the seasoning at room temp for 20 to 30 minutes.

3. Supply your smoker with wood pellets and follow the start-up procedure. Preheat the grill, with the lid closed, to 275° F.
4. Place the brisket fat side up on the grill grate. Cook until it reaches an internal temperature of 165℉, about 5 to 6 hours
5. Remove brisket and wrap tightly in Traeger Butcher Paper.
6. Place the wrapped brisket back on the grill and cook until it reaches an internal temperature of 204℉, about 3-4 hours. Grill: 275 ℉ Probe: 204 ℉
7. When the brisket reaches 204℉, remove from grill and let rest for 30 minutes. When ready to eat, unwrap brisket and slice against the grain. Enjoy!

Flavour Smoked Corned Beef Brisket Hash

Servings: 4
Cooking Time: 195 Minutes

Ingredients:
- 6 slices, chopped bacon
- 1 tsp black pepper
- 2 cups chicken stock
- 1, 2 lb. corned beef brisket
- 2 tbsp Italian parsley
- 1 ½ tsp   hickory bacon rub
- 1, chopped red bell pepper
- 1 tsp thyme, fresh, chopped
- 1, chopped yellow onion
- 1 ½ lbs yukon gold potatoes

Directions:
1. Remove corned beef brisket from packaging, rinse under cold water, and pat dry with paper towel.
2. Season brisket with included seasoning packet and coarse black pepper, then rest for 30 minutes.
3. Supply your smoker with wood pellets and follow the start-up procedure. Preheat the grill, with the lid closed, to 225° F. If using a gas or charcoal grill, set it up for low indirect heat.

4. Lay brisket directly on the grill grate and smoke for 2 ½ to 3 hours or until the internal temperature reaches 165°F.

5. Once this temperature is achieved, place the brisket in a 9 x 13 metal pan with potatoes and chicken stock.

6. Cover with foil and cook until brisket reaches an internal temperature of 202°F.

7. Remove brisket from grill and refrigerate overnight or until brisket and potatoes have fully cooled.

8. When ready to cook, peel and dice potatoes then chop up 1 lb. of brisket, reserving the remainder for future use.

9. Place a cast-iron skillet on the pellet grill and preheat to 400°F.

10. Once skillet is heated, add bacon and sauté for 8 to 10 minutes, until brown.

11. Remove with slotted spoon and place on paper towel-lined tray.

12. Add onion and red bell pepper to skillet with rendered bacon fat and sauté for 3 minutes, then add cooked brisket.

13. Add Hickory Bacon Rub, parsley and thyme and sauté another 3 minutes.

14. Add diced potatoes. Gently stir to incorporate and serve hot.

Beer Chili Bratwurst

Servings: 4
Cooking Time: 45 Minutes

Ingredients:
- 1 Chopped Chipotle In Adobo
- 3 - 4 Cans Of Beer, Any Brand
- 4 Bratwursts, Raw
- 4 Bratwurst Buns
- ½ Cup Prepared Nacho Cheese Sauce
- 1 Cup Chili, Prepared
- Caramelized Onions
- Sweet Rib Rub

Directions:
1. Supply your smoker with wood pellets and follow the start-up procedure. Preheat the grill, with the lid closed, to 350° F. If you're using charcoal or gas, set the temperature to medium high.

2. Place a pot filled with beer, Sweet Rib Rub, caramelized onions and raw brats. Place on grill and par-boil for 20 minutes.

3. Grill the brats for 7-10 minutes, or until internal temperature of the brats is 160°F. Remove the brats from the grill and allow them to rest for 5 minutes.

4. While the brats rest, place the chili in a sauce pan, and place the sauce pan on the grill. Heat the chili all the way through.

5. In a separate sauce pan, add the nacho cheese to the pan, add adobo chili peppers and a shake of Sweet Rib Rub. Place the saucepan on the grill and heat until warm all the way through.

6. Assemble the brats: place a brat in a bun, then top with a spoonful of chili and a spoonful of nacho cheese. Serve immediately.

Perfect Roast Prime Rib

Servings: 8-12
Cooking Time: 300minutes

Ingredients:
- 1 (3-bone) rib roast
- Salt
- Freshly ground black pepper
- 1 garlic clove, minced

Directions:
1. Supply your smoker with wood pellets and follow the start-up procedure. Preheat the grill, with the lid closed, to 360°F.

2. Season the roast all over with salt and pepper and, using your hands, rub it all over with the minced garlic.

3. Place the roast directly on the grill grate and smoke for 4 or 5 hours, until its internal temperature reaches 145°F for medium-rare.

4. Remove the roast from the grill and let it rest for 15 minutes, before slicing and serving.

Vietnamese Beef Jerky

Servings: 6
Cooking Time: 240 Minutes

Ingredients:
- 2 Pound lean bottom round, rump roast or sirloin
- 2 Large garlic, roughly chopped
- 1 Stalk fresh lemongrass, trimmed and white parts thinly sliced
- 1 1/2 inch fresh ginger, peeled and roughly chopped
- 1/2 Cup soy sauce or Bragg Liquid Aminos
- 3 Tablespoon water
- 3 Tablespoon sugar
- 2 Tablespoon fish sauce
- 2 Teaspoon red chile flakes, or more to taste
- 1/2 Teaspoon pink curing salt (optional)

Directions:
1. Remove any visible fat from the meat and slice it into thin strips against the grain with a sharp chef's knife. (This is easier if the meat is partially frozen.) Transfer to a large, sturdy resealable bag.
2. Make the Marinade: In a blender jar or food processor bowl, combine the garlic, lemongrass, ginger, soy sauce, water, sugar, fish sauce, chile flakes and pink curing salt, if using. Pulse until relatively smooth.
3. Pour over the meat and massage the bag so the meat strips are evenly coated with the marinade. Refrigerate for at least 8 hours, or overnight. Turn the bag once or twice to redistribute the juices.
4. Supply your smoker with wood pellets and follow the start-up procedure. Preheat the grill, with the lid closed, to 165° F.
5. Drain the meat (discard the marinade) and pat dry with paper towels. Arrange the meat strips directly on the grill grate, perpendicular to the bars in a single layer. If you like your jerky spicy, feel free to lightly sprinkle additional red chile flakes on the meat.
6. Smoke the jerky, turning once, until the jerky is dry, but still pliant, about 4 to 6 hours. Grill: 165 °F
7. Let cool completely, then transfer to a clean resealable bag. Store in the refrigerator for the longest shelf life. The jerky can also be frozen. Enjoy!

Smoked Spiced Pulled Beef Chuck Roast

Servings: 6-8
Cooking Time: 360 Minutes

Ingredients:
- 1 chuck roast (3-4 pounds)
- 1 yellow or white onion (sliced)
- 3 cups beef stock (divided use)
- SIMPLE BEEF RUB
- 2 Tablespoons kosher salt
- 2 Tablespoons coarse black pepper
- 2 Tablespoons garlic powder

Directions:
1. Supply your smoker with wood pellets and follow the start-up procedure. Preheat the grill, with the lid closed, to 225 °F.
2. Combine all of the ingredients for the rub in a small bowl and rub liberally onto your beef roast, using your hands to press the rub into every surface of the meat.
3. Put the roast directly on your grill grate, fat-side up, and cook for 3 hours. Spray with 1 cup of the beef stock every hour (reserve the other 2 cups of stock).
4. Turn up the heat after 3 hours. Place the sliced onions in the bottom of a large disposable aluminum foil pan and pour the remaining 2 cups of stock in the bottom of the pan. Transfer the roast into the pan on top of the onions and place the pan into the grill.
5. Increase your grill temperature to 250 degrees F, and cook until the internal temperature reaches 165 degrees F (about 3 more hours).
6. Cover the pan tightly with aluminum foil once your roast hits 165 degrees F, and continue cooking until thermometer inserted in the thickest part of the meat reads 200 to 202 degrees F (this step can take another 3 hours). Every roast will be done at a slightly different temperature, so look for your probe to slide into the meat like it is sliding into softened butter.
7. Remove the pan from the smoker and let rest for a few minutes. Separate the roast from the cooking liquid. Shred the roast and separate the fat from the cooking liquid. Moisten the roast with the remaining cooking liquid, or make it into jus for dipping, or turn it into gravy.

Grilled Bell Pepper Flank Steak Fajitas

Servings: 1
Cooking Time: 30 Minutes

Ingredients:

- 1 Green Bell Pepper, Sliced
- 3 Tbsp Olive Oil
- 1 Onion, Diced
- Sweet Heat Rub
- 1 Red Bell Peppers, Sliced
- 1 -16Oz Steak, Flank
- 8 Tortilla, Corn
- 1 Yellow Bell Pepper, Sliced

Directions:

1. Rub flank steak with 1 tbsp olive oil and Sweet Heat Rub Grill seasoning. Cover and marinate in the refrigerator for 1 hour.
2. Lightly brush peppers and onion with olive oil.
3. Supply your smoker with wood pellets and follow the start-up procedure. Preheat the grill, with the lid closed, to 400° F. Place pepper and onion on grill and cook 5 minutes per side. Watch carefully to ensure the peppers and onion do not burn.
4. Remove peppers and onion from grill and toss lightly with remaining olive oil in a medium sized bowl. Transfer peppers and onions to a cutting board and slice into strips. Set aside.
5. Place flank steak directly on grill. Cook until medium rare (an internal temperature of 165°F).
6. Remove flank steak from the grill and transfer to cutting board. Let meat rest for 5 minutes, then slice against the grain into strips.
7. Place flank steak, peppers, and onions in a platter and serve immediately with warm tortillas, salsa, guacamole, sour cream, shredded cheese, thinly sliced iceberg lettuce, or your favorite fajita toppings.

Cucumber Beef Kefta

Servings: 4
Cooking Time: 10 Minutes

Ingredients:

- bamboo skewers, soaked in warm water
- 1 tbsp blackened saskatchewan rub seasoning
- 3 tbsp cilantro, chopped
- for topping, cucumbers
- 1 tsp cumin
- 2 lbs ground beef
- 1 tsp paprika
- 3 tbsp parsley, chopped
- pitas
- 1 red onion, grated
- for topping, tomatoes
- to taste, tzatziki sauce

Directions:

1. In a mixing bowl, combine ground beef, onion, Blackened Saskatchewan, cumin, paprika, cilantro, and parsley. Mix well, then cover and refrigerate for 1 hour to allow the flavors to blend.
2. Supply your smoker with wood pellets and follow the start-up procedure. Preheat the grill, with the lid closed, to 425° F. If using a gas or charcoal grill, set it up for medium-high heat.
3. Prepare kebabs: take small amounts of ground beef kefta and shape into popsicle-size cylinders. Skewer the meat, squeezing it to mold it to the skewer.
4. Grill kefta 3 to 5 minutes per side, then remove from the grill and serve warm with pitas, tzatziki sauce, and your favorite fresh veggies.

Carne Asada Recipe

Servings: 4
Cooking Time: 15 Minutes

Ingredients:

- 2 Pound Flank Steak, or substitute skirt steak
- 1 Cup Carne Asada Marinade
- 1 lime, juiced
- 2 Clove garlic, minced
- 1 Teaspoon cumin
- 1 Teaspoon dried oregano, preferably Mexican
- 1 Chile Pepper in Adobo Sauce, minced

Directions:

1. Lay the flank steak in a baking dish large enough to hold it. In a small bowl, combine the Carne Asada Marinade, the lime juice, garlic, cumin, oregano, and chile in adobo sauce, if using. Pour the marinade over

the steak, turning to coat, then cover with plastic wrap and refrigerate for 2 to 4 hours.

2. Supply your smoker with wood pellets and follow the start-up procedure. Preheat the grill, with the lid closed, to High heat.

3. Lift the flank steak from the marinade (discard the marinade) and pat dry with paper towels.

4. Arrange the steak at a diagonal directly on the grill grate. Grill for 6 minutes, then turn with tongs. Continue grilling for 4 to 6 minutes more. (The exact time will depend on the thickness of your steak, but flank steak is best medium-rare.) Grill: 500 ℉

5. Transfer the steak to a cutting board and let rest for 5 minutes. Slice thinly on the diagonal across the grain. Arrange on a platter. Serve immediately with the tortillas and salsa. Enjoy!

Hot Coffee-rubbed Brisket

Servings: 8
Cooking Time: 240 Minutes

Ingredients:
- aluminum foil
- 12 lbs beef brisket, packer cut
- java chop house rub

Directions:

1. Inject the brisket with 1 cup of beef broth, being sure to inject with the grain, spacing 1 inch apart.

2. Season the whole brisket with Java Chophouse, then set aside.

3. Supply your smoker with wood pellets and follow the start-up procedure. Preheat the grill, with the lid closed, to 350° F. If using a gas or charcoal grill, set it up for medium heat.

4. Place the brisket, directly on the grill grate, fat side down, and cook for 1 hour. Begin spraying with broth (1 cup total) every 15 minutes until the internal temperature reaches 160 to 165° F (about 30 to 60 min).

5. Remove brisket from the grill and set on a foil-lined tray. Bring up the sides of the foil, then slowly pour the remaining cup of broth over the top of the brisket, giving time to allow broth to seep into the brisket. Wrap with foil, then set on a sheet tray and return to the grill.

6. Reduce temperature to 275°F and cook for an additional 1 ½ to 2 1/2 hours.

7. Begin checking the brisket for tenderness after 1 hour. Punch thermometer probe or skewer into brisket. Desired tenderness is achieved when the probe or skewer easily slides into the brisket, like butter. If the brisket is slightly tough, repeat this test every 30 minutes. The target temperature is between 206 and 210° F.

8. Remove the brisket from the grill, and cut foil to vent. Allow the brisket to rest for 30 to 45 minutes before slicing. Separate the point from the flat. Slice the flat against the grain, then cube the brisket point for burnt ends. Serve warm.

Bbq Brisket Tacos

Servings: 6
Cooking Time: 45 Minutes

Ingredients:
- 5 Pound leftover beef brisket
- 1/2 Cup beef broth
- 5 avocados
- 4 diced Roma tomatoes
- 1 jalapeño, minced
- 1/2 Cup sour cream
- 1 lime juice
- salt and pepper
- 20 flour tortillas

Directions:

1. Supply your smoker with wood pellets and follow the start-up procedure. Preheat the grill, with the lid closed, to 300° F.

2. If not already sliced, slice brisket against the grain to 1/4 inch slices. Place sliced brisket in a double layer of foil and add beef broth. Seal foil and place on grill for 45 to 60 minutes until warm. Grill: 300 ℉

3. If not using leftover brisket, see here for our favorite brisket recipe.

4. While brisket is warming up, make the guacamole. Mash the avocados and mix with tomatoes, jalapeño, onion, sour cream, lime juice and salt and pepper. Set aside.

5. Wrap the tortillas in foil and place in grill for 15 minutes or until warm. Grill: 300 °F

6. Remove brisket and tortillas from grill and assemble. Top with guacamole and your favorite toppings. Enjoy!

Smoked Red Wine Beef Roast

Servings: 8
Cooking Time: 180 Minutes

Ingredients:

- 12 oz beef broth
- 6 lbs eye of round beef roast
- 2 tbsp black pepper
- ½ tbsp celery salt
- ½ tbsp garlic powder
- 2 tbsp kosher salt
- ½ tbsp onion powder
- 2 cups red wine
- 1/3 cup Worcestershire sauce

Directions:

1. Supply your smoker with wood pellets and follow the start-up procedure. Preheat the grill, with the lid closed, to 225 °F.

2. Mix the beef broth, red wine, and Worcestershire sauce in a mixing bowl. Fill your meat injector with the mixture.

3. Mix the seasonings in a spice bottle and apply the rub all over the roast, making sure to coat the whole roast evenly.

4. Place the beef roast in the foil pan, fat side up. Using the meat injector, inject the liquid into all areas of the beef roast. Fill the bottom of the pan with the remaining liquid.

5. Place the pan in the smoker and let it cook for 3 hours, basting with the juices in the pan every hour or so.

6. After 3 hours, start checking the roast for the desired internal temperature (Rare: 135 °F, Medium Rare: 145 °F, Medium: 155 °F, Well Done: 170 °F).

7. Remove from the grill and the pan, and let the roast rest for 20 to 30 minutes before slicing.

8. Slice against the grain and enjoy!

Cheesy Skillet Shepherd's Pie

Servings: 4 - 6
Cooking Time: 40 Minutes

Ingredients:

- 2 Tbsp All-Purpose Flour
- 1 Cup Beef Broth
- ½ Tsp Black Pepper
- 2 Tbsp Butter
- 1 Cup Cheddar Cheese, Grated
- 4 Oz. Cream Cheese
- 3 Garlic Cloves, Minced
- 1 Lb. Ground Beef
- 1 Tbsp Italian Parsley
- 1 Tbsp Kosher Salt
- 1 Tbsp Olive Oil
- ½ Cup Minced Onion
- 1 ½ Cup Peas, Frozen
- 2 Tsp Pulled Pork Rub
- 1 Tsp Rosemary, Finely Chopped
- 1 ½ Lbs. Russet Potatoes, Peeled And Quartered

Directions:

1. Supply your smoker with wood pellets and follow the start-up procedure. Preheat the grill, with the lid closed, to 400° F. If using a gas or charcoal grill, set the temp to medium-high heat.

2. In a cast iron Dutch oven, bring potatoes and just enough water to cover to a boil. Add salt and cook until tender, 12 to 15 minutes. Drain potatoes, and return to pot. Add cream cheese, butter, ½ teaspoon salt, ½ teaspoon black pepper, and mash until smooth. Set aside.

3. Place cast iron skillet on grill and heat oil. Add onion and sauté 2 minutes, then add garlic and sauté until fragrant. Add ground beef, Pulled Pork Rub, and rosemary, and cook, stirring occasionally, breaking up the meat until browned.

4. Sprinkle flour over beef and stir until combined. Add the broth and cook, stirring until thickened, about 3 minutes.

5. Add a layer of peas over beef and sprinkle with parsley. Dollop mashed potatoes on top of peas and spread evenly.

6. Increase temperature to 450° F. Cover and cook for 5 minutes, then top with grated cheese. Cover and cook and additional 5 to 7 minutes, until cheese is melted, and edges of potatoes begin to brown. Serve hot.

Steak Tips With Mashed Potatoes

Servings: 4-6
Cooking Time: 60 Minutes

Ingredients:
- 1 Cup Beef Broth
- 1 Stick (Room Temperature) Butter, Unsalted
- 2 Tablespoon Flour, All-Purpose
- 1 Tablespoon Java Chophouse Seasoning
- 4 Tablespoon Java Chophouse Seasoning, Divided
- 2 Pounds Medium Russet Potatoes, Peeled And Cut (Large Chunks)
- 2 Pounds Strip Sirloin
- 1/2 To 1 Cup Whole Milk, Warm

Directions:

1. For the mashed potatoes: add the potatoes to a large pot and add enough cold water to cover the potatoes. Bring to a simmer over medium heat until the potatoes are tender enough to be pierced with a fork, about 40 minutes. Drain the potatoes.

2. Add the potatoes to a large mixing bowl. Add the butter, 1 tablespoon of Java Chop House and ½ cup of warm milk. Mash until smooth and lump free. If potatoes are too thick, add more milk, a tablespoon at a time, until you reach your desired consistency.

3. For the steak tips: Supply your smoker with wood pellets and follow the start-up procedure. Preheat the grill, with the lid closed, to 350° F. Season the steaks generously on both sides with 2 tablespoons of Java Chop House seasoning and grill for 8-10 minutes per side. When steaks are done, remove from grill, allow to rest for 15 minutes, then cut into chunks.

4. While the steak is resting, add the butter to a small saucepan over low heat. Once the butter is melted, whisk in the flour and cook for 2 minutes until the flour smells toasted. Slowly whisk in the beef broth and remaining 2 tablespoons of Java Chop House seasoning and cook the gravy over low heat until thickened. Remove from heat and toss the steak tips in the gravy.

5. Serve steak tips over mashed potatoes. Enjoy!

Savory Chili Mac And Cheese

Servings: 4
Cooking Time: 25 Minutes

Ingredients:
- 4 Cups Beef Stock
- 2 Teaspoons Chili Powder
- 2 Tbsp Chopped Fresh Parsley Leaves
- 2 Cloves Garlic, Minced
- 1 1/2 Teaspoon Cumin
- 10 Oz. Elbow Macaroni / Noodles
- 8 Oz Ground Beef
- 3/4 Cup Kidney Beans, Drained And Rinsed
- And Freshly Ground Black Pepper Kosher Salt
- 1 Tbs Olive Oil
- 1 Onion, Diced
- 1 Tbs Sweet Heat Rub
- 3/4 Cup Shredded Cheddar Cheese
- 1 (14.5-Ounce) Tomatoes, Canned And Diced

Directions:

1. Supply your smoker with wood pellets and follow the start-up procedure. Preheat the grill, with the lid open, to 350° F. If you're using a gas or charcoal grill, set it up for medium heat.

2. Heat olive oil in a Dutch oven or cast iron pan over medium-high heat. Add garlic, onion and ground beef, and cook until browned, about 3-5 minutes. Break up the beef as it cooks with a large wooden spoon or fork.

3. Stir in beef broth, tomatoes, beans, Sweet Heat, chili powder and cumin. Add salt and pepper to taste. Bring to a simmer and stir in pasta.

4. Transfer pot to the preheated grill and cover. Cook until pasta is cooked through, about 15-20 minutes. Remove from heat and top generously with shredded cheese, replace the cover to allow cheese to melt, about 2 minutes. Garnish with fresh parsley and serve immediately!

Salt & Pepper Dinosaur Bones

Servings: 3-4
Cooking Time: 480 Minutes

Ingredients:

- 1 rack of beef plate short ribs, about 4 to 5lb (1.8 to 2.3kg) total, or 3 bones
- coarse kosher salt
- freshly ground black pepper
- granulated garlic
- crushed red pepper flakes (optional)
- 1½ cups sugar-free dark-colored soda, sugar-free root beer, beef broth, or brewed coffee

Directions:

1. Supply your smoker with wood pellets and follow the start-up procedure. Preheat the grill, with the lid closed, to 250° F.
2. Place the ribs in an aluminum foil roasting pan. If the rack has a thick cap of fat on the meaty side, trim most of it off because that will impede the formation of a nice bark on the ribs.
3. Generously season the ribs on all sides with salt, pepper, garlic, and red pepper flakes (if using). Place the ribs bone side down on the grate and smoke for 3 hours.
4. Add the soda to a spray bottle and spritz the ribs. Continue to smoke the ribs until the internal temperature reaches 203°F (95°C), about 4 to 5 hours more, spritzing once an hour. (Insert the probe next to the middle rib, being careful not to touch the bone.) When the ribs are tender, the meat will feel gelatinous and springy and will have shrunk back from the ends of the bones by up to 2 inches (5cm).
5. Transfer the ribs to a clean sheet pan and wrap with heavy-duty aluminum foil. Let rest for 1 hour, preferably in an insulated cooler.
6. Slice the ribs apart or remove the meat from the bones and thinly slice before serving with additional salt and pepper.

Jalapeno Pepper Jack Cheese Bacon Burgers

Servings: 4
Cooking Time: 30 Minutes

Ingredients:

- 4 Slices, Raw Bacon
- 1/2 Cup Prepared Barbecue Sauce
- 1 Pound Ground Beef
- Hickory Bacon Seasoning, Plus More For Sprinkling
- 2 Thinly Sliced Jalapeno Peppers
- 1/2 Cup Olive Oil
- 4 Onion Burger Buns
- Onion, Crispy
- 4 Pepper Jack Cheese, Sliced

Directions:

1. Supply your smoker with wood pellets and follow the start-up procedure. Preheat the grill, with the lid closed, to 350° F. If using a gas or charcoal grill, set it up for medium high heat.
2. Make the burgers: in a large bowl, mix together the ground beef and Hickory Bacon seasoning until the seasoning is well incorporated. Use the Burger Press to make burger patties. Repeat until all the ground beef is gone.
3. In a small bowl, toss the sliced raw jalapenos with the olive oil and place them in the vegetable grill basket. Grill the jalapenos, stirring occasionally, until soft and charred in some spots. Remove from the grill and set aside.
4. Place the bacon on the vegetable grill basket and grill for 5-7 minutes, or until the bacon is crispy and brown. Remove from the grill and set aside.
5. Grill the burgers: place the burger patties on the grill and, if desired, sprinkle more Hickory Bacon seasoning on the patties. Grill the burgers for 5 minutes on one side, then flip and top with a slice of pepper jack cheese and grill for another 5-7 minutes, or until the internal temperature of the burgers is 135-140°F.
6. Remove the burgers from the grill and place on an onion bun. Top with the bacon, grilled jalapenos, crisped onions, and a spoonful of barbecue sauce.

The Boss Beef Burger

Servings: 10
Cooking Time: 85 Minutes

Ingredients:
- 4 Lbs Beef, Ground
- 1 Loaf Bread, Sourdough Round
- 1/2 Cup Butter
- Condiments (Ketchup, Mustard, Relish, Etc.)
- Lettuce
- 3 Cups Mushroom
- 3 Onion, Chopped
- Kansas City BBQ Sauce
- Mandarin Habanero Spice
- 1 Lbs Pork, Ground
- Red Onion, Chopped
- 1 Bag Shredded Cheddar Cheese
- Tomato, Sliced

Directions:
1. Supply your smoker with wood pellets and follow the start-up procedure. Preheat the grill, with the lid closed, to 300° F.
2. In a large bowl, mix together the ground beef, ground pork, eggs, barbecue sauce, and seasoning until combined. Do not over mix as this will cause the meat to be tough after cooking. Split the mixture into two equal parts.
3. Melt the butter in a pan over medium heat and sauté the onion mushrooms until golden.
4. In a cast iron pan, flatten one half of the meat mixture into the bottom, taking care to work meat slightly up the sides of the pan. Sprinkle in half of the bag of cheese. Pour in onion mixture and top with the rest of the cheese.
5. On a clean work surface, mold the second half of the meat mixture into a circle and cover the filling to complete the burger. Make sure that the top and bottom meat patties are secured together so that the filling cannot be seen.
6. Place the cast iron pan in the Grill for 1 hour - 1 hour 15 minutes, or until the internal temperature reaches 160°F. Crank up the to "HIGH" and open the flame broiler. Flip the burger out of the cast iron pan onto the grates and sear each side for 5 minutes, to get those beautiful grill marks.
7. To serve: You can make an enormous burger like we did, or you can cut it like a pie into slices to be served on regular hamburger buns with your desired condiments.

Lemon Tomahawk Steak

Servings: 2 – 4
Cooking Time: 215 Minutes

Ingredients:
- Apple Corer Or Metal Spoon
- 3 Lbs Gala Apples
- 1 Lemon
- Chop House Steak Rub
- 1 Tbsp Tennessee Apple Butter Rub
- Sugar
- 4 Cups Water

Directions:
1. Supply your smoker with wood pellets and follow the start-up procedure. Preheat the grill, with the lid closed, to 400° F. If using a gas or charcoal grill, set heat to medium-high heat.
2. Core and halve the apples. Place apples skin-side down on a sheet tray and season with Tennessee Apple Butter and set aside.
3. In a cast iron pot, combine the apple cores with the juice and zest from one lemon. Cover the mixture with water, transfer to the grill and bring to a boil. Reduce heat to 225° F. Place the apples directly on the grill grate (skin-side down) and cook for 1 hour.
4. After 1 hour, remove cast iron pot from the grill. Strain liquid, discard cores, return liquid to pot, and whisk in sugar. Cover with lid and return to grill. Allow to simmer for another hour.
5. Add smoked apples to the pot and continue to simmer for 20 minutes. Remove pot from grill and purée apple mixture in a blender. Pour apple purée back into pot and return to grill. Increase heat to 375° F and simmer for 20 minutes. Remove from grill and allow to cool slightly.
6. Reduce heat on grill to 225° F. Season the tomahawk steak with   Chop House Steak Rub on both

sides. Place the steak on the grill grates, insert a temperature probe, and grill, undisturbed, for 45 minutes, or until the steak reaches an internal temperature of 120°F

7. Remove steak from grill and set aside. Open the Sear Slide on your   and increase temperature to 400°F. Return tomahawk to grill and sear over open flames, about 2-3 minutes per side.

8. Pull the steak off the grill and allow it to rest for 10 minutes. Ladle reserved apple butter over steak and serve.

Teriyaki Bbq Beef Skewers

Servings: 8
Cooking Time: 8 Minutes

Ingredients:
*   2 Pound Top Round Steak, boneless, cut into 1/4" slices
*   3/4 Cup light brown sugar
*   1/2 Cup soy sauce
*   1/4 Cup Pineapple Juice (optional)
*   1/4 Cup water
*   Cup vegetable oil
*   1 Clove Garlic (Large), finely chopped

Directions:
1. Slice the beef into 1-1/2 - 2" wide strips.
2. Whisk brown sugar, soy sauce, pineapple juice, water, vegetable oil, and garlic together.
3. Pour the marinade into a large zip-top bag and drop beef slices into the mixture. Marinate beef in refrigerator for 24 hours.
4. Remove beef from the marinade, shaking to remove any excess liquid. Discard marinade. Thread beef slices in a zig-zag onto the skewers.
5. Supply your smoker with wood pellets and follow the start-up procedure. Preheat the grill, with the lid closed, to 325° F.
6. Cook skewers on preheated grill until the beef is cooked through, about 3 minutes per side. Enjoy! Grill: 325 °F

Chorizo Cheese Stuffed Burgers

Servings: 2

Cooking Time: 45 Minutes

Ingredients:
*   2 Pound ground beef, 80% lean
*   4 Ounce Prime Rib Rub
*   12 Ounce Chorizo
*   2 Slices cheddar cheese
*   4 Whole Brioche Bun
*   Tomatoes, sliced
*   red onion, sliced
*   lettuce, sliced

Directions:
1. Mix 2 lb of 80/20 ground beef in mixing bowl with Traeger Prime Rib Rub.
2. Divide the ground beef into eight 1/4 lb patties. Make one patty the base, lay down 1/4 of a cheese slice, add 3 oz. of chorizo and top with another 1/4 cheese slice. Apply another patty on top and pinch the ends all the way around the burger to seal together the two patties.
3. Repeat until all 4 patties are done.
4. Supply your smoker with wood pellets and follow the start-up procedure. Preheat the grill, with the lid closed, to 325° F.
5. Place burgers on the Traeger for 15 minutes on each side. If desired, top each burger with slice of Cheddar cheese, let melt. Remove from Traeger and let rest for 10 minutes tented with foil.
6. While burgers are resting, brush the brioche buns with melted better and toast for 30-45 seconds on the grill.
7. Remove buns from grill and assemble burger with toppings. Enjoy!

Smoked Black Pepper Beef Back Ribs

Servings: 2 – 4
Cooking Time: 260 Minutes

Ingredients:
*   2 racks beef back ribs
*   ½ tbsp black pepper
*   ⅓ cup chop house steak seasoning

Directions:

1. Supply your smoker with wood pellets and follow the start-up procedure. Preheat the grill, with the lid closed, to 250° F. If using a gas or charcoal grill, set it up for low heat.

2. Place the ribs on a sheet tray, then remove the membrane from the back of the ribs: Take a butter knife and wedge it just underneath the membrane to loosen it. Using your hands, or a paper towel to grip, pull the membrane up and off the bone. Rub each rack generously with Chop House Steak seasoning and black pepper.

3. Place the ribs on the grill and smoke for 2 hours. Increase the temperature to 300°F and cook an additional 45 to 60 minutes, or until the ribs reach an internal temperature of 205° F. Be sure and flip the ribs halfway to achieve good bark.

4. Remove ribs from the grill and wrap in butcher paper. Allow ribs to rest for 20 minutes, then slice and serve hot.

Sweet And Spicy Beef Sirloin Tip Roast

Servings: 8
Cooking Time: 120 Minutes

Ingredients:
- 3 Pound beef sirloin tip roast
- 2 Tablespoon Beef Rub
- 1/2 Cup 'Que BBQ Sauce
- 1/4 Cup chili sauce

Directions:
1. Season sirloin tip roast evenly with Traeger Beef Rub on all sides. Let roast rest at room temperature for 30 minutes.

2. Supply your smoker with wood pellets and follow the start-up procedure. Preheat the grill, with the lid closed, to 275° F.

3. Place the roast on the Traeger and cook for about 75 minutes or until the internal temperature reaches 130°F. Grill: 275 °F Probe: 130 °F

4. In a small bowl, combine Traeger 'Que and chili sauce. Once meat has reached 130°F, brush the roast with 1/4 cup of the bbq chili sauce.

5. Continue cooking until internal temperature reaches 140°F. Grill: 275 °F Probe: 140 °F

6. Remove from the grill and place on a cutting board then tent with foil. Let stand 10 minutes or until internal temperature reaches 145°F.

7. Slice roast across the grain into thin slices and brush each slice with remaining sauce. Serve, enjoy!

Bacon-swiss Cheesesteak Meatloaf

Servings: 4
Cooking Time: 120 Minutes

Ingredients:
- 1 tablespoon canola oil
- 2 garlic cloves, finely chopped
- 1 medium onion, finely chopped
- 1 poblano chile, stemmed, seeded, and finely chopped
- 2 pounds extra-lean ground beef
- 2 tablespoons Montreal steak seasoning
- 1 tablespoon A.1. Steak Sauce
- ½ pound bacon, cooked and crumbled
- 2 cups shredded Swiss cheese
- 1 egg, beaten
- 2 cups breadcrumbs
- ½ cup Tiger Sauce

Directions:
1. On your stove top, heat the canola oil in a medium sauté pan over medium-high heat. Add the garlic, onion, and poblano, and sauté for 3 to 5 minutes, or until the onion is just barely translucent

2. Supply your smoker with wood pellets and follow the start-up procedure. Preheat, with the lid closed, to 225°F.

3. In a large bowl, combine the sautéed vegetables, ground beef, steak seasoning, steak sauce, bacon, Swiss cheese, egg, and breadcrumbs. Mix with your hands until well incorporated, then shape into a loaf.

4. Put the meatloaf in a cast iron skillet and place it on the grill. Close the lid and smoke for 2 hours, or until a meat thermometer inserted in the loaf reads 165°F.

5. Top with the meatloaf with the Tiger Sauce, remove from the grill, and let rest for about 10 minutes before serving.

Savory Cheese Steak Rolls With Puff Pastry

Servings: 4
Cooking Time: 25 Minutes

Ingredients:
- 4 oz american or jack cheese, shredded, divided
- 2 tbsp butter
- to taste, chop house steak rub
- to taste, chop house steak rub (for sauce)
- 3 oz cream cheese
- 1 egg, beaten
- 1 tbsp flour
- 1 tbsp flour (for sauce)
- 1 puff pastry sheet, thawed
- 1 lb sandwich steak, shaved/sliced thin
- 1 tbsp vegetable oil
- 1 cup yellow onion, sliced thin
- 2/3 cup milk

Directions:
1. Supply your smoker with wood pellets and follow the start-up procedure. Preheat the grill, with the lid closed, to 400° F. If using a gas or charcoal grill, set it up for medium-high heat. Preheat the griddle to medium flame.
2. Add oil to the griddle, then cook steak for 2 to 3 minutes, turning with a spatula. Add onions, season with Chop House and cook another minute to soften. Transfer steak and onions to a bowl, then set aside to cool.
3. Meanwhile, melt butter in a sauté pan on the griddle. Stir in flour, then cook for 1 minute. Whisk in milk, then add cream cheese, and 2 ounces of shredded cheese. Whisk until smooth, then remove from the griddle to cool slightly. Use half of the sauce in the pastry, and the other half for serving/dipping once baked.
4. Flour your rolling surface, then set the pastry sheet on top of the flour. Roll the pastry sheet into a 10 to 12 inch square, then cut into 4 squares.
5. Spoon cheese sauce on each pastry square, then divide the steak and onion mixture among the pastries. Top each with remaining shredded cheese, brush sides with beaten egg, then fold pastries over, corner to corner.

Secure the seams by pressing down with a fork. Brush the top with beaten egg, then place on a sheet tray.
6. Place the sheet tray on the grill and bake for 18 to 20 minutes, until golden. Remove from the grill, cool for 5 minutes, then cut in half and serve warm with cheese sauce.

Smoked Corned Beef & Cabbage

Servings: 6
Cooking Time: 300 Minutes

Ingredients:
- 1 (3-5 lb) corned beef brisket
- 1 Quart chicken stock
- 12 Ounce (12 oz) beer, preferably pilsner or lager
- 1/4 Teaspoon garlic salt
- 1/2 Cup (1 stick) butter, cut into slices
- 2 Cup baby carrots
- 1 Pound baby or fingerling potatoes
- 1 Head cabbage, cut into wedges
- 2 Tablespoon fresh chopped dill

Directions:
1. Soak the corned beef in water for about 8 hours, changing water every 2 hours.
2. Supply your smoker with wood pellets and follow the start-up procedure. Preheat the grill, with the lid closed, to 180° F.
3. Remove brisket from water and pat dry. Place directly on the grill grate and smoke for 2 hours. Grill: 180 °F
4. Transfer brisket from grill and place in a roasting pan. Increase grill temperature to 325°F and preheat, lid closed. Grill: 325 °F
5. Sprinkle seasoning packet on top of brisket and pour chicken stock and dark beer over the roast.
6. Cover roasting pan with foil and place on the grill. Cook for 2 hours or until beef is fork tender. Grill: 325 °F
7. Remove foil and add carrots and potatoes to the roasting pan. Cover meat and vegetables with garlic salt and butter slices. Grill: 325 °F
8. Recover with foil and cook for an additional hour or until carrots and potatoes are just tender. Add cabbage,

cover and return to grill for 20 minutes more. Grill: 325 °F

9.   Remove vegetables from the pan to a bowl or serving platter. Slice beef and serve with potatoes, cabbage and carrots. Garnish with fresh dill and thyme if desired. Enjoy!

Kansas City Cheese Brisket Burger

Servings: 4
Cooking Time: 30 Minutes

Ingredients:

- 1/2 Cup Barbecue Sauce
- 4 Brioche Burger Buns
- 4 Slices Brisket
- 1 Lbs Ground Beef
- 8 Onion Rings
- 4 Tablespoons Sweet Rib Rub
- 4 Slices Smoked Guoda Cheese, Sliced

Directions:

1.   In a large bowl, sprinkle the   Sweet Rib Rub over the ground beef and mix well to combine. Shape the ground beef into 4 patties and set aside.

2.   Supply your smoker with wood pellets and follow the start-up procedure. Preheat the grill, with the lid closed, to 350° F. Grill your burgers for 8-10 minutes, or until desired degree of doneness.

3.   Halfway through cooking, top each burger patty with a slice of smoked Guoda cheese.

4.   Remove the burgers from the grill and assemble the burgers. Place each burger on a bun and top with 2 tablespoons of barbecue sauce, 2 onion rings and a slice of brisket, then serve and enjoy!

Traditional Tomahawk Steak

Servings: 4-6
Cooking Time: 120 Minutes

Ingredients:

- 1 tomahawk ribeye steak (2 1/2 to 3 1/2 lbs)
- 5 garlic cloves, minced
- 2 tbsp kosher salt
- 1 bundle fresh thyme
- 2 tbsp ground black pepper

- 8 oz butter stick
- 1 tbsp garlic powder
- 1/8 cup olive oil

Directions:

1.   Mix rub ingredients (salt, black pepper, and garlic powder) in a small bowl. Use this mixture to season all sides of the ribeye steak generously. You can also substitute your favorite steak seasoning. After applying seasoning, let the steak rest at room temperature for at least 30 minutes.

2.   While the steak rests, preheat your pellet grill to 450°F - 550°F for searing

3.   Sear the steak for 5 minutes on each side. Halfway through each side (so after 2 1/2 minutes), rotate the steak 90° to form grill marks on the tomahawk

4.   After the tomahawk steak has seared for 5 minutes on each side (10 minutes total), move the steak to a raised rack

5.   Adjust your pellet grill's temperature to 250°F and turn up smoke setting if applicable. Leave the lid open for a moment to help allow some heat to escape

6.   Stick your probe meat thermometer into the very center of the cut to measure internal temperature.

7.   Place butter stick, garlic cloves, olive oil, and thyme in the aluminum pan. Then place the aluminum pan under the steak to catch drippings. After a few minutes, the steak drippings and ingredients will mix together

8.   Baste the steak with the aluminum pan mixture every 10 minutes until the tomahawk steak reaches your desired doneness

9.   Once the steak reaches its desired doneness, remove from the grill and place on a cutting board or serving dish. The steak should rest for 10-15 minutes before cutting/serving.

Smoked Beef Ribs

Servings: 4-8
Cooking Time: 360 Minutes

Ingredients:

- 2 (2- or 3-pound) racks beef ribs
- 2 tablespoons yellow mustard
- 1 batch Sweet and Spicy Cinnamon Rub

Directions:

1. Supply your smoker with wood pellets and follow the start-up procedure. Preheat the grill, with the lid closed, to 225°F.

2. Remove the membrane from the backside of the ribs. This can be done by cutting just through the membrane in an X pattern and working a paper towel between the membrane and the ribs to pull it off.

3. Coat the ribs all over with mustard and season them with the rub. Using your hands, work the rub into the meat.

4. Place the ribs directly on the grill grate and smoke until their internal temperature reaches between 190°F and 200°F.

5. Remove the racks from the grill and cut them into individual ribs. Serve immediately.

Grilled Skirt Steak Quesadillas

Servings: 4
Cooking Time: 15 Minutes

Ingredients:

- 2 Tablespoon chili powder
- 2 Teaspoon kosher salt
- 1 Teaspoon ground cumin
- 1/2 Teaspoon Chipotle Chili Powder
- 1/2 Teaspoon cayenne pepper
- 1 Teaspoon lime zest
- 1 1/2 Pound skirt steak
- 12 Whole Corn Tortillas, 6 inch
- 1 vegetable oil
- 1/2 Cup shredded pepper jack cheese

Directions:

1. For the skirt steak, combine the chili powder, salt, cumin, chipotle powder, cayenne and lime zest in a small bowl.

2. Rub the spice mixture over entire skirt steak and let marinate in a zip-top bag at least 20 to 25 minutes.

3. Supply your smoker with wood pellets and follow the start-up procedure. Preheat the grill, with the lid closed, to 400° F.

4. Place skirt steak on grill 3-4 minutes per side. Let rest for 20 minutes before cutting into bite sized pieces. Grill: 400 °F

5. For the quesadillas, take the tortillas and fill with cheese and grilled skirt steak. Cook on a grill pan or in a sauté pan with extra oil to prevent burning.

6. Serve with guacamole, sour cream or salsa. Enjoy!

Bbq Bacon Meatballs

Servings: 4
Cooking Time: 60 Minutes

Ingredients:

- 1 Pound ground beef
- 1 egg
- 1/4 Cup milk
- 1/2 Cup breadcrumbs
- 2 Tablespoon Beef Rub
- 4 Strips bacon, cut in half
- 1/4 Cup Rub
- 1/2 Cup Apricot BBQ Sauce

Directions:

1. Mix beef, egg, milk, breadcrumbs and Traeger Beef Rub in a large bowl by hand. Once well mixed, make 2 ounce meatballs until complete.

2. Wrap each meatball with a half slice of bacon and slide toothpick all the way through.

3. Put Traeger Rub in a small bowl and roll each meatball in the rub until well coated.

4. Supply your smoker with wood pellets and follow the start-up procedure. Preheat the grill, with the lid closed, to 180° F.

5. Place the meatballs on the grate, close the lid and smoke for 1 hour. Grill: 180 °F

6. Increase the Traeger temperature to 350°F and preheat, lid closed for 15 minutes. Cook meatballs for another 20 to 30 minutes or until the internal temperature reaches 160°F to 165°F. Grill: 350 °F Probe: 160 °F

7. About 10 minutes before the meatballs are ready, brush with Traeger Apricot BBQ Sauce and allow it to caramelize.

8. Remove from grill and allow to rest for 5 minutes. Enjoy!

Roasted Duck

Servings: 4
Cooking Time: 180 Minutes

Ingredients:
- 1 (5-6 lb) duck, defrosted
- Pork & Poultry Rub
- 1 Small onion, peeled and quartered
- 1 orange, quartered
- fresh herbs, such as parsley, sage or rosemary

Directions:
1. Remove the giblets and discard or save for another use. Trim any loose skin at the neck and remove excess fat from around the main cavity. Remove the wing tips if desired.
2. Rinse the duck under cold running water, inside and out, and dry with paper towels.
3. Prick the skin all over with the tip of a knife or the tines of a fork; do not pierce the meat. This helps to render the fat and crisp the skin.
4. Season the bird, inside and out, with Traeger Pork and Poultry Rub. Tuck the onion, orange, and fresh herbs into the cavity.
5. Tie the legs together with butcher's string.
6. Supply your smoker with wood pellets and follow the start-up procedure. Preheat the grill, with the lid closed, to 225° F.
7. Place the duck directly on the grill grate. Roast for 2-1/2 to 3 hours, or until the skin is brown and crisp. The internal temperature should register 160°F in the thigh (be sure to avoid the bone as this will give you an inaccurate reading). Grill: 225 °F Probe: 160 °F
8. If the duck is not browned to your liking, increase the grill temperature to 375°F and roast for several minutes at the higher temperature. Grill: 375 °F
9. Tent the duck loosely with foil and allow it to rest for 30 minutes.
10. Remove the butcher's twine and carve. Enjoy!

Flavour Reverse Seared T-bone Steak

Servings: 1 - 2
Cooking Time: 64 Minutes

Ingredients:
- Java Chop House Rub
- 1 Steak, T-Bone

Directions:
1. Supply your smoker with wood pellets and follow the start-up procedure. Preheat the grill, with the lid closed, to 250° F.
2. As the is preheating to the perfect temperature, spice the T-bone with your favorite steak rub.
3. Lay the steak on the grill for roughly 60 minutes or until the steaks reach an internal temperature of 105 to 110°F. Remove the steaks and set aside.
4. Crank up the heat to 450°F and open the flame broiler.
5. Place the steak over the flame broiler and sear for about 2 minutes a side, 4 minutes in total. You know when your steak is done once the internal temperature reaches 130 to 135°F (for medium-rare). Follow the below internal temperature for your cooking preference:
6. Rare: 125°F
7. Medium Rare: 130°F
8. Medium: 140°F
9. Well Done: 160°F
10. Once reached for personal preference, take the steaks off the grill and eat! Enjoy!

Smoked Meatball Egg Sandwiches

Servings: 4
Cooking Time: 25 Minutes

Ingredients:
- 3/4 Cup Breadcrumbs
- 2 Cloves Garlic, Minced
- 1 & 1/2 Lb. Ground Chuck
- 1 Jar Of Your Favorite Marinara Sauce
- 1 Large Eggs
- ¼ Cup Onion
- ¼ Cup Parsley, Minced Fresh
- ½ Tsp Pepper
- 1 Tbsp Chop House Steak Seasoning
- Provolone Cheese, Sliced
- ½ Tsp Salt
- Shredded Mozzarella Cheese
- 4 Sub Rolls Or Baguettes (6"), Sliced

- 2 Tbsp Worcestershire

Directions:

1. In a larger mixing bowl, combine the ground chuck, onions, garlic, Chop House Steak seasoning, salt, pepper, fresh parsley, Worcestershire, and egg. Add the breadcrumb mixture and parmesan cheese to the bowl and fold it into meat until well combined.

2. Supply your smoker with wood pellets and follow the start-up procedure. Preheat the grill, with the lid closed, to 400° F. If you're using a gas or charcoal grill, set it up for medium high heat and add your cast iron pan to the grill to warm up.

3. Roll the meat mixture into balls about 1 ½ inches wide, roughly the size of golf balls. Place meatballs into the cast iron skillet. Cook for 15 minutes or until meatballs are fully cooked and beginning to brown.

4. Pour full jar of marinara into the cast iron pan and gently stir to coat meatballs. Let simmer for 10-15 minutes.

5. Tear off four sheets of aluminum foil and place a sliced bun in the center of each. Divide the meatballs with sauce among the rolls. Top each roll with provolone cheese slices and mozzarella, and wrap entire sandwich tightly in foil. Return to the grill and cook an additional 10 minutes or until cheese is melty and bread has toasted. Serve immediately and enjoy!

Citrus Grilled Lamb Chops

Servings: 4 - 6
Cooking Time: 15 Minutes

Ingredients:

- 2 Tablespoons Chophouse Steak Seasoning
- 4 Finely Garlic Clove, Minced
- 2 Pounds Thick Cut Rib Chops Or Lamb Loin
- Juice From 1/2 Lemon
- Juice From 1/2 Lime
- ¼ Cup Olive Oil
- 3 Tablespoons Orange Juice
- ¼ Cup Red Wine Vinegar

Directions:

1. In a mixing bowl, whisk together all the ingredients and 2 tbsp Chophouse Steak. Place the lamb chops in a glass baking pan and pour the marinade over the top. Flip the chops over a few times to make sure that they are completely coated.

2. Cover the glass pan in aluminum foil and allow the lamb chops to marinade for 4-12 hours. Once the meat has finished marinating, drain off the excess marinade and discard.

3. Supply your smoker with wood pellets and follow the start-up procedure. Preheat the grill, with the lid closed, to 400° F. If you're using a gas or charcoal grill, set it up for medium high heat. Grill the chops for 5-7 minutes per side, then lower the temperature to 350°F or medium heat, and flip and grill for another 5-7 minutes.

4. Remove the lamb chops from the grill, cover in foil, and allow to rest for 5 minutes before serving.

Smoked Chicken Steak Sandwiches

Servings: 6
Cooking Time: 270 Minutes

Ingredients:

- 1 1/2 tsp black pepper, ground
- 3 lbs brisket flat
- 1 tbsp butter
- 1 1/2 cups chicken stock
- 1/4 cup chop house steak rub
- for topping, dill pickles
- 2 tsp garlic powder
- 8 oz maple cure
- 2 tsp mustard powder
- 1 onion, sliced
- 1 1/2 tbsp pickling spice
- pumpernickel rye, sliced
- to taste, sauerkraut
- to taste, spicy brown mustard
- 6 swiss cheese, sliced
- 2 qts water, cold

Directions:

1. Set the brisket flat on a cutting board, then trim off excess fat and silver skin.

2. Whisk together water and maple cure, until dissolved.

3. Lay brisket in a large container, season with pickling spice, then cover with brine/cure. The meat must be completely immersed. Cover and place in the refrigerator for 3 to 4 days.

4. Remove brisket flat from brine/cure. It will be pale grey in color, which is normal. Discard the cure and replace with plain water. Allow brisket to soak 1-2 hours.

5. Combine all ingredients for the rub in a bowl. Remove the brisket from the water and blot dry with paper towel.

6. Season the brisket well with the rub, pushing and massaging it into the surface. Place the brisket back into the refrigerator, uncovered, overnight.

7. Supply your smoker with wood pellets and follow the start-up procedure. Preheat the grill, with the lid closed, to 250° F. If using a gas or charcoal grill, set it up for low, indirect heat.

8. Transfer the brisket flat directly on the grill grate, fat side down, over indirect heat. Smoke for 2 hours, flipping after 1 hour.

9. Remove the brisket from the grill and place it in a cast iron skillet, or foil-lined aluminum pan with chicken stock and onions. Cover with a lid, or foil and return to the grill.

10. Increase temperature to 275° F, and cook an additional 1 hour, then check the brisket to see if enough liquid remains. If reducing too quickly, add 1 cup of water. Cook the brisket for another 1 hour, or until the brisket is probe tender

11. Remove from the grill and rest for at least 30 minutes, prior to slicing thin.

12. Preheat the griddle over low flame.

13. Grease griddle with 1 tablespoon of butter, then spread mustard on 4 slices of rye, then set on griddle. Add 2 portions of sliced pastrami. Warm pastrami 1 to 2 minutes, then flip. Top pastrami with sauerkraut and cheese, then close the griddle lid for 1 minute to crisp up the underside of the pastrami and melt the cheese.

14. Brush rye with mustard then set pastrami on every other slice. Set remaining toasted rye on top complete the smoked pastrami sandwich.

15. Remove from the griddle, then repeat. Slice each sandwich on the bias and serve warm with dill pickles.

Flavour Texas Smoke Beef

Servings: 8
Cooking Time: 315 Minutes

Ingredients:

- 1 Cup Strong Brewed Coffee or Espresso, Cold
- 1 Cup Cola
- 1/2 Cup Soy Sauce
- 1/4 Cup Worcestershire Sauce
- 1/4 Cup Brown Sugar
- 1 Tablespoon Morton Tender Quick Home Meat Cure
- 1 1/2 Teaspoon Freshly Ground Black Pepper
- 1 Tablespoon Hot Sauce
- 2 Pound Trimmed Beef Top Or Bottom Round

Directions:

1. Plan ahead! This recipe requires marinating time overnight. In a mixing bowl, combine the coffee, cola, soy sauce, Worcestershire sauce, brown sugar, curing salt (if using), pepper, and hot sauce.

2. With a sharp knife, slice the beef into 1/4" thick slices against the grain. (This is easier if the meat is partially frozen.)

3. Trim any fat or connective tissue.

4. Put the beef slices in a large resealable plastic bag.

5. Pour the marinade mixture over the beef, and massage the bag so that all the slices get coated with the marinade.

6. Seal the bag and refrigerate for several hours, or overnight.

7. Supply your smoker with wood pellets and follow the start-up procedure. Preheat the grill, with the lid closed, to 180 °F.

8. Remove the beef from the marinade and discard the marinade.

9. Dry the beef slices between paper towels. Arrange the meat in a single layer directly on the grill grate.

10. Smoke for 4 to 5 hours, or until the jerky is dry but still chewy and somewhat pliant when you bend a piece.

Pulled Beef

Servings: 5-8
Cooking Time: 840 Minutes

Ingredients:

- 1 (4-pound) top round roast
- 2 tablespoons yellow mustard
- 1 batch Espresso Brisket Rub
- ½ cup beef broth

Directions:

1. Supply your smoker with wood pellets and follow the start-up procedure. Preheat the grill, with the lid closed, to 225°F.
2. Coat the top round roast all over with mustard and season it with the rub. Using your hands, work the rub into the meat.
3. Place the roast directly on the grill grate and smoke until its internal temperature reaches 160°F and a dark bark has formed.
4. Pull the roast from the grill and place it on enough aluminum foil to wrap it completely.
5. Increase the grill's temperature to 350°F.
6. Fold in three sides of the foil around the roast and add the beef broth. Fold in the last side, completely enclosing the roast and liquid. Return the wrapped roast to the grill and cook until its internal temperature reaches 195°F.
7. Pull the roast from the grill and place it in a cooler. Cover the cooler and let the roast rest for 1 or 2 hours.
8. Remove the roast from the cooler and unwrap it. Pull apart the beef using just your fingers. Serve immediately.

Grilled Bison Rib Eye Kabobs

Servings: 4
Cooking Time: 20 Minutes

Ingredients:

- 3 Tablespoon Prime Rib Rub
- 3 Tablespoon Rosemary, finely chopped
- 2 Teaspoon salt
- 2 Tablespoon pepper
- 4 Clove garlic, minced

- 3 Pound Bison, Rib Eye, Trimmed and Cut into 1.25" Cubes

Directions:

1. In a small bowl, mix together Traeger Prime Rib Rub, rosemary, garlic, black pepper, and salt. Place bison cubes in a large Ziploc bag and pour in marinade.
2. Toss bison in marinade to coat the meat well and transfer to the refrigerator for 45 minutes to an hour. Remove bison from marinade draining any excess liquid that has gathered.
3. Thread bison pieces on a skewer and set aside.
4. Supply your smoker with wood pellets and follow the start-up procedure. Preheat the grill, with the lid closed, to 375° F.
5. Place kabobs directly on the grill grate and cook for 8-10 minutes per side or until internal temperature reaches 135°F for medium-rare. Grill: 375 °F Probe: 135 °F
6. Remove from grill and let rest 5 minutes before serving. Finish with additional chopped herbs if desired. Enjoy

Slow Smoked Spiced Beef

Servings: 6
Cooking Time: 360 Minutes

Ingredients:

- 3 lb beef (roast, rump, sirloin, top, or chuck)
- 1 1/2 tsp salt
- 1 tsp pepper
- 1 tsp garlic powder
- 1 tsp smoked paprika
- 1/2 tsp onion powder
- Worcestershire sauce to rub down

Directions:

1. Supply your smoker with wood pellets and follow the start-up procedure. Preheat the grill, with the lid closed, to 215 °F.
2. Start by mixing the salt, pepper, smoked paprika, garlic, and onion powders together.
3. Give the roast a good rub down with Worcestershire sauce, and then apply the spice rub.

4. Cook it in a smoker at around 215°F for 4 to 6 hours. The roast is ready to come out when its internal temperature is between 145°F to 155 °F.

5. Before slicing, let the roast rest for 20 minutes, covered with foil.

6. To help brighten up the beef's flavors, sprinklea little salt on the slices.

7. Serve and enjoy.

Smoked Beer Corned Beef

Servings: 6

Cooking Time: 240 Minutes

Ingredients:

- 6 lb corned beef brisket raw
- 2 tbsp black pepper
- 8 oz light beer

Directions:

1. Supply your smoker with wood pellets and follow the start-up procedure. Preheat the grill, with the lid closed, to 275 °F.

2. Cut open packaging of corned beef and drain off liquid. Be sure to grab the spice packet included with the brisket. Gently rinse off corned beef and then pat dry with a paper towel.

3. Open the spice packet included with your corned beef and sprinkle contents over the brisket, then sprinkle a light dusting of black pepper according to your preference.

4. Once pellet grill has reached temperature, insert probes into corned beef brisket pieces. If you only have a single probe, insert that probe in the center of the smallest piece because it will cook the fastest.

5. Smoke for 3 to 4 hours until corned beef reaches an internal temperature of 175 degrees F. Next transfer briskets to an aluminum pan and pour just enough beer in to cover the bottom of the pan. Cover with foil leaving one corner open to let out steam.

6. Continue cooking for another 2-3 hours until internal temperature reaches about 205 degrees F. Use an instant read thermometer and poke different parts of the brisket checking for tenderness. If probe goes into the

meat with very little tension than it is done. If not, continue cooking until it becomes tender.

7. Once meat is tender and fully cooked, remove pan from pellet grill and let the corned beef rest for about 30 minutes still covered with one corner open to prevent overcooking.

8. Slice corned beef into 1/8 inch slices cutting against the grains of the brisket. If brisket crumbles make slices a little thicker.

Greek Leg Of Lamb

Servings: 12-16

Cooking Time: 25 Minutes

Ingredients:

- 2 tablespoons finely chopped fresh rosemary
- 1 tablespoon ground thyme
- 5 garlic cloves, minced
- 2 tablespoons sea salt
- 1 tablespoon freshly ground black pepper
- Butcher's string
- 1 whole boneless (6- to 8-pound) leg of lamb
- ¼ cup extra-virgin olive oil
- 1 cup red wine vinegar
- ½ cup canola oil

Directions:

1. In a small bowl, combine the rosemary, thyme, garlic, salt, and pepper; set aside.

2. Using butcher's string, tie the leg of lamb into the shape of a roast. Your butcher should also be happy to truss the leg for you.

3. Rub the lamb generously with the olive oil and season with the spice mixture. Transfer to a plate, cover with plastic wrap, and refrigerate for 4 hours.

4. Remove the lamb from the refrigerator but do not rinse.

5. Supply your smoker with wood pellets and follow the start-up procedure. Preheat, with the lid closed, to 325°F.

6. In a small bowl, combine the red wine vinegar and canola oil for basting.

7. Place the lamb directly on the grill, close the lid, and smoke for 20 to 25 minutes per pound (depending on

desired doneness), basting with the oil and vinegar mixture every 30 minutes. Lamb is generally served medium-rare to medium, so it will be done when a meat thermometer inserted in the thickest part reads 140°F to 145°F.

8.   Let the lamb rest for about 15 minutes before slicing to serve.

Irish Pasties

Servings: 4
Cooking Time: 20 Minutes

Ingredients:
- 1 Pound Roast Beef, cubed & browned
- 4 Whole Potatoes, cooked & cut into 1/2" cubes
- salt and pepper
- 1 Piecrust
- milk
- 2 Cup Beef Gravy

Directions:
1.   Supply your smoker with wood pellets and follow the start-up procedure. Preheat the grill, with the lid closed, to 425° F.
2.   Mix the beef, potatoes, salt, and pepper in a large mixing bowl. Unroll the piecrust, and cut in half. Put a good amount of filling in each half, fold over, and seal shut. Brush with a little milk.
3.   Place on a greased basking sheet, and poke a few holes in the top of each pasty. Bake for 16-20 minutes, or until the crust is golden brown. Grill: 425 °F
4.   Remove from the Traeger, brush with butter, and serve with gravy. Enjoy!

Spicy Beer Beef Jerky

Servings: 4-6
Cooking Time: 240 Minutes

Ingredients:
- 1 12 Oz Bottle Dark Beer
- 1/4 Cup Brown Sugar
- 2 Tbsp Coarse Black Pepper
- 4 Tbsp Garlic Salt
- 2 Tbsp Hot Sauce
- 2 Tablespoons, Divided   Sweet Heat Rub

- 1 Tablespoon Quick Curing Salt
- 1 Cup Soy Sauce
- 2 Pounds Trimmed Flank Steak
- ¼ Worcestershire Sauce

Directions:
1.   When you are ready to smoke your jerky, remove the beef from the marinade and discard the marinade.
2.   Supply your smoker with wood pellets and follow the start-up procedure. Preheat the grill, with the lid closed, to 200° F. If using a sawdust or charcoal smoker, set it up for medium low heat.
3.   Arrange the meat in a single layer directly on the smoker grate. Smoke the beef for 4-5 hours, or until the jerky is dry but still chewy and still bends somewhat.
4.   Remove the jerky from the grill with tongs and transfer to a resealable plastic bag while still warm. Let the jerky rest for 1 hour at room temperature.
5.   Squeeze any air out of the resealable plastic bag and refrigerate the jerky. It will keep for several weeks. Enjoy!

Savory Whiskey Grilled Elk Steaks

Servings: 4
Cooking Time: 10 Minutes

Ingredients:
- ¼ Cup Brown Sugar
- 1 Tbsp Chop House Steak Seasoning
- 1 Tbsp Coarse Ground Pepper
- 4 Elk Steaks
- ½ Cup Olive Oil
- ½ Cup Soy Sauce
- ½ Cup Whiskey, Such As Jack Daniel'S
- ¼ Cup Yellow Mustard

Directions:
1.   In a large mixing bowl, add the whiskey, soy sauce, olive oil, brown sugar, yellow mustard, and Chophouse Steak seasoning to a large mixing bowl and whisk until everything is well combined. Pour the marinade into a large, resealable plastic bag or glass baking dish, then add the elk steaks. Seal the bag and turn the steaks once to coat. Place the bag in the refrigerator and marinate for 4-12 hours.

2. Supply your smoker with wood pellets and follow the start-up procedure. Preheat the grill, with the lid open, to 425° F. If you're using a gas or charcoal grill, set it up for medium heat. Remove the elk steaks from the bag and discard the excess marinade. Insert a temperature probe into one of the elk steaks and place on the grill.

3. Grill the steaks for 7-10 minutes per side, or until the steaks reach an internal temperature of 135°F. Remove the steaks from the grill and allow the steaks to rest for 10 minutes before serving.

Bistecca Alla Fiorentina With Mushroom Ragout

Servings: 3
Cooking Time: 25 Minutes

Ingredients:
- 2 sprigs of fresh sage
- 2 sprigs of fresh rosemary
- 2 sprigs of fresh thyme
- 1 porterhouse steak, about 2½lb (1.25kg)
- extra virgin olive oil
- coarse salt
- fresh coarsely ground black pepper
- for the ragout
- 3 tbsp unsalted butter
- 3 shallots or 1 white onion, peeled and chopped
- 2 garlic cloves, peeled and minced
- 2lb (1kg) wild mushrooms, cleaned, destemmed, and sliced or chopped
- coarse salt
- freshly ground black pepper
- 2 tbsp Cognac or brandy
- ½ cup low-salt beef broth, plus more
- 2 tsp light soy sauce
- 2 tsp chopped fresh thyme or 1 tsp dried thyme
- ½ cup heavy whipping cream, plus more
- freshly squeezed lemon juice
- freshly chopped chives

Directions:
1. Place a cast iron skillet or cast iron griddle on the grate. Supply your smoker with wood pellets and follow the start-up procedure. Preheat the grill, with the lid closed, to 450° F.

2. In a large skillet on the stovetop over medium heat, begin making the ragout by melting the butter. Add the shallots and sauté until they soften, about 2 to 3 minutes, stirring often. Add the garlic and mushrooms. Season with salt and pepper. Cook until the mushrooms give up their liquid and begin to brown, about 5 minutes. Add the Cognac and cook for 1 minute. Stir in the broth, soy sauce, and thyme. Cook until the liquid reduces slightly, about 5 minutes. Remove the skillet from the stovetop and set aside.

3. Tie the sprigs of sage, rosemary, and thyme together with butcher's twine. Place the steak on a rimmed sheet pan and use the herb brush to generously brush both sides with olive oil. Season with salt and pepper.

4. Place the steak on the skillet and grill until the internal temperature reaches 125°F (52°C), about 8 to 10 minutes per side, occasionally using the herb brush to brush the steak with olive oil. If your grill has enough clearance, stand the porterhouse upright, resting on the bone, and continue to cook for a few minutes more.

5. Transfer the meat to a cutting board and brush it one final time with olive oil. Let rest for 5 minutes.

6. Add the cream to the ragout and reheat over medium-high heat until the mixture boils. Taste for seasoning, adding salt and pepper. If the ragout seems dry, add more cream or broth. If the flavors need brightening, stir in 1 or 2 teaspoons of lemon juice. Transfer the ragout to an attractive serving bowl and top with chives.

7. Carve off the strip steak and filet mignon. Slice them on a diagonal, keeping the slices in order. Place the bone on a platter and then place the slices around the bone. Serve immediately with the mushroom ragout.

Garlic Standing Rib Roast

Servings: 4
Cooking Time: 240 Minutes

Ingredients:
- 1 tbsp cracked black pepper
- 1/2 tbsp granulated garlic

- 1/2 tbsp granulated onion
- 2 tbsp kosher salt
- 1 tbsp olive oil
- 2 tsp oregano, dried
- 1/2 tbsp parsley, dried
- 5 1/2 lbs prime rib roast, bone-in
- 2 tsp smoked paprika

Directions:

1. Place the roast in a glass baking dish. In a small mixing bowl, combine the salt, pepper, granulated garlic, granulated onion, parsley, oregano and smoked paprika. Season the entire roast with the spice blend, then cover and refrigerate overnight.

2. One hour prior to cooking, remove roast from the refrigerator, uncover, and let it sit out at room temperature.

3. Supply your smoker with wood pellets and follow the start-up procedure. Preheat the grill, with the lid closed, to 225° F. If using a gas or charcoal grill, set it up for low, indirect heat.

4. Place seasoned roast on a cast iron skillet, drizzle with olive oil, and transfer to the grill. Smoke the roast for 1 hour 45 minutes, or until internal temperature reaches 120° F. Remove from the grill and allow roast to rest for 15 minutes.

5. Increase the grill temperature to 450 F, then return roast to grill for an additional 10 to 15 minutes. Allow roast to rest for 15 minutes, slice and serve warm.

Smoked New York Steaks

Servings: 4
Cooking Time: 120 Minutes

Ingredients:

- 4 (1-inch-thick) New York steaks
- 2 tablespoons olive oil
- Salt
- Freshly ground black pepper

Directions:

1. Supply your smoker with wood pellets and follow the start-up procedure. Preheat the grill, with the lid closed, to 180°F.

2. Rub the steaks all over with olive oil and season both sides with salt and pepper.

3. Place the steaks directly on the grill grate and smoke for 1 hour.

4. Increase the grill's temperature to 375°F and continue to cook until the steaks' internal temperature reaches 145°F for medium-rare.

5. Remove the steaks and let them rest 5 minutes, before slicing and serving.

Smoked Bourbon Jerky

Servings: 6
Cooking Time: 360 Minutes

Ingredients:

- 3 Pound flank steak
- 1 Cup bourbon
- 1/2 Cup brown sugar
- 1/4 Cup Jerky Rub
- 1 Can chipotle peppers in adobo sauce
- 3 Tablespoon Worcestershire sauce
- 1/2 Cup apple cider vinegar

Directions:

1. Roll flank steak up parallel to the grain. Slice, with the grain, into 1/4 inch thick slices.

2. Combine all ingredients for marinade in a medium bowl and mix well. Place sliced flank steak in a large zip top bag and pour marinade over steak.

3. Place in refrigerator and marinate overnight.

4. Supply your smoker with wood pellets and follow the start-up procedure. Preheat the grill, with the lid closed, to 180° F.

5. Remove flank from the marinade, discard marinade and lay slices on a jerky rack or directly on the grill grate. Grill: 180 °F

6. Smoke for about 6 hours or until jerky has dried out but is still pliable. Grill: 180 °F

7. Remove from grill and let cool at room temperature, lightly covered for 1 hour.

8. Store in an airtight container or zip top bag in the refrigerator. Enjoy!

Grilled Rosemary Rack Of Lamb

Servings: 8
Cooking Time: 30 Minutes

Ingredients:
- 2 Tablespoons Dijon Mustard
- 1 Tablespoon Fresh Parsley, Chopped
- Chop House Steak Rub
- 2 Chine Bones Removed, And Excess Fat Trimmed Racks Of Lamb
- 1 Teaspoon Rosemary, Finely Chopped

Directions:
1. Place the racks of lamb on a flat work surface, then generously brush the lamb all over with Dijon mustard.
2. Season the meat on all sides with Chophouse Steak seasoning and sprinkle with parsley and rosemary.
3. Supply your smoker with wood pellets and follow the start-up procedure. Preheat the grill, with the lid closed, to 400° F.
4. If you're using a gas or charcoal grill, set it up for high heat.
5. Insert a temperature probe into the thickest part of the rack of lamb and sear the rack, meaty side down for about 6 minutes.
6. Remove the lamb from the grill and turn the temperature down to 300°F.
7. Return the lamb to the grill and lean the two racks against each other so that they stand up, and grill for another 20 minutes, or until the internal temperature reaches 130°F.
8. Remove the racks from the grill and allow to rest for 10 minutes before carving and serving.

Duck Fat Fries (confit)

Servings: 6
Cooking Time: 180 Minutes

Ingredients:
- 1/4 Cup sea salt
- 12 Whole black peppercorn
- 2 Sprig thyme sprigs
- 2 Clove garlic, crushed
- 1 Whole bay leaves
- 6 Whole Duck Leg Quarters, (leg with thigh attached), preferallb moulard
- olive oil

Directions:
1. Combine the salt and the water in a large resealable plastic bag (or a large bowl) and stir until the salt crystals dissolve.
2. Add the peppercorns, thyme, garlic, bay leaf, coriander, if using, and duck leg quarters. Seal the bag, put in a pan or bowl (to contain any potential leaks) and refrigerate for 24 hours.
3. Drain the duck leg quarters (discard the brine) and rinse under cold running water. Pat dry with paper towels. Prick the skin all over with a darning needle or sharp fork, being careful not to nick the meat. (It helps if you go in at an angle.) This creates channels for the fat to escape, making for crispier skin.
4. Supply your smoker with wood pellets and follow the start-up procedure. Preheat the grill, with the lid closed, to 400° F.
5. Meanwhile add enough olive oil to a large cast iron skillet or roasting pan to film the bottom. Arrange the duck leg quarters in the skillet or roasting pan in a single layer, skin-side down.
6. Put the skillet or roasting pan on the grill grate. Roast the duck for 30 minutes, or until the duck fat begins to render. Reduce the temperature to 300F (150C). Turn the duck legs so they are skin-side up. Cover the skillet or roasting pan tightly with foil. Grill: 300 °F
7. Continue to roast the duck for 2 hours. Uncover the duck and roast for an additional hour, or until the skin is crisp and golden brown. Remove the duck, shred, and serve immediately. (Alternatively, you can refrigerate the duck for up to a week. Re-crisp the skin by grilling the duck, skin-side down, in a hot cast iron skillet or on your Traeger.) Serve with brown butter french fries.
8. Strain the remaining duck fat through cheesecloth or a fine-mesh kitchen strainer and transfer to a covered container; refrigerate for up to 6 months. Use the flavorful fat to saut potatoes or sturdy greens.

Texas-style Smoked Beef Brisket By Doug Scheiding

Servings: 6
Cooking Time: 1080 Minutes

Ingredients:
- 1 (12-15 lb) brisket
- 2/3 Cup Butcher BBQ Prime Brisket Injection
- 2 Cup water
- 2 Tablespoon canola oil
- 1 1/2 Cup apple juice
- 1 Cup Prime Rib Rub
- 1 Cup Coffee Rub
- 4 Tablespoon ground black pepper

Directions:

1. Trim fat cap off the top of brisket and remove all silverskin. Trim off any brown areas such as on the side of the brisket. Make a long cut with the grain on the flat (thin side) of the brisket and a short cut again on the flat to show direction of cuts after cooking. Trim bottom fat cap to about 1/4 inch thickness.

2. Combine Butcher BBQ Prime Brisket Injection and water. Inject into the brisket with the grain in a checkerboard fashion. Rub entire brisket with canola oil then spritz with apple juice and let sit for 30 minutes.

3. Combine both Traeger rubs and season brisket liberally. Season the top with the black pepper.

4. Supply your smoker with wood pellets and follow the start-up procedure. Preheat the grill, with the lid closed, to 180° F.

5. Place brisket directly on the grill grate and cook 8 to 12 hours fat side down. Spritz with apple juice every 30 to 45 minutes after the first 3 hours. Grill: 180 °F Probe: 160 °F

6. After 8 hours, begin taking the temperature by inserting about two-thirds of the way up into the thickest part. It should register between 150°F to 160°F. Once the brisket registers 160°F, wrap with two sheets of aluminum foil leaving one end open. Pour in remaining brisket injection and seal foil packet. Increase the temperature on the grill to 225°F and place wrapped brisket directly on grill grate. Cook for another 3 to 4 hours until internal temperature registers 204°F. Grill: 225 °F Probe: 204 °F

7. Remove from the grill and place in a cooler wrapped in a towel to rest for at least 2 hours. When ready to serve, cut slices about the thickness of a pencil against the grain. If desired, separate cooking liquid from fat and pour juices over cut slices of brisket. Enjoy!

Grilled Garlic Tomahawk Steak

Servings: 1 - 2
Cooking Time: 60 Minutes

Ingredients:
- 3 Tablespoons Unsalted Butter
- 2 Tablespoons Chophouse Steak Seasoning
- 2 Garlic, Cloves
- Kosher Salt
- 1 Sprig Rosemary, Fresh
- 1, 2-Inch Thick Bone-In Tomahawk Ribeye

Directions:

1. Supply your smoker with wood pellets and follow the start-up procedure. Preheat the grill, with the lid closed, to 225° F.

2. Generously coat the tomahawk steak with kosher salt on all sides.

3. Allow the steak to sit at room temperature for one hour. After an hour, wipe off the salt and pat the steak dry.

4. Season the tomahawk steak with Chophouse Steak on both sides.

5. Place the steak on the grill grates, insert a temperature probe, and grill, undisturbed, for 45 minutes, or until the steak reaches an internal temperature of 120°F.

6. Remove the steak from the grill, tent with aluminum foil and allow it to rest for 10 minutes.

7. Place a cast iron skillet on the grill and increase the temperature of the to 450°F. Allow the pan to get as hot as possible.

8. Place the steak in the cast iron pan with the butter, garlic cloves, and rosemary sprig. Immediately begin spooning the butter over the steak as it melts.

9. Sear on one side for 1 minute.

10. Flip the steak, place the garlic and rosemary on top of the steak, and continue to baste the steak with the butter for another minute.

11. Pull the steak off the grill and allow it to rest for 10 minutes until the temperature rises to 130-135°F.

12. Pour the melted butter from the pan over the steak, slice, and serve immediately.

Italian Beef Pinwheels

Servings: 6
Cooking Time: 45 Minutes

Ingredients:
- 3 Pound skirt steak
- Prime Rib Rub
- 2 Cup spinach
- 4 Slices havarti cheese
- 4 Slices provolone cheese
- 1 Cup sun-dried tomatoes

Directions:
1. Supply your smoker with wood pellets and follow the start-up procedure. Preheat the grill, with the lid closed, to 375° F.

2. Season skirt steak generously with Traeger Prime Rib Rub. Lay your skirt steak flat and add a layer of spinach. Depending on the size of the steak, add up to the full 2 cups. Then add a layer of cheese and lastly the sun-dried tomatoes.

3. Tightly roll the meat up and insert toothpicks to hold it together.

4. Place meat roll directly on the grill grate and cook for 45 minutes. After 45 minutes, remove from the grill and let rest for 10 minutes before slicing. Grill: 375 °F

5. Serve with a large helping of mashed potatoes or your favorite side dish. Enjoy!

Rosemary-smoked Lamb Chops

Servings: 4
Cooking Time: 125 Minutes

Ingredients:
- 4½ pounds bone-in lamb chops
- 2 tablespoons olive oil
- Salt

- Freshly ground black pepper
- 1 bunch fresh rosemary

Directions:
1. Supply your smoker with wood pellets and follow the start-up procedure. Preheat the grill, with the lid closed, to 180°F.

2. Rub the lamb chops all over with olive oil and season on both sides with salt and pepper.

3. Spread the rosemary directly on the grill grate, creating a surface area large enough for all the chops to rest on. Place the chops on the rosemary and smoke until they reach an internal temperature of 135°F.

4. Increase the grill's temperature to 450°F, remove the rosemary, and continue to cook the chops until their internal temperature reaches 145°F.

5. Remove the chops from the grill and let them rest for 5 minutes before serving.

Spatchcocked Quail With Smoked Fruit

Servings: 4
Cooking Time: 60 Minutes

Ingredients:
- 4 quail, spatchcocked
- 2 teaspoons salt
- 2 teaspoons freshly ground black pepper
- 2 teaspoons garlic powder
- 4 ripe peaches or pears
- 4 tablespoons (½ stick) salted butter, softened
- 1 tablespoon sugar
- 1 teaspoon ground cinnamon

Directions:
1. Supply your smoker with wood pellets and follow the start-up procedure. Preheat, with the lid closed, to 225°F.

2. Season the quail all over with the salt, pepper, and garlic powder.

3. Cut the peaches (or pears) in half and remove the pits (or the cores).

4. In a small bowl, combine the butter, sugar, and cinnamon; set aside.

5. Arrange the quail on the grill grate, close the lid, and smoke for about 1 hour, or until a meat thermometer inserted in the thickest part reads 145°F.

6. After the quail has been cooking for about 15 minutes, add the peaches (or pears) to the grill, flesh-side down, and smoke for 30 to 40 minutes.

7. Top the cooked peaches (or pears) with the cinnamon butter and serve alongside the quail.

Santa Maria Tri-tip

Servings: 4
Cooking Time: 60 Minutes

Ingredients:
- 2 teaspoons sea salt
- 2 teaspoons freshly ground black pepper
- 2 teaspoons onion powder
- 2 teaspoons garlic powder
- 2 teaspoons dried oregano
- 1 teaspoon cayenne pepper
- 1 teaspoon ground sage
- 1 teaspoon finely chopped fresh rosemary
- 1 (1½ – to 2-pound) tri-tip bottom sirloin

Directions:
1. Supply your smoker with wood pellets and follow the start-up procedure. Preheat the grill, with the lid closed, to 425°F.

2. In a small bowl, combine the salt, pepper, onion powder, garlic powder, oregano, cayenne pepper, sage, and rosemary to create a rub.

3. Season the meat all over with the rub and lay it directly on the grill.

4. Close the lid and smoke for 45 minutes to 1 hour, or until a meat thermometer inserted in the thickest part of the meat reads 120°F for rare, 130°F for medium-rare, or 140°F for medium, keeping in mind that the meat will come up in temperature by about another 5°F during the rest period.

5. Remove the tri-tip from the heat, tent with aluminum foil, and let rest for 15 minutes before slicing against the grain.

Reverse Sear Tomahawk Chop

Servings: 4
Cooking Time: 60 Minutes

Ingredients:
- 2 Tbsp Coarsely Ground Black Peppercorns
- 1 Melted Stick Butter, Salted
- 2 Tablespoons Chophouse Steak Seasoning
- 2 Tbsp Sea Salt
- 2 Tsp Sprigs Fresh Thyme, Minced
- 2 Steaks, Tomahawk

Directions:
1. In a small mixing bowl, add the black peppercorns, sea salt, Chophouse Seasoning, and fresh thyme. Mix together and reserve half the seasoning.

2. Place your Tomahawk Steaks onto a sheet pan covered with butcher paper, foil, or parchment paper. Generously season the steaks with the seasoning mixture and rub it into the steaks. Let steaks sit for 1-2 hours if you would like the seasoning to penetrate the meat.

3. Supply your smoker with wood pellets and follow the start-up procedure. Preheat the grill, with the lid closed, to 225° F. If you're using a gas or charcoal grill, set it up for low, indirect heat. Insert a temperature probe into the thickest part of one of the tomahawk chops and place them in the center of the grill. If you have 2 temperature probes insert another into the other steak. Grill until the internal temperature of the steaks reaches 110°F, about 30-40 minutes.

4. Once the steaks reach their internal temperature, remove them from the grill and set aside. Increase the grill temperature to 450-500°F. While the grill is heating up melt one stick of butter and add the reserved seasoning to the melted butter. Mix together and brush the steaks with the butter making sure to evenly coat both sides of the steaks.

5. Place the steaks back on the grill over an open flame and sear for 3-5 min per side to reach 130°F-140°F. Remove the steaks from the grill, let them rest for 5 minutes and slice and serve immediately.

Smoked Burgers

Servings: 8
Cooking Time: 120 Minutes

Ingredients:

- 2 Pound ground beef
- 1 Tablespoon Worcestershire sauce
- 2 Tablespoon Beef Rub

Directions:

1. Mix ground beef with Worcestershire sauce and Traeger Beef rub.
2. Form beef mixture into 8 hamburger patties.
3. Supply your smoker with wood pellets and follow the start-up procedure. Preheat the grill, with the lid closed, to 180° F.
4. Place patties directly on the grill grate and smoke for 2 hours. Grill: 180 °F
5. After 2 hours, remove from grill and serve with your favorite toppings. Enjoy!

Grilled Lemon Skirt Steak

Servings: 1-2
Cooking Time: 5 Minutes

Ingredients:

- 2 Cloves Garlic, Chopped
- 1 Lemon, Juice
- 2 Tablespoons Mustard, Grainy
- 1/4 Cup Olive Oil
- 2 Tablespoons Java Chophouse Seasoning
- 2 Pounds Skirt Steak, Trimmed
- 1 Tablespoon Worcestershire Sauce

Directions:

1. In a small bowl, mix together the Java Chophouse Seasoning, oil, garlic, lemon juice, and Worcestershire. Generously rub the mixture all over the skirt steak and allow to marinate for 45 minutes.
2. Supply your smoker with wood pellets and follow the start-up procedure. Preheat the grill, with the lid closed, to 400° F.
3. Grill the skirt steaks for 3-5 minutes on each side or until the steak is done to the desired degree of doneness.

4. Remove the steaks from the grill and allow to rest for 5 minutes before slicing and serving.

3-2-1 Bbq Beef Cheeks

Servings: 8
Cooking Time: 480 Minutes

Ingredients:

- 2 (2 lb) beef cheeks, silverskin trimmed
- Beef Rub
- 1/4 Cup liquid of choice (beef stock, dark beer, etc.)
- 2 Tablespoon honey, brown sugar or other sweetener

Directions:

1. Make sure the beef cheeks are trimmed of all silverskin. Season liberally with Traeger Beef rub.
2. Supply your smoker with wood pellets and follow the start-up procedure. Preheat the grill, with the lid closed, to 180° F.
3. Place beef cheeks directly on the grill grate and cook until they reach an internal temperature of 165°F, about 3 hours. Remove from grill and place the cheeks in a small rimmed baking dish. Grill: 180 °F Probe: 165 °F
4. Increase grill temperature to 225°F.
5. In a small bowl, combine liquid and sweetener and stir until sweetener is dissolved. Pour mixture into the baking dish and return the cheeks to the grill to cook for an additional two hours. Grill: 225 °F
6. Remove cheeks from the grill and cover with foil. Return to the grill to cook for an additional hour or until the internal temperature reaches 205°F. Grill: 225 °F Probe: 205 °F
7. Remove from the grill and allow the steam to escape. Wrap with foil again and let rest for 30 minutes before shredding or slicing. Enjoy!

Smoked Beer Brisket

Servings: 16
Cooking Time: 420 Minutes

Ingredients:

- 1 15 lb brisket
- Brisket Baste:
- 1 cup beer
- 1/4 cup apple cider vinegar

- 1/4 cup beef stock
- 5 tbsp butter, melted
- Brisket Rub:
- 2 tbsp garlic powder
- 2 tbsp onion powder
- 2 tbsp paprika
- 2 tbsp chili powder
- 2 tbsp kosher salt
- 2 tbsp coarse ground black pepper
- 1 tbsp brown sugar

Directions:

1. Supply your smoker with wood pellets and follow the start-up procedure. Preheat the grill, with the lid closed, to 225 °F.
2. In a small bowl, mix together garlic powder, onion powder, paprika, chili pepper, kosher salt, and pepper.
3. Rub the seasonings on all sides of the brisket.
4. Place the brisket on the grill grate, fat side down.
5. Cook the brisket until it reaches an internal temperature of 160 °F(about 3 to 4 hours).
6. When brisket reaches an internal temperature of 160 °F, remove it from the grill.
7. Double wrap the meat in aluminum foil and add the beef broth to the foil packet.
8. Return brisket to the grill grate and cook until it reaches an internal temperature of 204 °F(about 3 hours more).
9. Once finished, remove the brisket from the grill, unwrap from foil and let it rest for 15 minutes.
10. Cut against the grain and serve. Enjoy!

Bbq Burnt End Sandwich

Servings: 2
Cooking Time: 480 Minutes

Ingredients:
- 1 point cut brisket
- Beef Rub
- 1/2 Cup beef broth
- 1 Cup Texas Spicy BBQ Sauce
- 4 Slices Monterey Jack cheese
- 4 burger buns

Directions:

1. Supply your smoker with wood pellets and follow the start-up procedure. Preheat the grill, with the lid closed, to 250° F.
2. Trim excess fat off brisket point. Season brisket point liberally with Traeger Beef rub.
3. Place brisket point directly on the grill grate. Cook until it reaches an internal temperature of 170℉, approximately 4 to 5 hours. Grill: 250 °F
4. Remove brisket from grill and cut into 1-inch cubes. Add the beef broth to the pan with the cubed brisket. Cover pan with aluminum foil.
5. Place pan in grill and cook for 90 minutes. Grill: 250 °F
6. Remove the foil and add Traeger Texas Spicy BBQ sauce. Stir and put back on the grill, uncovered, for an additional 45 minutes. Remove from grill. Grill: 250 °F
7. Top each bun with the burnt ends, cheese, and additional BBQ sauce. Enjoy!

Grilled Loco Moco Burger

Servings: 4
Cooking Time: 10 Minutes

Ingredients:
- Ounce ground beef, 80% lean
- 3 Tablespoon kosher salt
- 2 Tablespoon black pepper
- Cup Beef Gravy
- 2 Cup Rice, Cooked
- 4 eggs
- burger buns
- 2 Cup Hawaiian Pasta Salad

Directions:

1. Supply your smoker with wood pellets and follow the start-up procedure. Preheat the grill, with the lid closed, to 375° F.
2. Divide the ground beef into four, 6 oz portions and shape into patties. Season the patties with salt and pepper.
3. Place the patties on the grill and flip after six minutes cook time.

4. Check the internal temperature of the patties. Burgers are done when they reach an internal temperature of 165°F. Probe: 165 °F

5. While the patties are cooking, heat the gravy and the rice. Cook the eggs over easy.

6. To assemble the burger: Start with the bottom of the bun, 1/4 cup rice, 1/4 cup pasta salad, a hamburger patty, gravy, a fried egg, and the top of the bun.

7. Serve while hot. Enjoy!

Grilled Tomahawk Steak

Servings: 4
Cooking Time: 60 Minutes

Ingredients:
- 2 Large tomahawk steaks
- 2 Tablespoon kosher salt
- 2 Tablespoon ground black pepper
- 1 Tablespoon paprika
- 1/2 Tablespoon garlic powder
- 1/2 Tablespoon onion powder
- 1/2 Tablespoon brown sugar
- 1 Teaspoon ground mustard
- 1/4 Teaspoon cayenne pepper

Directions:
1. In a small bowl, combine all ingredients for the rub. Season the steaks liberally with the rub and set steaks aside while the grill preheats.

2. Supply your smoker with wood pellets and follow the start-up procedure. Preheat the grill, with the lid closed, to 225° F.

3. Place the steaks directly on the grill grate and smoke for 45 minutes to 1 hour, until the internal temperature reaches 120°F. Grill: 225 °F

4. Remove steaks from the grill and set aside to rest.

5. Increase the grill temperature to 450°F. Grill: 450 °F

6. Place the steaks directly on the grill grate and cook 7 to 10 minutes per side, or until the internal temperature reaches 130°F. Grill: 450 °F Probe: 130 °F

7. Remove from grill and let rest 5 minutes before serving. Enjoy!

Flavour Bbq Brisket Burnt Ends

Servings: 6-8
Cooking Time: 420 Minutes

Ingredients:
- 1 Brisket Point
- Georgia Style BBQ Sauce (Mustard Base)
- As Needed Chop House Steak Rub

Directions:
1. Supply your smoker with wood pellets and follow the start-up procedure. Preheat the grill, with the lid closed, to 250° F.

2. Place your brisket on the grates, cook for 6 to 7 hours or until the internal temperature reaches 190°F

3. Remove from the grill and cut into 1-inch cubes. Toss brisket cubes with seasoning and your favorite BBQ sauce into a pan.

4. Place the pan in the grill for 2 hours, stirring halfway through.

Korean Style Bbq Prime Ribs

Servings: 5
Cooking Time: 480 Minutes

Ingredients:
- 3 lbs beef short ribs
- 2 tbsp sugar
- 3/4 cup water
- 1 tbsp ground black pepper
- 3 tbsp white vinegar
- 2 tbsp sesame oil
- 3 tbsp soy sauce
- 6 cloves garlic, minced
- 1/3 cup light brown sugar
- 1/2 yellow onion, finely chopped

Directions:
1. Combine soy sauce, water, and vinegar in a bowl. Mix and whisk in brown sugar, white sugar, pepper, sesame oil, garlic, and onion. Whisk until the sugars have completely dissolved

2. Pour marinade into large bowl or baking pan with high sides. Dunk the short ribs in the marinade, coating completely. Cover marinaded short ribs with plastic wrap

and refrigerate for 6 to 12 hours3. Preheat pellet grill to 225°F.

3. Remove plastic wrap from ribs and pull ribs out of marinade. Shake off any excess marinade and dispose of the contents left in the bowl.

4. Place ribs on grill and cook for about 6-8 hours, until ribs reach an internal temperature of 203°F. Measure using a probe meat thermometer

5. Once ribs reach temperature, remove from grill and allow to rest for about 20 minutes. Slice, serve, and enjoy!

Smoked Longhorn Brisket

Servings: 8
Cooking Time: 420 Minutes

Ingredients:
- 1 (12-14 lb) whole packer brisket, trimmed
- 1/4 Cup Prime Rib Rub
- 2 Tablespoon coffee grounds

Directions:
1. Supply your smoker with wood pellets and follow the start-up procedure. Preheat the grill, with the lid closed, to 250° F.

2. Rub brisket with Traeger Prime Rib Rub and coffee grounds.

3. Place brisket on the grill grate fat-side down and smoke until it reaches an internal temperature of 160°F, this should take about 4 to 5 hours. Grill: 250 °F Probe: 160 °F

4. Remove brisket from grill and double wrap in foil. Return wrapped brisket to grill and cook until brisket reaches an internal temperature of 204°F, about 2-1/2 to 3 hours. Grill: 250 °F Probe: 204 °F

5. Once finished, remove from grill, unwrap and let rest for 15 minutes. Slice against the grain and serve. Enjoy!

Smoked Garlic Prime Rib Roast

Servings: 12
Cooking Time: 60 Minutes

Ingredients:
- 1 10 pounds Prime Rib Roast (the bones cut off and tied back on)

- 1/2 cup horseradish mustard
- 2 tablespoons Worcestershire sauce
- 4 cloves garlic (minced)
- Coarse ground salt and black pepper (to taste)

Directions:
1. Supply your smoker with wood pellets and follow the start-up procedure. Preheat the grill, with the lid closed, to 225 °F.

2. Prepare your roast while the grill is heating. Trim any excess fat from the top of the roast down to 1/4 inch thick.

3. In a small bowl, combine the mustard, Worcestershire sauce,and garlic. Slather the entire roast with the mustard mixture and season liberally with salt and pepper.

4. Place the roast on the grill grate and close the lid. Smoke until the internal temperature of the roast reaches 120 °F for Rare or 130 °F for Medium. For a rare, bone-in roast, plan on 35 minutes per pound of prime rib.

5. Remove the roast to a cutting board, cover the roast with foil, and allow it to rest for 20 minutes.

6. While the roast is resting, increase the temperature of your grill to 400 °F.

7. Once the grill temperature reaches 400 °F, return the roast to the grill and sear until it reaches your desired internal temperature. Pull the roast off at 130 °F for rare, 135 °F for medium rare, 140 °F for medium. This process should go quickly, so keep an eye on your temperature.

8. Remove your roast to the cutting board and let the meat rest for at least 15 minutes.

9. Slice and serve.

Kalbi-style Steak Wraps

Servings: 4
Cooking Time: 8 Minutes

Ingredients:
- 1 flat iron steak, about 1½lb (680g)
- 1 tbsp toasted sesame seeds
- 2 scallions, trimmed, white and green parts thinly sliced on a sharp diagonal
- for the marinade

- 1 small white onion, peeled and coarsely grated
- 4 garlic cloves, peeled and smashed with a chef's knife
- ½ Asian pear, decored and coarsely grated
- ½ cup light soy sauce
- ½ cup low-carb beer or distilled water
- 2 tbsp light brown sugar or low-carb substitute
- 2 tbsp rice vinegar or apple cider vinegar
- 2 tbsp toasted sesame oil
- 1 tbsp peeled and grated fresh ginger
- 1 tsp freshly ground black pepper

Directions:

1. In a large bowl, make the marinade by combining the ingredients. Stir until the sugar dissolves. Place the steaks in a resealable plastic bag and add the marinade, massaging the bag to thoroughly coat the meat. Refrigerate for 8 hours or overnight, turning the bag once or twice.

2. Supply your smoker with wood pellets and follow the start-up procedure. Preheat the grill, with the lid closed, to 450° F.

3. Remove the steaks from the marinade and remove any solids. (Discard the marinade.) Pat dry with paper towels. Place the steaks on the cast iron pan and grill until the internal temperature reaches 125 to 130°F (52 to 54°C), about 3 to 4 minutes per side, turning once.

4. Transfer the steaks to a cutting board and let rest for 2 minutes. Thinly slice each steak on a sharp diagonal and place on a platter. Scatter the sesame seeds and scallions over the top.

5. Place leaf lettuce, thinly sliced jalapeños, fresh cilantro leaves, kimchi (optional), and thinly sliced garlic on a separate platter. Place gochujang (Korean chili paste) in a small ramekin and add that to the platter.

6. Place the two platters on the table. Advise each diner to assemble the lettuce wraps to their desire. Serve with Asian beer, sake, or Korean soju.

Grilled Garlic Tri Tip

Servings: 2
Cooking Time: 20 Minutes

Ingredients:

- 4 Tablespoons Beef & Brisket Rub
- 1/3 Cup Brown Sugar
- 1 Stick Unsalted Softened Butter
- 1/2 Tsp Cayenne Pepper
- 1 Garlic Clove, Minced
- 2 Tablespoons Olive Oil
- Juice From 1 Orange
- 1 Tbsp Paprika, Powder
- 1/3 Cup Soy Sauce
- 3 - 4 Pounds Trimmed Tri Tip Roast
- 2 Tablespoons Worcestershire Sauce

Directions:

1. Add the brown sugar, orange juice, Worcestershire sauce, minced garlic and soy sauce to a resealable plastic bag. Add the tri tip to the bag, seal it, and massage the meat to help coat it evenly with the marinade. Place the bag in the refrigerator and allow the tri tip to marinate for 2 hours.

2. Remove the bag from the refrigerator and drain the marinade. Remove the steak from the bag and pat dry with paper towels.

3. In a small mixing bowl, combine the softened butter with 2 tablespoons of Beef & Brisket Seasoning, paprika, and cayenne. Mix the butter until well combined. Set aside.

4. Rub the tri tip down with the olive oil and season generously with the remaining Beef & Brisket Seasoning.

5. Supply your smoker with wood pellets and follow the start-up procedure. Preheat the grill, with the lid closed, to 450° F. If you're using a gas or charcoal grill, set it up for high heat. Insert a temperature probe into the thickest part of the steak and place it on the grill. Sear the tri tip on the grill for 3-5 minutes, then flip it and sear for another 3-5 minutes.

6. Turn the temperature down to 250°F, then grill the tri tip for 15 more minutes until the internal temperature reaches 135°F.

Bbq Burnt Ends

Servings: 6
Cooking Time: 540 Minutes

Ingredients:

- 1 (4-6 lb) point cut brisket
- 2 Cup beef broth
- 12 Ounce Texas Spicy BBQ Sauce
- Beef Rub

Directions:

1. Supply your smoker with wood pellets and follow the start-up procedure. Preheat the grill, with the lid closed, to 250° F.
2. Combine broth and sauce in small bowl and set aside. Trim excess fat off brisket point and rub brisket with Traeger Beef Rub.
3. Place brisket on the grill grate and cook until the internal temperature reaches 190°F (approximately 6 to 7 hours). Remove brisket from grill and cut into 1 inch cubes. Grill: 250 °F Probe: 190 °F
4. Toss brisket cubes with sauce mixture in a pan and cover the pan with aluminum foil. Place pan in grill and cook for 1 hour. Grill: 250 °F
5. Stir the burnt ends and cook for an additional hour. Enjoy!

Tuscan Cheesesteaks

Servings: 8
Cooking Time: 20 Minutes

Ingredients:

- 2 tbsp extra virgin olive oil, plus more
- 12oz (340g) mixed wild or cremini mushrooms, cleaned and chopped
- 1 red bell pepper, trimmed, deseeded, and cut into ¼-inch (.5cm) strips
- 1 green bell pepper, trimmed, deseeded, and cut into ¼-inch (.5cm) strips
- 1 white onion, peeled and diced
- 3 garlic cloves, peeled and minced
- 1 center-cut beef tenderloin, about 4lb (1.8kg), trimmed
- coarse salt
- freshly ground black pepper

- ½ cup pesto, plus more
- 1 cup grated or shaved Parmigiano-Reggiano cheese
- 12 sun-dried tomatoes packed in olive oil, roughly chopped
- 12oz (340g) thinly sliced provolone cheese, preferably aged

Directions:

1. Supply your smoker with wood pellets and follow the start-up procedure. Preheat the grill, with the lid closed, to 450° F.
2. In a large skillet on the stovetop over medium heat, warm the olive oil. Add the mushrooms and sauté until tender, about 8 minutes, stirring as needed. Transfer the mushrooms to a bowl.
3. Add the bell peppers, onion, and garlic to the skillet and cook until softened, about 5 to 6 minutes. Stir the mushrooms into the vegetable mixture. Remove the skillet from the heat and let the vegetables cool.
4. Place the tenderloin on a rimmed sheet pan. Make a lengthwise cut from one end to the other, but don't cut all the way through. (This is called "butterflying.") Open like a book and season the inside with salt and pepper. Spread the pesto on the inside of the meat with a small rubber spatula. Sprinkle the Parmigiano-Reggiano over the sauce. Place the tomatoes in a line in the center. Top with the vegetable mixture and provolone.
5. Cut five 12-inch (30.5cm) lengths of butcher's twine and place them at evenly spaced intervals under and perpendicular to the tenderloin. Bring the meat up over the stuffing and tie the pieces of twine together, snipping any loose ends. Coat the outside of the tenderloin with olive oil and season with salt and pepper.
6. Place the tenderloin on the grate at an angle to the bars. Grill until the cheese oozes out and the internal temperature reaches 125 to 130°F (52 to 54°C), about 4 to 5 minutes per side, turning with tongs.
7. Transfer the tenderloin to a cutting board and let rest for 3 minutes. Slice the tenderloin into 1-inch-thick (2.5cm) slices before serving.

Smoked Bacon Brisket Flat

Servings: 4
Cooking Time: 480 Minutes

Ingredients:

- 1/2 lbs bacon
- 4 lbs brisket flat, trimmed
- tt lonestar brisket rub

Directions:

1. Supply your smoker with wood pellets and follow the start-up procedure. Preheat the grill, with the lid open, to 250° F. If using a gas or charcoal grill, set it up for low, indirect heat.
2. Place the brisket in a foil-lined aluminum pan. Season the fat side of the brisket with Lonestar Brisket Rub, then flip and season the meat side with additional rub.
3. Transfer the brisket to the grill and smoke for 1 hour.
4. Use tongs to flip the brisket over, so the fat side is up, then drape half the bacon slices over the brisket. Smoke for 2 hours, then remove the browned bacon, and set aside.
5. Lay the remaining raw bacon strips over the brisket, and continue cooking until these new bacon strips are browned and the internal temperature of the brisket reads 202°F, which will likely take an additional 3 to 4 hours cook time.
6. Remove the brisket from the grill, and rest for 1 hour, then slice thin. Serve warm.

Braised Onion Chuck Roast Beef Sandwiches

Servings: 4
Cooking Time: 540 Minutes

Ingredients:

- 3 cups beef stock, divided
- 2 lbs chuck roast
- 4 hoagie rolls, sliced lengthwise
- to taste, lone star brisket rub
- 1 yellow onion

Directions:

1. Place chuck roast in a glass baking dish. Season with Lone Star Brisket Rub, then cover with plastic wrap and refrigerate overnight.
2. The next day, remove chuck roast from the refrigerator. Supply your smoker with wood pellets and follow the start-up procedure. Preheat the grill, with the lid closed, to 225° F. If using a gas or charcoal grill, set it up for low, indirect heat.
3. Place chuck roast directly on the grill grate, then close the lid and smoke for 3 hours, spraying with 1 cup of beef stock every hour.
4. Slice the onion and place in a cast iron skillet, then pour the remaining cup of stock over the onions and set roast on top of onions.
5. Increase temperature to 275° F and cook an additional 2 ½ to 3 hours, or until internal temperature reaches 165° F.
6. Cover the roast with a cast iron lid or aluminum foil, and cook for another 2 ½ to 3 hours, or until the internal temperature reaches 200° F.
7. Remove chuck roast from the grill. Allow the roast to rest for 10 minutes, then remove from the skillet and shred.
8. Serve pulled roast beef in a hoagie roll with braised onions and pan jus.

Smoked Corned Beef Brisket

Servings: 4
Cooking Time: 300 Minutes

Ingredients:

- 1 (3 lb) flat cut corned beef brisket, fat cap at least 1/4 inch thick
- 1 Bottle Apricot BBQ Sauce
- 1/4 Cup Dijon mustard

Directions:

1. Remove the corned beef brisket from its packaging and discard the spice packet, if any. Soak the corned beef in water for at least 8 hours changing the water every 2 hours.
2. Supply your smoker with wood pellets and follow the start-up procedure. Preheat the grill, with the lid closed, to 275° F.

3. Put the brisket directly on the grill grate, fat side up and cook for 2 hours. Grill: 275 °F

4. Meanwhile, combine the Traeger Apricot BBQ Sauce and the Dijon mustard in a medium bowl, whisking to mix.

5. Pour half of the BBQ sauce-mustard mixture in the bottom of a disposable aluminum foil pan. With tongs, transfer the brisket to the pan, fat-side up. Pour the remainder of the BBQ sauce-mustard mixture over the top of the brisket, using a spatula to spread the sauce evenly. Cover the pan tightly with aluminum foil.

6. Return the brisket to the grill and continue to cook for 2 to 3 hours, or until the brisket is tender. The internal temperature should be 203°F on an instant-read meat thermometer. Probe: 203 °F

7. Remove from the grill and allow the meat to rest for 15 to 20 minutes at room temperature. Slice across the grain into 1/4 inch slices with a sharp knife and serve immediately. Enjoy!

Beef Brisket With Chophouse Steak Rub

Servings: 12
Cooking Time: 480 Minutes

Ingredients:
- As Needed, Chop House Steak Rub
- 1, 10 To 12 Lb Whole Beef Brisket

Directions:
1. Supply your smoker with wood pellets and follow the start-up procedure. Preheat the grill, with the lid closed, to 250° F.

2. While the grill is heating up, trim your brisket of excess fat, score the meat against the grain and season with Chop House Steak Rub or your favorite seasoning.

3. Place your brisket on the grates, fat side up and cook for 7-8 hours or until the internal temperature reaches 190°F. If the meat is not probe tender, keep cooking until your temperature probe can easily slide into the meat with little to no resistance.

4. Remove from the grill and allow to rest for 20-30 minutes.

5. Slice against the grain and enjoy!

Smoked Cheese Beef Burgers

Servings: 4
Cooking Time: 66 Minutes

Ingredients:
- 1 ½ pounds ground beef chuck 80/20
- 4 slices cheddar cheese optional
- 4 burger buns
- Assorted burger toppings
- Smoked Burger Seasoning
- 1 Tablespoon Kosher salt
- 1 Tablespoon coarse ground black pepper
- 1 Tablespoon garlic powder

Directions:
1. Supply your smoker with wood pellets and follow the start-up procedure. Preheat the grill, with the lid closed, to 225 °F.

2. Shape your ground beef into 4 patties, about 1/2 inch larger in diameter than your burger buns.

3. In a small bowl combine the burger seasoning and sprinkle on both sides of your burger patties.

4. Place the seasoned patties on the grill and smoke for up to 1 hour, or until the internal temperature of your burgers reads 135 °F.

5. Increase the heat of your grill to the high setting (at least 400 °F). Sear the burger patties for about 2-3 minutes on both sides. Add cheese after the first flip, if desired.

6. Check the temperature of your burger patties for desired doneness. The FDA recommends 165 °F for a well done burger.

7. Remove the burger patties and toast the buns over high heat. Assemble your smoked burgers on your toasted buns with any desired toppings and serve immediately.

Pastrami

Servings: 6-8
Cooking Time: 960 Minutes

Ingredients:
- 1 (8-pound) corned beef brisket
- 2 tablespoons yellow mustard
- 1 batch Espresso Brisket Rub

- Worcestershire Mop and Spritz, for spritzing

Directions:

1. Supply your smoker with wood pellets and follow the start-up procedure. Preheat the grill, with the lid closed, to 225°F.

2. Coat the brisket all over with mustard and season it with the rub. Using your hands, work the rub into the meat. Pour the mop into a spray bottle.

3. Place the brisket directly on the grill grate and smoke until its internal temperature reaches 195°F, spritzing it every hour with the mop.

4. Pull the corned beef brisket from the grill and wrap it completely in aluminum foil or butcher paper. Place the wrapped brisket in a cooler, cover the cooler, and let it rest for 1 or 2 hours.

5. Remove the corned beef from the cooler and unwrap it. Slice the corned beef and serve.

Grilled Lemon Steak Pinwheels

Servings: 4
Cooking Time: 30 Minutes

Ingredients:

- 2 Tablespoons Chophouse Steak Seasoning
- Zest From 2 Lemons
- ¾ Cup Finely Parsley, Chopped
- 1 Pkg Provolone Cheese, Sliced
- 6 Oz Washed Spinach
- 1 Whole 1 ½ Pound Trimmed Hanger, Skirt, Or Steak, Flank

Directions:

1. Cut the steak into two even size pieces. Lay the steak out on a flat work surface and cover with plastic wrap. Using a meat mallet, gently pound the steak until it's at least 4 inches wide and no more than 1/3 inch thick.

2. Season both sides of each steak with Chophouse Seasoning. Lay the provolone cheese first followed by spinach. Beginning at the thinnest end of the steak, roll the steak up around the filling. Repeat with the second steak.

3. Tie a length of butcher's twin around the middle, then one piece around the ends. Cut the rolls in half, then slice the wheels again at the twine. Repeat this process with the second steak.

4. Supply your smoker with wood pellets and follow the start-up procedure. Preheat the grill, with the lid closed, to 400° F.If you're using a gas or charcoal grill, set it up for high heat.

5. Cook the pinwheels cut-side down, flipping once, or until browned on both sides and cooked to your liking, about 10-15 minutes each side for medium rare (135°F). Let the pinwheels rest for 5 minutes before serving.

APPETIZERS AND SNACKS

Chicken Wings With Teriyaki Glaze

Servings: 4
Cooking Time: 50 Minutes

Ingredients:

- 16 large chicken wings, about 3lb (1.4kg) total
- 1 to 1½ tbsp toasted sesame oil
- for the glaze
- ½ cup light soy sauce or tamari
- ¼ cup sake or sugar-free dark-colored soda
- ¼ cup light brown sugar or low-carb substitute
- 2 tbsp mirin or 1 tbsp honey
- 1 garlic clove, peeled, minced or grated
- 2 tsp minced fresh ginger
- 1 tsp cornstarch mixed with 1 tbsp distilled water (optional)
- for serving
- 1 tbsp toasted sesame seeds
- 2 scallions, trimmed, white and green parts sliced sharply diagonally

Directions:

1. Supply your smoker with wood pellets and follow the start-up procedure. Preheat the grill, with the lid closed, to 350° F.
2. Place the chicken wings in a large bowl, add the sesame oil, and turn the wings to coat thoroughly.
3. Place the wings on the grate at an angle to the bars. Grill for 20 minutes and then turn. Continue to cook until the wings are nicely browned and the meat is no longer pink at the bone, about 20 minutes more.
4. To make the glaze, in a saucepan on the stovetop over medium-high heat, combine the ingredients and bring the mixture to a boil. Reduce the glaze by 1/3, about 6 to 8 minutes. If you prefer your glaze to be glossy and thick, add the cornstarch and water mixture to the glaze and cook until it coats the back of a spoon, about 1 to 2 minutes more.
5. Transfer the wings to an aluminum foil roasting pan. Pour the glaze over them, turning to coat thoroughly.

Place the pan on the grate and cook the wings until the glaze sets, about 5 to 10 minutes.
6. Transfer the wings to a platter. Scatter the sesame seeds and scallions over the top. Serve with plenty of napkins.

Bacon-wrapped Jalapeño Poppers

Servings: 12
Cooking Time: 30 Minutes

Ingredients:

- 8 ounces cream cheese, softened
- ½ cup shredded Cheddar cheese
- ¼ cup chopped scallions
- 1 teaspoon chipotle chile powder or regular chili powder
- 1 teaspoon garlic powder
- 1 teaspoon salt
- 18 large jalapeño peppers, stemmed, seeded, and halved lengthwise
- 1 pound bacon (precooked works well)

Directions:

1. Supply your smoker with wood pellets and follow the start-up procedure. Preheat, with the lid closed, to 350°F. Line a baking sheet with aluminum foil.
2. In a small bowl, combine the cream cheese, Cheddar cheese, scallions, chipotle powder, garlic powder, and salt.
3. Stuff the jalapeño halves with the cheese mixture.
4. Cut the bacon into pieces big enough to wrap around the stuffed pepper halves.
5. Wrap the bacon around the peppers and place on the prepared baking sheet.
6. Put the baking sheet on the grill grate, close the lid, and smoke the peppers for 30 minutes, or until the cheese is melted and the bacon is cooked through and crisp.
7. Let the jalapeño poppers cool for 3 to 5 minutes. Serve warm.

Bacon Pork Pinwheels (kansas Lollipops)

Servings: 4-6

Cooking Time: 20 Minutes

Ingredients:

- 1 Whole Pork Loin, boneless
- To Taste salt and pepper
- To Taste Greek Seasoning
- 4 Slices bacon
- To Taste The Ultimate BBQ Sauce

Directions:

1. When ready to cook, start the smoker and set temperature to 500F. Preheat, lid closed, for 10 to 15 minutes.

2. Trim pork loin of any unwanted silver skin or fat. Using a sharp knife, cut pork loin length wise, into 4 long strips.

3. Lay pork flat, then season with salt, pepper and Cavender's Greek Seasoning.

4. Flip the pork strips over and layer bacon on unseasoned side. Begin tightly rolling the pork strips, with bacon being rolled up on the inside.

5. Secure a skewer all the way through each pork roll to secure it in place. Set the pork rolls down on grill and cook for 15 minutes.

6. Brush BBQ Sauce over the pork. Turn each skewer over, then coat the other side. Let pork cook for another 5-10 minutes, depending on thickness of your pork. Enjoy!

Bayou Wings With Cajun Rémoulade

Servings: 8

Cooking Time: 40 Minutes

Ingredients:

- 16 large whole chicken wings or 32 drumettes and flats, about 3lb (1.4kg) total
- for the rub
- 1 tbsp kosher salt
- 1 tsp freshly ground black pepper
- 1 tsp paprika
- ½ tsp ground cayenne, plus more
- ½ tsp garlic powder
- ½ tsp celery salt
- ½ tsp dried thyme
- 2 tbsp vegetable oil
- for the rémoulade
- 1¼ cups reduced-fat mayo
- ¼ cup Creole-style or whole grain mustard
- 2 tbsp horseradish
- 2 tbsp pickle relish
- 1 tbsp freshly squeezed lemon juice
- 1 tsp paprika, plus more
- 1 tsp hot sauce, plus more
- 1 tsp Worcestershire sauce
- coarse salt
- for serving
- lemon wedges
- pickled okra (optional)

Directions:

1. Supply your smoker with wood pellets and follow the start-up procedure. Preheat the grill, with the lid closed, to 350° F.

2. If using whole wings, cut through the two joints, separating them into drumettes, flats, and wing tips. (Discard the wing tips or save them for chicken stock.) Alternatively, leave the wings whole. Place the chicken in a resealable plastic bag.

3. In a small bowl, make the rub by combining the ingredients. Mix well. Pour the rub over the wings and toss them to thoroughly coat. Refrigerate for 2 hours.

4. In a small bowl, make the Cajun rémoulade by whisking together the mayo, mustard, horseradish, pickle relish, lemon juice, paprika, hot sauce, and Worcestershire. Season with salt to taste. The mixture should be highly seasoned. Transfer to a serving bowl and lightly dust with paprika. Cover and refrigerate until ready to serve.

5. Remove the wings from the refrigerator and allow the excess marinade to drip off. Place the wings on the grate at an angle to the bars. Grill for 20 minutes and then turn. (They'll brown more evenly but will also have less of a tendency to stick.) Continue to cook until the wings are nicely browned and the meat is no longer pink at the bone, about 20 minutes more.

6. Remove the wings from the grill and pile them on a platter. Serve with the Cajun rémoulade, lemon wedges, and pickled okra (if using).

Pulled Pork Loaded Nachos

Servings: 4
Cooking Time: 10 Minutes

Ingredients:

- 2 cups leftover smoked pulled pork
- 1 small sweet onion, diced
- 1 medium tomato, diced
- 1 jalapeño pepper, seeded and diced
- 1 garlic clove, minced
- 1 teaspoon salt
- 1 teaspoon freshly ground black pepper
- 1 bag tortilla chips
- 1 cup shredded Cheddar cheese
- ½ cup The Ultimate BBQ Sauce, divided
- ½ cup shredded jalapeño Monterey Jack cheese
- Juice of ½ lime
- 1 avocado, halved, pitted, and sliced
- 2 tablespoons sour cream
- 1 tablespoon chopped fresh cilantro

Directions:

1. Supply your smoker with wood pellets and follow the start-up procedure. Preheat, with the lid closed, to 375°F.
2. Heat the pulled pork in the microwave.
3. In a medium bowl, combine the onion, tomato, jalapeño, garlic, salt, and pepper, and set aside.
4. Arrange half of the tortilla chips in a large cast iron skillet. Spread half of the warmed pork on top and cover with the Cheddar cheese. Top with half of the onion-jalapeño mixture, then drizzle with ¼ cup of barbecue sauce.
5. Layer on the remaining tortilla chips, then the remaining pork and the Monterey Jack cheese. Top with the remaining onion-jalapeño mixture and drizzle with the remaining ¼ cup of barbecue sauce.
6. Place the skillet on the grill, close the lid, and smoke for about 10 minutes, or until the cheese is melted and bubbly. (Watch to make sure your chips don't burn!)
7. Squeeze the lime juice over the nachos, top with the avocado slices and sour cream, and garnish with the cilantro before serving hot.

Citrus-infused Marinated Olives

Servings: 6
Cooking Time: 30 Minutes

Ingredients:

- 1½ cups mixed brined olives, with pits
- ½ cup extra virgin olive oil
- 1 tbsp freshly squeezed lemon juice
- 1 garlic clove, peeled and thinly sliced
- 1 tsp smoked Spanish paprika
- 2 sprigs of fresh rosemary
- 2 sprigs of fresh thyme
- 2 bay leaves, fresh or dried
- 1 small dried red chili pepper, deseeded and flesh crumbled, or ¼ tsp crushed red pepper flakes
- 3 strips of orange zest
- 3 strips of lemon zest

Directions:

1. Supply your smoker with wood pellets and follow the start-up procedure. Preheat the grill, with the lid closed, to 180° F.
2. Drain the olives, reserving 1 tablespoon of brine. Spread the olives in a single layer in an aluminum foil roasting pan. Place the pan on the grate and cook the olives for 30 minutes, stirring the olives or shaking the pan once or twice.
3. In a small saucepan on the stovetop over low heat, warm the olive oil. Whisk in the lemon juice and the reserved 1 tablespoon of brine. Stir in the garlic and paprika. Add the rosemary, thyme, bay leaves, chili pepper, and orange and lemon zests. Warm over low heat for 10 minutes. Remove the saucepan from the heat.
4. Transfer the olives and olive oil mixture to a pint jar. Tuck the aromatics around the sides of the jar. Let cool and then cover and refrigerate for up to 5 days. Let the olives come to room temperature before serving.

Chorizo Queso Fundido

Servings: 4-6
Cooking Time: 20 Minutes

Ingredients:

- 1 poblano chile
- 1 cup chopped queso quesadilla or queso Oaxaca

118

- 1 cup shredded Monterey Jack cheese
- ¼ cup milk
- 1 tablespoon all-purpose flour
- 2 (4-ounce) links Mexican chorizo sausage, casings removed
- ⅓ cup beer
- 1 tablespoon unsalted butter
- 1 small red onion, chopped
- ½ cup whole kernel corn
- 2 serrano chiles or jalapeño peppers, stemmed, seeded, and coarsely chopped
- 1 tablespoon minced garlic
- 1 tablespoon freshly squeezed lime juice
- 1 teaspoon ground cumin
- 1 teaspoon salt
- 1 teaspoon freshly ground black pepper
- 1 tablespoon chopped fresh cilantro
- 1 tablespoon chopped scallions
- Tortilla chips, for serving

Directions:

1. Supply your smoker with wood pellets and follow the start-up procedure. Preheat, with the lid closed, to 350°F.

2. On the smoker or over medium-high heat on the stove top, place the poblano directly on the grate (or burner) to char for 1 to 2 minutes, turning as needed. Remove from heat and place in a closed-up lunch-size paper bag for 2 minutes to sweat and further loosen the skin.

3. Remove the skin and coarsely chop the poblano, removing the seeds; set aside.

4. In a bowl, combine the queso quesadilla, Monterey Jack, milk, and flour; set aside.

5. On the stove top, in a cast iron skillet over medium heat, cook and crumble the chorizo for about 2 minutes.

6. Transfer the cooked chorizo to a small, grill-safe pan and place over indirect heat on the smoker.

7. Place the cast iron skillet on the preheated grill grate. Pour in the beer and simmer for a few minutes, loosening and stirring in any remaining sausage bits from the pan.

8. Add the butter to the pan, then add the cheese mixture a little at a time, stirring constantly.

9. When the cheese is smooth, stir in the onion, corn, serrano chiles, garlic, lime juice, cuvmin, salt, and pepper. Stir in the reserved chopped charred poblano.

10. Close the lid and smoke for 15 to 20 minutes to infuse the queso with smoke flavor and further cook the vegetables.

11. When the cheese is bubbly, top with the chorizo mixture and garnish with the cilantro and scallions.

12. Serve the chorizo queso fundido hot with tortilla chips.

Grilled Guacamole

Servings: 6
Cooking Time: 30 Minutes

Ingredients:

- 3 large avocados, halved and pitted
- 1 lime, halved
- ½ jalapeño, deseeded and deveined
- ½ small white or red onion, peeled
- 2 garlic cloves, peeled and skewered on a toothpick
- 1 tsp coarse salt, plus more
- 1½ tbsp reduced-fat mayo
- 2 tbsp chopped fresh cilantro
- 2 tbsp crumbled queso fresco (optional)
- tortilla chips

Directions:

1. Supply your smoker with wood pellets and follow the start-up procedure. Preheat the grill, with the lid closed, to 225° F.

2. Place the avocados, lime, jalapeño, and onion cut sides down on the grate. Use the toothpicks to balance the garlic cloves between the bars. Smoke for 30 minutes. (You want the vegetables to retain most of their rawness.)

3. Transfer everything to a cutting board. Remove the garlic cloves from the toothpick and roughly chop. Sprinkle with the salt and continue to mince the garlic until it begins to form a paste. Scrape the garlic and salt into a large bowl.

4. Scoop the avocado flesh from the peels into the bowl. Squeeze the juice of ½ lime over the avocado. Mash the avocados but leave them somewhat chunky. Finely dice the jalapeño. Dice 2 tablespoons of onion. (Reserve the

remaining onion for another use.) Add the jalapeño, onion, mayo, and cilantro to the bowl. Stir gently to combine. Taste for seasoning, adding more salt, lime juice, and jalapeño as desired.

5.   Transfer the guacamole to a serving bowl. Top with the queso fresco (if using). Serve with tortilla chips.

Pigs In A Blanket

Servings: 4-6
Cooking Time: 15 Minutes

Ingredients:
- 2 Tablespoon Poppy Seeds
- 1 Tablespoon Dried Minced Onion
- 2 Teaspoon garlic, minced
- 2 Tablespoon Sesame Seeds
- 1 Teaspoon salt
- 8 Ounce Original Crescent Dough
- 1/4 Cup Dijon mustard
- 1 Large egg, beaten

Directions:
1.   When ready to cook, start your smoker at 350 degrees F, and preheat with lid closed, 10 to 15 minutes.
2.   Mix together poppy seeds, dried minced onion, dried minced garlic, salt and sesame seeds. Set aside.
3.   Cut each triangle of crescent roll dough into thirds lengthwise, making 3 small strips from each roll.
4.   Brush the dough strips lightly with Dijon mustard. Put the mini hot dogs on 1 end of the dough and roll up.
5.   Arrange them, seam side down, on a greased baking pan. Brush with egg wash and sprinkle with seasoning mixture.
6.   Bake in smoker until golden brown, about 12 to 15 minutes.
7.   Serve with mustard or dipping sauce of your choice. Enjoy!

Simple Cream Cheese Sausage Balls

Servings: 5
Cooking Time: 30 Minutes

Ingredients:
- 1 pound ground hot sausage, uncooked
- 8 ounces cream cheese, softened

- 1 package mini filo dough shells

Directions:
1.   Supply your smoker with wood pellets and follow the start-up procedure. Preheat, with the lid closed, to 350°F.
2.   In a large bowl, using your hands, thoroughly mix together the sausage and cream cheese until well blended.
3.   Place the filo dough shells on a rimmed perforated pizza pan or into a mini muffin tin.
4.   Roll the sausage and cheese mixture into 1-inch balls and place into the filo shells.
5.   Place the pizza pan or mini muffin tin on the grill, close the lid, and smoke the sausage balls for 30 minutes, or until cooked through and the sausage is no longer pink.
6.   Plate and serve warm.

Deviled Eggs With Smoked Paprika

Servings: 6
Cooking Time: 30 Minutes

Ingredients:
- 6 large eggs
- 3 tbsp reduced-fat mayo, plus more
- 1 tsp Dijon or yellow mustard
- ½ tsp Spanish smoked paprika or regular paprika, plus more
- dash of hot sauce
- coarse salt
- freshly ground black pepper
- for garnishing
- small sprigs of fresh parsley, dill, tarragon, or cilantro
- chopped chives
- minced scallions
- Mustard Caviar
- sliced green or black olives
- celery leaves
- sliced radishes
- diced bell peppers
- sliced cherry tomatoes
- fresh or pickled jalapeños
- sliced or diced pickles

- slivers of sun-dried tomatoes
- bacon crumbles
- smoked salmon
- Hawaiian black salt
- Caviar

Directions:

1. Supply your smoker with wood pellets and follow the start-up procedure. Preheat the grill, with the lid closed, to 180° F.

2. On the stovetop over medium-high heat, bring a saucepan of water to a boil. (Make sure there's enough water in the saucepan to cover the eggs by 1 inch [5cm].) Use a slotted spoon to gently lower the eggs into the water. Lower the heat to maintain a simmer. Set a timer for 13 minutes.

3. Prepare an ice bath by combining ice and cold water in a large bowl. Carefully transfer the eggs to the ice bath when the timer goes off.

4. When the eggs are cool enough to handle, gently tap them all over to crack the shell. Carefully peel the eggs. Rinse under cold running water to remove any clinging bits of shell, but don't dry the eggs. (A damp surface will help the smoke adhere to the egg whites.)

5. Place the eggs on the grate and smoke until the eggs take on a light brown patina from the smoke, about 25 minutes. Transfer the eggs to a cutting board, handling them as little as possible.

6. Slice each egg in half lengthwise with a sharp knife. Wipe any yolk off the blade before slicing the next egg. Gently remove the yolks and place them in a food processor. Pulse to break up the yolks. Add the mayo, mustard, paprika, and hot sauce. Season with salt and pepper to taste. Pulse until the filling is smooth. Add additional mayo 1 teaspoon at a time if the mixture is a little dry. (It shouldn't be too loose either.)

7. Spoon the filling into each egg half or pipe it in using a small resealable plastic bag. You can also use a pastry bag fitted with a fluted tip.

8. Place the eggs on a platter and lightly dust with paprika. Accompany with one or more of the suggested garnishes.

Smoked Cashews

Servings: 6
Cooking Time: 60 Minutes

Ingredients:

- 1 pound roasted, salted cashews

Directions:

1. Supply your smoker with wood pellets and follow the start-up procedure. Preheat the grill, with the lid closed, to 120°F.

2. Pour the cashews onto a rimmed baking sheet and smoke for 1 hour, stirring once about halfway through the smoking time.

3. Remove the cashews from the grill, let cool, and store in an airtight container for as long as you can resist.

Pig Pops (sweet-hot Bacon On A Stick)

Servings: 24
Cooking Time: 30 Minutes

Ingredients:

- Nonstick cooking spray, oil, or butter, for greasing
- 2 pounds thick-cut bacon (24 slices)
- 24 metal skewers
- 1 cup packed light brown sugar
- 2 to 3 teaspoons cayenne pepper
- ½ cup maple syrup, divided

Directions:

1. Supply your smoker with wood pellets and follow the start-up procedure. Preheat, with the lid closed, to 350°F.

2. Coat a disposable aluminum foil baking sheet with cooking spray, oil, or butter.

3. Thread each bacon slice onto a metal skewer and place on the prepared baking sheet.

4. In a medium bowl, stir together the brown sugar and cayenne.

5. Baste the top sides of the bacon with ¼ cup of maple syrup.

6. Sprinkle half of the brown sugar mixture over the bacon.

7. Place the baking sheet on the grill, close the lid, and smoke for 15 to 30 minutes.

8. Using tongs, flip the bacon skewers. Baste with the remaining ¼ cup of maple syrup and top with the remaining brown sugar mixture.

9. Continue smoking with the lid closed for 10 to 15 minutes, or until crispy. You can eyeball the bacon and smoke to your desired doneness, but the actual ideal internal temperature for bacon is 155°F

10. Using tongs, carefully remove the bacon skewers from the grill. Let cool completely before handling.

Chuckwagon Beef Jerky

Servings: 6
Cooking Time: 300 Minutes

Ingredients:

- 2½lb (1.2kg) boneless top or bottom round steak, sirloin tip, flank steak, or venison
- 1 cup sugar-free dark-colored soda
- 1 cup cold brewed coffee
- ½ cup light soy sauce
- ¼ cup Worcestershire sauce
- 2 tbsp whiskey (optional)
- 2 tsp chili powder
- 1½ tsp garlic salt
- 1 tsp onion powder
- 1 tsp pink curing salt

Directions:

1. Slice the meat into ¼-inch-thick (.5cm) strips, trimming off any visible fat or gristle. (Slice against the grain for more tender jerky and with the grain for chewier jerky.) Place the meat in a large resealable plastic bag.

2. In a small bowl, whisk together the soda, coffee, soy sauce, Worcestershire sauce, whiskey (if using), chili powder, garlic salt, onion powder, and curing salt (if using). Whisk until the salt dissolves. Pour the mixture over the meat and reseal the bag. Refrigerate for 24 to 48 hours, turning the bag several times to redistribute the brine.

3. Supply your smoker with wood pellets and follow the start-up procedure. Preheat the grill, with the lid closed, to 150° F.

4. Drain the meat and discard the brine. Place the strips of meat in a single layer on paper towels and blot any excess moisture.

5. Place the meat in a single layer on the grate and smoke for 4 to 5 hours, turning once or twice. (If you're aware of hot spots on your grate, rotate the strips so they smoke evenly.) To test for doneness, bend one or two pieces in the middle. They should be dry but still somewhat pliant. Or simply eat a piece to see if it's done to your liking.

6. For the best texture, when you remove the meat from the grill, place the still-warm jerky in a resealable plastic bag and let rest for 30 minutes. (You might see condensation form on the inside of the bag, but the moisture will be reabsorbed by the meat.) Or let the meat cool completely and then store in a resealable plastic bag or covered container. The jerky will last a few days at room temperature but will last longer (up to 2 weeks) if refrigerated.

Smoked Cheese

Servings: 4
Cooking Time: 150 Minutes

Ingredients:

- 1 (2-pound) block medium Cheddar cheese, or your favorite cheese, quartered lengthwise

Directions:

1. Supply your smoker with wood pellets and follow the start-up procedure. Preheat the grill, with the lid closed, to 90°F.

2. Place the cheese directly on the grill grate and smoke for 2 hours, 30 minutes, checking frequently to be sure it's not melting. If the cheese begins to melt, try flipping it. If that doesn't help, remove it from the grill and refrigerate for about 1 hour and then return it to the cold smoker.

3. Remove the cheese, place it in a zip-top bag, and refrigerate overnight.

4. Slice the cheese and serve with crackers, or grate it and use for making a smoked mac and cheese.

Roasted Red Pepper Dip

Servings: 8
Cooking Time: 45 Minutes

Ingredients:

- 4 red bell peppers, halved, destemmed, and deseeded
- 1 cup English walnuts, divided
- 1 small white onion, peeled and coarsely chopped
- 2 garlic cloves, peeled and smashed with a chef's knife
- ¼ cup extra virgin olive oil, plus more
- 1 tbsp balsamic vinegar or balsamic glaze
- 1 tsp honey (eliminate if using balsamic glaze)
- 1 tsp coarse salt, plus more
- 1 tsp ground cumin
- 1 tsp smoked paprika
- ½ to 1 tsp Aleppo red pepper flakes, plus more
- ¼ cup fresh white breadcrumbs (optional)
- distilled water (optional)
- assorted crudités or wedges of pita bread

Directions:

1. Supply your smoker with wood pellets and follow the start-up procedure. Preheat the grill, with the lid closed, to 400° F.
2. Place the peppers skin side down on the grate and grill until the skins blister and the flesh softens, about 30 minutes. Transfer the peppers to a bowl and cover with plastic wrap. Let cool to room temperature. Remove the skins with a paring knife or your fingers. Coarsely chop or tear the peppers.
3. Place ¾ cup of walnuts in an aluminum foil roasting pan. Place the pan on the grate and toast for 10 to 15 minutes, stirring twice. Remove the pan from the grill and let the walnuts cool.
4. Place the peppers, onion, garlic, and walnuts in a food processor fitted with the chopping blade. Pulse several times. Add the olive oil, balsamic vinegar, honey, salt, cumin, paprika, and red pepper flakes. Process until the mixture is fairly smooth. Taste for seasoning, adding more salt or red pepper flakes (if desired). (If the mixture is too loose, add breadcrumbs until the texture is to your liking. If it's too thick, add olive oil or water 1 tablespoon at a time.)

5. Transfer the dip to a serving bowl. Use the back of a spoon to make a shallow depression in the center. Top with the remaining ¼ cup of walnuts and drizzle olive oil in the depression. Serve with crudités or pita bread.

Delicious Deviled Crab Appetizer

Servings: 30
Cooking Time: 10 Minutes

Ingredients:

- Nonstick cooking spray, oil, or butter, for greasing
- 1 cup panko breadcrumbs, divided
- 1 cup canned corn, drained
- ½ cup chopped scallions, divided
- ½ red bell pepper, finely chopped
- 16 ounces jumbo lump crabmeat
- ¾ cup mayonnaise, divided
- 1 egg, beaten
- 1 teaspoon salt
- 1 teaspoon freshly ground black pepper
- 2 teaspoons cayenne pepper, divided
- Juice of 1 lemon

Directions:

1. Supply your smoker with wood pellets and follow the start-up procedure. Preheat, with the lid closed, to 425°F.
2. Spray three 12-cup mini muffin pans with cooking spray and divide ½ cup of the panko between 30 of the muffin cups, pressing into the bottoms and up the sides. (Work in batches, if necessary, depending on the number of pans you have.)
3. In a medium bowl, combine the corn, ¼ cup of scallions, the bell pepper, crabmeat, half of the mayonnaise, the egg, salt, pepper, and 1 teaspoon of cayenne pepper.
4. Gently fold in the remaining ½ cup of breadcrumbs and divide the mixture between the prepared mini muffin cups.
5. Place the pans on the grill grate, close the lid, and smoke for 10 minutes, or until golden brown.
6. In a small bowl, combine the lemon juice and the remaining mayonnaise, scallions, and cayenne pepper to make a sauce.
7. Brush the tops of the mini crab cakes with the sauce and serve hot.

Smoked Turkey Sandwich

Servings: 1
Cooking Time: 15 Minutes

Ingredients:

- 2 slices sourdough bread
- 2 tablespoons butter, at room temperature
- 2 (1-ounce) slices Swiss cheese
- 4 ounces leftover Smoked Turkey
- 1 teaspoon garlic salt

Directions:

1. Supply your smoker with wood pellets and follow the start-up procedure. Preheat the grill, with the lid closed, to 375°F.
2. Coat one side of each bread slice with 1 tablespoon of butter and sprinkle the buttered sides with garlic salt.
3. Place 1 slice of cheese on each unbuttered side of the bread, and then put the turkey on the cheese.
4. Close the sandwich, buttered sides out, and place it directly on the grill grate. Cook for 5 minutes. Flip the sandwich and cook for 5 minutes more. Remove the sandwich from the grill, cut it in half, and serve.

Sriracha & Maple Cashews

Servings: 10
Cooking Time: 60 Minutes

Ingredients:

- 2 tbsp unsalted butter
- 3 tbsp pure maple syrup
- 1 tbsp sriracha
- 1 tsp coarse salt (use only if nuts are unsalted)
- 2½ cups unsalted cashews

Directions:

1. Supply your smoker with wood pellets and follow the start-up procedure. Preheat the grill, with the lid closed, to 250° F.
2. In a small saucepan on the stovetop over low heat, melt the butter. Add the maple syrup, sriracha, and salt (if using). Stir until combined. Add the nuts and stir gently to coat thoroughly.
3. Spread the nuts in a single layer in an aluminum foil roasting pan coated with cooking spray. Place the pan on

the grate and smoke the nuts until they're lightly toasted, about 1 hour, stirring once or twice.
4. Remove the pan from the grill and let the nuts cool for 15 minutes. They'll be sticky at first but will crisp up. Break them up with your fingers and store at room temperature in an airtight container, such as a lidded glass jar.

Jalapeño Poppers With Chipotle Sour Cream

Servings: 8
Cooking Time: 45 Minutes

Ingredients:

- 3 strips of thin-sliced bacon
- 12 large jalapeños, red, green, or a mix
- 8oz (225g) light cream cheese, at room temperature
- 1 cup shredded pepper Jack, Monterey Jack, or Cheddar cheese
- 1 tsp chili powder
- ½ tsp garlic salt
- smoked paprika
- for the sour cream
- 1¼ cups light sour cream
- juice of ½ lime
- ½ to 1 canned chipotle peppers in adobo sauce, finely minced, plus 1 tsp of sauce, plus more
- 1 tbsp minced fresh cilantro leaves
- ½ tsp coarse salt, plus more

Directions:

1. Supply your smoker with wood pellets and follow the start-up procedure. Preheat the grill, with the lid closed, to 375° F.
2. Line a rimmed sheet pan with aluminum foil and place a wire rack on top. Place the bacon in a single layer on the wire rack. Place the pan on the grate and grill until the bacon is crisp and golden brown, about 20 minutes. Transfer the bacon to paper towels to cool and then crumble. Set aside.
3. In a small bowl, make the chipotle sour cream by whisking together the ingredients. Add more salt, chipotle peppers, or adobe sauce to taste. Cover and refrigerate.

4. Slice the jalapeños lengthwise through their stems. Scrape out the veins and seeds with the edge of a small metal spoon.

5. In a small bowl, beat together the cream cheese, shredded cheese, chili powder, and garlic salt. Stir in the crumbled bacon. Mound the cream cheese mixture in the jalapeño halves. Line another rimmed sheet pan with aluminum foil and place a wire rack on top. Place the jalapeños filled side up in a single layer on the wire rack.

6. Place the sheet pan on the grate and roast the jalapeños until the filling has melted and the peppers have softened, about 20 to 25 minutes. (They should no longer look bright in color.) Remove the pan from the grill and let the peppers rest for 5 minutes.

7. Transfer the poppers to a platter and lightly dust with paprika. Serve with the chipotle sour cream.

Cold-smoked Cheese

Servings: 6
Cooking Time: 180 Minutes

Ingredients:
- 2lb (1kg) well-chilled hard or semi-hard cheese, such as:
- Edam
- Gouda
- Cheddar
- Monterey Jack
- pepper Jack
- goat cheese
- fresh mozzarella
- Muenster
- aged Parmigiano-Reggiano
- Gruyère
- blue cheese

Directions:
1. Unwrap the cheese and remove any protective wax or coating. Cut into 4-ounce (110g) portions to increase the surface area.

2. If possible, move your smoker to a shady area. Place 1 resealable plastic bag filled with ice on top of the drip pan. This is especially important on a warm day because you want to keep the interior temperature of the grill between 70 and 90°F (21 and 32°C) or below.

3. Place a grill mat on one side of the grate. Place the cheese on the mat and allow space between each piece.

4. Fill your smoking tube or pellet maze (see Cast Iron Skillets and Grill Pans) with pellets or sawdust and light according to the manufacturer's instructions. Place the smoking tube on the grate near—but not on—the grill mat. When the tube is smoking consistently, close the grill lid.

5. Smoke the cheese for 1 to 3 hours, replacing the pellets or sawdust and ice if necessary. Monitor the temperature and make sure the cheese isn't beginning to melt. Carefully lift the mat with the cheese to a rimmed baking sheet and let the cheese cool completely before handling.

6. Package the smoked cheese in cheese storage paper or bags or vacuum-seal the cheese, labeling each. (While you can wrap the cheese tightly in plastic wrap, the cheese will spoil faster.) Let the cheese rest for at least 2 to 3 days before eating. It will be even better after 2 weeks.

POULTRY RECIPES

Smoked Chicken With Apricot Bbq Glaze

Servings: 4
Cooking Time: 60 Minutes

Ingredients:

- 2 Whole Chickens, halved
- 4 Tablespoon Chicken Rub
- 1 Cup Apricot BBQ Sauce

Directions:

1. Supply your smoker with wood pellets and follow the start-up procedure. Preheat the grill, with the lid closed, to 375° F.
2. Season chicken with Chicken Rub and place on grill meat side up. Cook 1 hour or until internal temperature has reached 160°F in the breast and 175°F in the leg. Grill: 375 °F Probe: 160 °F
3. Baste each chicken half with a bit of the Apricot BBQ glaze and return to grill for 10 minutes. Grill: 375 °F
4. Remove chicken from the grill and allow to rest 5-10 minutes. Portion each half by removing the leg and cutting each breast in half leaving you with four legs and 8 breast pieces. Serve with your favorite vegetables or sides. Enjoy!

Roasted Tin Foil Dinners

Servings: 4
Cooking Time: 25 Minutes

Ingredients:

- 4 boneless, skinless chicken breast
- Chicken Rub
- 1/2 Pound new potatoes, quartered
- 8 Ounce cremini mushrooms, cleaned and quartered
- salt and pepper
- 1/2 Pound green beans, ends trimmed
- 1 Medium lemon, cut into 3/4 inch slices

Directions:

1. Supply your smoker with wood pellets and follow the start-up procedure. Preheat the grill, with the lid closed, to 400° F.
2. Season chicken breast with salt, pepper and Traeger Chicken Rub. Place the potatoes, mushrooms and chicken in the middle of a large sheet of foil, season with more salt and pepper as needed, and wrap up tightly.
3. Place foil pack directly on the grill grate and cook for 15 minutes. Grill: 400 °F
4. Open up the foil pack and add green beans, lemon and additional salt and pepper, if needed. Wrap back up and return to the Traeger for an additional 10 minutes. Grill: 400 °F
5. Remove from the Traeger, open packet and enjoy!

Buffalo Chicken

Servings: 6
Cooking Time: 90 Minutes

Ingredients:

- 1 1/2 Tbsp Apple Cider Vinegar
- 3 Tbsp Bleu Cheese, Crumbled
- 1/4 Cup Buffalo Sauce
- 1/2 Cup Butter, Unsalted, Cubed
- 1/4 Tsp Cayenne Pepper
- 3 Celery Stalks, Cut Into Sticks
- 1 Cup Cheddar Jack Cheese, Shredded
- 1 Lb Chicken Breast, Boneless, Skinless
- 3 Oz Cream Cheese, Softened
- 1/8 Tsp Garlic, Granulated
- 2/3 Cup Hot Pepper Sauce
- 12 Jalapeno Peppers
- Mason Jar(S)
- 1/4 Red Bell Pepper, Chopped
- 2 Scallions, Sliced Thin
- Shredded Chicken
- 3 Tbsp Sour Cream
- To Taste, Sweet Heat Rub
- 1/2 Tsp Sweet Heat Rub (For Sauce)
- 1/4 Tsp Worcestershire Sauce

Directions:

1. Supply your smoker with wood pellets and follow the start-up procedure. Preheat the grill, with the lid open, to 200° F. If using a gas or charcoal grill, set it up for low, indirect heat.

2. Season chicken breasts with Sweet Heat, then place on the grill. Smoke for 1 hour, then remove from the grill, and set aside to rest.

3. While the chicken is resting, prepare the Buffalo sauce: Set a small cast iron pan or saucepan on the grill. Open the sear slide and increase the grill temperature to 350° F. Add the hot pepper sauce, apple cider vinegar, Worcestershire sauce, Sweet Heat, cayenne, and granulated garlic to the skillet, and whisk to combine. When the sauce begins to bubble, remove the skillet from the grill and whisk in butter. Transfer the sauce to a mason jar.

4. Shred the chicken with 2 forks in the sauce skillet. Set aside.

5. Prepare the filling: In a mixing bowl, use a hand mixer to blend cream cheese, bleu cheese, Buffalo sauce and sour cream. Fold in scallions, red bell pepper, and shredded chicken.

6. Prepare the peppers: Cut each jalapeño in half, lengthwise. Use a paring knife or teaspoon to scrape out the seeds and membrane, then place in a cast iron skillet (might need to divide between 2 skillets). Stuff the mixture into the jalapeño halves, then top with shredded cheese.

7. Transfer peppers to the grill, with the sear slide closed. Close the lid and cook for 15 to 20 minutes, until peppers begin to soften and cheese has melted.

8. Remove the peppers from the grill, transfer to a serving board or platter, and serve warm with extra Buffalo sauce.

Roasted Duck With Cherry Salsa

Servings: 2-3
Cooking Time: 180 Minutes

Ingredients:

- 1 whole Long Island (Pekin) duck, about 5 to 6lb (2.3 to 2.7kg), thawed if frozen
- coarse salt
- freshly ground black pepper
- 1 white onion, peeled and quartered
- 1 orange, quartered
- 4 garlic cloves, peeled and quartered
- 3 sprigs of fresh thyme or fresh rosemary, plus more for the salsa
- 2 cups dark red cherries, washed, destemmed, pitted, and coarsely chopped
- 1 scallion, trimmed, white and green parts sliced crosswise
- 1 jalapeño, destemmed, deseeded, and finely diced
- 1 tbsp granulated sugar, plus more
- 1 tbsp port wine (optional)
- 2 tsp freshly squeezed lime juice
- 2 tsp freshly squeezed orange juice
- 1½ tsp finely chopped orange zest

Directions:

1. Supply your smoker with wood pellets and follow the start-up procedure. Preheat the grill, with the lid closed, to 350° F.

2. In a small bowl, make the salsa by combining the ingredients. Slightly bruise some of the cherries to release their juices. Set aside.

3. Use kitchen shears to cut off the wing tips and trim any excessive neck skin from the duck. Use a sharp knife to score the skin of the breasts in the classic diamond pattern, making the cuts about 1 inch (2.5cm) apart, but don't penetrate the meat. Use a fork with sharp tines to prick the skin on the thighs. Rinse the bird inside and out with cold running water and pat dry with paper towels.

4. Season the duck inside and out with the salt and pepper. Tuck the onion, orange, garlic, and thyme in the cavity. Pull the excess skin over the opening and tie the legs together with butcher's twine.

5. Place a wire rack in a shallow roasting pan and place the duck breast side up on top of the rack. Place the roasting pan on the grate and roast the duck for 1 hour. Use tongs to turn the bird breast side down. Roast for 1 hour more and then turn again, finishing breast side up. Roast until the skin is nicely browned and the internal temperature in the thickest part of a breast reaches 170°F (77°C), about 30 minutes to 1 hour more. (There should

also be quite a bit of duck fat in the bottom of the pan. Save in a covered container and refrigerate or freeze for another use.)

6. Remove the pan from the grill and let the duck rest for 15 minutes. Transfer the duck to a cutting board and carve.

7. Place the duck meat on a platter and scatter the fresh thyme over the top. Serve with the cherry salsa.

Loaded Chicken Fries

Servings: 4

Cooking Time: 20 Minutes

Ingredients:

- 8 Slices Bacon, Cooked And Diced
- 1 12 Oz Bag Cheese, Shredded
- 1 Bag Fries, Frozen
- 2 Tablespoons Green Onions, Diced
- ¼ Cup White Barbecue Sauce

Directions:

1. Supply your smoker with wood pellets and follow the start-up procedure. Preheat the grill, with the lid open, to 400° F.

2. Bake the fries on the baking sheet in your according to the manufacturer's instructions. Once the fries are done, remove them from the grill and reduce the temperature to 350°F.

3. Top the fries with the cheese, chicken and bacon. Place the fries back on the grill and cook for another 5-7 minutes, or until the chicken is warmed through and the cheese is melted. Remove the fries from the grill.

4. Top the fries with the white barbecue sauce and green onions and serve immediately.

Duck Breast With Pomegranate Sauce

Servings: 4

Cooking Time: 13 Minutes

Ingredients:

- 4 duck breasts, each about 6oz (170g), skin on
- for the rub
- 2 tsp coarse salt
- 1 tsp ground cumin
- 1 tsp ground coriander
- 1 tsp freshly ground black pepper
- ½ tsp ground cinnamon
- ½ tsp ground fennel
- for the sauce
- 1 shallot, peeled and minced
- 1 cup pomegranate juice
- 1 tbsp sherry vinegar or balsamic vinegar
- 1 tsp cornstarch
- ¼ cup chicken stock or chicken broth
- 1 tbsp chilled unsalted butter, cut into 4 pieces
- ¼ cup fresh pomegranate seeds (optional)
- 1 tbsp minced fresh chives

Directions:

1. Place a cast iron skillet on the grate. Supply your smoker with wood pellets and follow the start-up procedure. Preheat the grill, with the lid closed, to 400° F.

2. In a small bowl, make the rub by combining the ingredients. Use a sharp knife to diagonally score the skin of each duck breast—but don't nick the flesh. Lightly season the scored side of each breast.

3. Place the duck breasts skin side down in the skillet and sear until the skin is crisp and golden brown, about 8 to 10 minutes. Turn the breasts and cook until the internal temperature in the thickest part of a breast reaches 130°F (54°C), about 2 to 3 minutes more. Transfer the breasts to a plate.

4. In a large saucepan on the stovetop over medium heat, make the sauce by heating 1 tablespoon of duck fat from the skillet. (Reserve the remainder for another use.) Add the shallot and sauté until soft, about 2 to 3 minutes.

5. Add the pomegranate juice and bring the mixture to a boil over medium-high heat. Reduce the sauce by half, about 3 to 5 minutes. Add the vinegar and lower the heat to medium low.

6. Whisk together the cornstarch and chicken stock until smooth. Whisk into the sauce and cook until the sauce thickens, about 1 to 2 minutes. Whisk in the butter and stir in the pomegranate seeds (if using).

7. Place the duck breasts on a warm platter. Drizzle the pomegranate sauce over the top. Scatter the chives around the platter before serving.

Thai Chicken Satays

Servings: 4
Cooking Time: 10 Minutes

Ingredients:

- 1½lb (680g) boneless, skinless chicken breasts
- for the marinade
- ½ cup unsweetened canned light coconut milk
- 2 garlic cloves, peeled and coarsely chopped
- ¼ cup loosely packed fresh cilantro leaves
- 1-inch (2.5cm) piece of fresh ginger, peeled and coarsely chopped
- 2 tbsp light soy sauce
- 1 tbsp Asian fish sauce
- 1 tbsp light brown sugar or low-carb substitute
- 2 tsp sambal oelek (optional)
- 1 tsp Thai-style curry powder
- 1 tsp ground cumin
- 1 tsp ground turmeric
- 1 tsp coarse salt
- 2 tbsp vegetable oil
- for serving
- butter lettuce leaves, washed and dried
- cherry tomatoes
- Peanut Sauce

Directions:

1. Use a sharp knife to slice the chicken breasts lengthwise into strips, each about 1 inch (2.5cm) wide. (If the chicken breasts are unusually thick, butterfly them before cutting them into strips.) Place the breasts in a resealable plastic bag.

2. In a blender, make the marinade by combining the ingredients. Blend until fairly smooth. Pour the marinade over the chicken, turning and massaging the bag to thoroughly coat the chicken. Refrigerate for 2 hours.

3. Supply your smoker with wood pellets and follow the start-up procedure. Preheat the grill, with the lid closed, to 450° F.

4. Remove the chicken from the marinade and let any excess drip off. (Discard the marinade.) Thread each chicken strip on a bamboo skewer, pushing the point in one side of the chicken and out the other as if sewing.

Leave very little of the tip exposed because it will burn easily.

5. Place the skewers on the grate perpendicular to the bars. Grill until the chicken has grill marks and is fully cooked, about 3 to 5 minutes per side.

6. Remove the skewers from the grill. Place the lettuce leaves on a platter. Place the satays atop the leaves. Scatter cherry tomatoes over the top. Serve with the peanut sauce.

Chile Chicken Thighs

Servings: 4
Cooking Time: 35 Minutes

Ingredients:

- 2 Tablespoon soy sauce
- 1/4 Cup honey
- 2 Clove garlic, minced
- 1/4 Teaspoon red pepper flakes
- 4 boneless, skinless chicken thighs
- 2 Tablespoon olive oil
- 2 Teaspoon Chicken Rub
- ancho chile powder
- 1/4 Teaspoon coarse ground black pepper

Directions:

1. Supply your smoker with wood pellets and follow the start-up procedure. Preheat the grill, with the lid closed, to 400° F.

2. In a small bowl, combine honey, soy sauce, garlic and red pepper chili flakes; blend well with wire whisk. Set aside.

3. Drizzle the chicken thighs with olive oil and season generously on both sides with the Traeger Chicken Rub and black pepper, then give each thigh a few shakes of ancho chili powder on both sides.

4. Place the seasoned chicken thighs directly on the grill grate and cook for about 15 minutes per side or until the internal temperature registers 165°F on an instant-read thermometer. Grill: 400 °F Probe: 165 °F

5. Brush with chili-honey glaze. Remove from grill. Serve with additional sauce. Enjoy!

Smoked Chicken Vermicelli Noodles

Servings: 4 – 6
Cooking Time: 120 Minutes

Ingredients:

- 2 Cup Broccoli
- ¼ Cup Chicken Stock
- 6 - 8 Chicken Thighs, Boneless, Skinless
- 1 Tbsp Chili Flakes
- 1 Tsp Cornstarch
- 4, Chopped Garlic Cloves
- 3 Tbsp Hoisin Sauce, Divided
- Knob Of Fresh Ginger, Grated
- 1, Thin Red Bell Peppers, Sliced
- 1 Tbsp Rice Wine Vinegar
- 8 Scallions, Sliced
- 1 ½ Tbsp Sesame Oil, Divided
- 1 Tbsp, Toasted Sesame Seeds
- 3.5 Oz Shitake Mushrooms, Sliced Thin
- 8 Oz Snow Peas
- 3 Tbsp Soy Sauce
- 2 Tbsp Sweet Chili Sauce
- 3 Tbsp Vegetable Oil
- 1 Lb Vermicelli Noodles, Or Linguini, Cooked And Drained

Directions:

1. In a large bowl, whisk together rice wine vinegar, 1 tablespoon of Hoisin sauce, and 1 tablespoon of sesame oil. Toss chicken to coat and allow to marinate for 1 hour.

2. Supply your smoker with wood pellets and follow the start-up procedure. Preheat the grill, with the lid open, to 225° F. If using a gas or charcoal grill, set it for low, indirect heat. Place chicken directly on the grill grate and smoke for 1 ½ to 2 hours, or until the internal temperature reaches 165° F. Remove it from the smoker, cover with foil, and rest for 10 minutes, then slice thin and set aside.

3. In a glass measuring cup whisk together 2 tablespoons of Hoisin sauce, soy sauce, sweet chili sauce, chicken stock, ½ tablespoon of sesame oil, and cornstarch. Set aside.

4. Preheat griddle to medium flame, then add oil. Working quickly, sauté ginger and garlic for 15 seconds, then add bell pepper and mushrooms and continue cooking for another minute, then add in snow peas and slaw. Toss in cooked pasta, chicken, scallions, and pour sauce over. Cook for one minute until sauce thickens and is well incorporated.

5. Transfer to platter and serve hot. Sprinkle with chili flakes and sesame seeds, if desired.

Garlic Sriracha Buffalo Chicken Wings

Servings: 6-8
Cooking Time: 160 Minutes

Ingredients:

- 1 Cup Buffalo Sauce
- 6 Lbs Chicken Wings
- 2 Tbsp Garlic Powder
- 1 Tsp Pepper
- Divided By 2 Tbsp And ½ Tbsp Sweet Heat Rub
- 1 Tsp Salt
- ⅓ Cup, Divided Sriracha Sauce

Directions:

1. In a non-stick sauce pot, add the remaining Sriracha and buffalo sauce. Stir to combine and set aside.

2. Supply your smoker with wood pellets and follow the start-up procedure. Preheat the grill, with the lid open, to 250° F. If using a gas or charcoal grill, set it to low heat with indirect heat. Place marinated wings directly on grill grate and cook (covered) for 1 hour 15 minutes.

3. Flip wings and baste each piece with Sriracha sauce. Season with additional Sweet Heat Rub, cover, and continue to grill for an additional 1 hour 15 minutes.

4. Remove wings from grill and place on sheet tray. Baste with additional sauce, then open Sear Slide and return wings to the grill. Grill for 3-5 minutes, rotating often, until wings begin to char lightly.

5. Transfer wings to a serving tray, baste with remaining sauce and serve!

Whole Roasted Chicken

Servings: 4
Cooking Time: 60 Minutes

Ingredients:

- 1 Whole fresh young chicken
- 1 Bottle Chicken Rub
- water
- 1/2 Tablespoon kosher salt
- 1 Tablespoon chopped sage
- 1 Tablespoon chopped thyme
- 1/2 Cup butter, softened
- 1/2 Tablespoon coarse ground black pepper

Directions:

1. Remove whole chicken from packaging and wipe dry with a paper towel.

2. Mix water and chicken rub to create a brine. Place the chicken and brine in a container that's large enough to submerge the entire chicken.

3. Set in fridge for 4-12 hours.

4. Supply your smoker with wood pellets and follow the start-up procedure. Preheat the grill, with the lid closed, to 375° F.

5. Take chicken out of brine, do not rinse.

6. Mix together thyme, sage, salt, pepper and butter. Smear the outside of the chicken with the butter mixture. Put any of the remaining butter in the cavity of the chicken.

7. Place chicken directly on the grill grate. Cook chicken until it reaches an internal temperature of 165 degrees F (about 60 mins) with an instant-read thermometer between the leg and thigh joint. Grill: 375 °F Probe: 165 °F

8. Also check the internal temperature of the breast to ensure it registers at least 165 degrees F. Once chicken is done, let it rest for 15-20 minutes. Enjoy!

Wood-fired Chicken Breasts

Servings: 2-4
Cooking Time: 45 Minutes

Ingredients:

- 2 (1-pound) bone-in, skin-on chicken breasts
- 1 batch Chicken Rub

Directions:

1. Supply your smoker with wood pellets and follow the start-up procedure. Preheat the grill, with the lid closed, to 350°F.

2. Season the chicken breasts all over with the rub. Using your hands, work the rub into the meat.

3. Place the breasts directly on the grill grate and smoke until their internal temperature reaches 170°F. Remove the breasts from the grill and serve immediately.

Buffalo Chicken Wings

Servings: 4
Cooking Time: 20 Minutes

Ingredients:

- 1 1/2 Tbsp Apple Cider Vinegar
- 1/2 Cup Butter, Unsalted, Cubed
- 1/4 Tsp Cayenne Pepper
- 3 Lbs Chicken Wings, Split
- 2 Tsp Chives, Minced (Garnish)
- 1/8 Tsp Garlic, Granulated
- 2/3 Cup Hot Pepper Sauce
- 1 Tbsp Ranch Seasoning
- To Taste, Sweet Heat Rub
- 1/2 Tsp Sweet Heat Rub (For Sauce)
- 1/4 Tsp Worcestershire Sauce

Directions:

1. Supply your smoker with wood pellets and follow the start-up procedure. Preheat the grill, with the lid open, to 425° F. If using a gas or charcoal grill, set it up for medium-high heat.

2. Place chicken wings in a large mixing bowl. Season with Sweet Heat.

3. Prepare sauce: Set a small cast iron pan or saucepan on the grill. Add the hot pepper sauce, apple cider vinegar, Worcestershire sauce, Sweet Heat, cayenne, and granulated garlic to the skillet, and whisk to combine. When the sauce begins to bubble, remove the skillet from the grill and whisk in butter. Transfer the sauce to a mason jar.

4. Combine 1 cup of the buffalo sauce with ranch seasoning. Set aside.

5. Place wings on the grill and cook for 20 minutes, flipping and rotating every 3 to 5 minutes.

6. Remove wings from the grill when an internal temperature of 165° F is reached. Transfer to a mixing bowl, then pour sauce over. Toss to evenly coat. Garnish with fresh chives and serve warm.

Oktoberfest Pretzel Mustard Chicken

Servings: 4
Cooking Time: 25 Minutes

Ingredients:
- 1/4 Pound pretzel sticks
- 3 Tablespoon Dijon mustard
- 3 Tablespoon apple cider or brown ale
- 1 Tablespoon honey
- 1 1/2 Teaspoon fresh thyme, plus more for garnish
- 4 boneless, skinless chicken breasts

Directions:
1. Pulse the pretzel sticks in a food processor or crush by hand in a resealable bag until they've turned into a powder the texture of panko breadcrumbs.

2. Transfer the crumbs to a wide, shallow bowl.

3. In separate shallow bowl, whisk mustard, beer or cider, honey and thyme together.

4. Spray a wire rack with cooking spray and place atop a sheet tray. Dip each chicken breast in the mustard mixture, then dredge in the pretzel crumbs to coat evenly and place on the wire rack. Spray the top of each chicken breast lightly with cooking spray.

5. Supply your smoker with wood pellets and follow the start-up procedure. Preheat the grill, with the lid closed, to 375° F.

6. Place the pan on the Traeger and bake for about 20 to 25 minutes, until the chicken breasts are fully cooked and register 165°F on an instant-read thermometer. Grill: 375 °F Probe: 165 °F

7. Let chicken rest for 5 minutes. Garnish with fresh thyme if desired. Enjoy!

Savory Smoked Turkey Legs

Servings: 4
Cooking Time: 150 Minutes

Ingredients:
- 1 Cup Chicken Stock
- 2 Tbsp Blackened Sriracha Rub
- 4 Turkey Legs (Drumsticks)

Directions:
1. Fire up your pellet grill on SMOKE mode. With the lid open, let it run for 10 minutes.

2. Supply your smoker with wood pellets and follow the start-up procedure. Preheat the grill, with the lid closed, to 225° F. If using a gas or charcoal grill, set it up for low, indirect heat.

3. Combine turkey stock with 2 teaspoons of Blackened Sriracha Rub.

4. Place turkey legs on a sheet tray, then inject each with seasoned stock. Season the outside of the legs with remaining Blackened Sriracha.

5. Place turkey legs directly on the grate of the smoking cabinet, and cook for 1 ½ hours.

6. Increase temperature to 325°F, then transfer turkey legs to the bottom grill and cook for another 45 to 60 minutes, until the internal temperature reaches 170°F.

7. Remove turkey from the grill, allow to rest for 10 minutes, then serve warm.

Grilled Honey Garlic Wings

Servings: 4
Cooking Time: 60 Minutes

Ingredients:
- 2 1/2 Pound chicken wings
- Pork & Poultry Rub
- 4 Tablespoon butter
- 3 Clove garlic, minced
- 1/4 Cup honey
- 1/2 Cup hot sauce
- 1 1/2 Cup blue cheese or ranch dressing

Directions:
1. Start by segmenting the wings into three pieces, cutting through the joints. Discard the wing tips or save them to make a stock.

2. Lay out the remaining pieces on a rimmed baking sheet lined with nonstick foil or parchment paper. Season well with Traeger Pork & Poultry Rub.

3. Supply your smoker with wood pellets and follow the start-up procedure. Preheat the grill, with the lid closed, to 350° F.

4. Place the baking sheet with wings directly on the grill grate and cook for 45 to 50 minutes or until they are no longer pink at the bone. Grill: 350 °F

5. To make the sauce: Melt butter in a small saucepan. Add the garlic and sauté for 2 to 3 minutes. Add in the honey and hot sauce and cook for a few minutes until completely combined. Keep sauce warm while the wings are cooking.

6. After 45 minutes, pour the spicy honey-garlic sauce over the wings, turning with tongs to coat.

7. Place wings back on the grill and cook for an additional 10 to 15 minutes to set the sauce. Grill: 350 °F

8. Serve with ranch or blue cheese dressing. Enjoy!

Savory-sweet Turkey Legs

Servings: 4
Cooking Time: 300 Minutes

Ingredients:

- 1 gallon hot water
- 1 cup curing salt (such as Morton Tender Quick)
- ¼ cup packed light brown sugar
- 1 teaspoon freshly ground black pepper
- 1 teaspoon ground cloves
- 1 bay leaf
- 2 teaspoons liquid smoke
- 4 turkey legs
- Mandarin Glaze, for serving

Directions:

1. In a large container with a lid, stir together the water, curing salt, brown sugar, pepper, cloves, bay leaf, and liquid smoke until the salt and sugar are dissolved; let come to room temperature.

2. Submerge the turkey legs in the seasoned brine, cover, and refrigerate overnight.

3. When ready to smoke, remove the turkey legs from the brine and rinse them; discard the brine.

4. Supply your smoker with wood pellets and follow the start-up procedure. Preheat, with the lid closed, to 225°F.

5. Arrange the turkey legs on the grill, close the lid, and smoke for 4 to 5 hours, or until dark brown and a meat thermometer inserted in the thickest part of the meat reads 165°F.

6. Serve with Mandarin Glaze on the side or drizzled over the turkey legs.

Smoked Whiskey Peach Pulled Chicken

Servings: 6-8
Cooking Time: 45 Minutes

Ingredients:

- 3-4 pound whole chicken
- 1 cup peach juice
- 1/4 cup whiskey
- 1/4 cup melted butter
- 1/4 cup Hey Grill Hey's Sweet BBQ Rub
- 1/2 cup Whiskey Peach BBQ sauce

Directions:

1. Supply your smoker with wood pellets and follow the start-up procedure. Preheat the grill, with the lid closed, to 225°F, using a mild fruit wood like a peach.

2. Remove any giblets or neck from inside of the chicken and pat dry.

3. In a jar, combine the peach juice, whiskey, and melted butter. Inject this mixture into your chicken in several spots. Be sure to inject in at least 3 different places in each breast, 2 places in the thighs, and 1 time in each leg.

4. Season your chicken generously on all sides with the Sweet BBQ Rub. Place in the middle of your grill and close the lid. Smoke for 45 minutes per pound of chicken.

5. Brush liberally with the whiskey peach BBQ sauce once the internal temperature of your meat reaches 150 degrees.

6. Check the temperature in both the thighs and the breasts and when your internal temperature reads consistently 160 degrees F, remove the chicken to a rimmed serving platter or baking sheet and cover tightly with foil to allow the chicken to come up to 165 degrees F and rest for 20 minutes.

7. Shred the chicken and set it onto your serving platter. Discard the carcass or save for homemade stock. Drizzle your smoked pulled chicken with more of the Whiskey Peach Barbecue Sauce and serve on toasted buns.

Roasted Honey Bourbon Glazed Turkey

Servings: 8
Cooking Time: 240 Minutes

Ingredients:
- 1 Whole (18-20 lb) turkey
- 1/4 Cup Fin & Feather Rub
- 1/2 Cup bourbon
- 1/2 Cup honey
- 1/4 Cup brown sugar
- 3 Tablespoon apple cider vinegar
- 1 Tablespoon Dijon mustard
- salt and pepper

Directions:
1. Supply your smoker with wood pellets and follow the start-up procedure. Preheat the grill, with the lid closed, to 375° F. Truss the turkey legs together. Season the exterior of the bird and the cavity with Traeger Fin and Feather Rub.
2. Place the turkey directly on the grill grate and cook for 20-30 minutes at 375°F or until the skin begins to brown. Grill: 375 °F
3. After 30 minutes, reduce the temperature to 325°F and continue to cook until internal temperature registers 165°F when an instant read thermometer is inserted into the thickest part of the breast, about 3-4 hours. Grill: 325 °F Probe: 165 °F
4. For the Whiskey Glaze: Combine all ingredients in a small saucepan and bring to a boil. Reduce the temperature and let simmer 15-20 minutes or until thick enough to coat the back of a spoon. Remove from heat and set aside.
5. During the last ten minutes of cooking, brush the glaze on the turkey while on the grill and cook until the glaze is set, about 10 minutes. Remove from grill and let rest 10-15 minutes before carving. Enjoy! *Cook times will vary depending on set and ambient temperatures.

Bourbon Chicken Waffles

Servings: 8
Cooking Time: 30 Minutes

Ingredients:
- 1 Shot Of Bourbon
- 3 Cups Bread Crumbs
- 4 Horizontally Half Sliced Boneless, Skinless Chicken Breast
- Butter Flavored Cooking Spray
- 3 Eggs
- 1 Tsp Garlic Powder
- 1 Tsp Paprika, Powder
- Red Velvet Cake Mix
- 16 Oz. Reduced Fat Sour Cream
- Sweet Rib Rub
- ¼ Cup Vegetable Oil
- 1 ¼ Cup Water
- 1 Tbsp Worcestershire Sauce

Directions:
1. Supply your smoker with wood pellets and follow the start-up procedure. Preheat the grill, with the lid closed, to 350° F. If you're using a gas or charcoal grill, set up the grill for medium heat.
2. In a large bowl, combine the sour cream, bourbon, Worcestershire sauce, paprika, garlic powder, and Sweet Rib Rub seasoning. Add the chicken, turn the chicken breasts to coat, and cover the bowl. Refrigerate for 4-12 hrs.
3. Remove the chicken from the refrigerator and drain the marinade from the chicken. Mix together 3 cups bread crumbs and 2 tbsp Sweet Rib Rub. Mix the coating together and bread the chicken breasts.
4. Moisten a paper towel with cooking oil and using a pair of tongs, lightly grease the grill rack.
5. Grill or smoke until the internal temperature of the chicken reaches 170°F and the chicken is crispy and golden brown.
6. While the chicken is cooking, mix the eggs, vegetable oil, water, and red velvet cake mix in a bowl with the electric mixer.
7. Add the mix into the waffle iron and cook. Make as many waffles as the mix allows.
8. On a plate, place the cooked chicken on top of the waffles and top with maple syrup or honey.

Bbq Chicken Breasts

Servings: 6
Cooking Time: 25 Minutes

Ingredients:

- 6 boneless, skinless chicken breast
- 1 1/2 Cup Sweet & Heat BBQ Sauce
- salt and pepper
- 1 Tablespoon chopped parsley, for garnish

Directions:

1. Place chicken breasts and 1 cup of Traeger Sweet & Heat BBQ Sauce in a resealable bag or large bowl, and gently turn to cover chicken evenly in the sauce. Marinate in the refrigerator overnight.
2. Supply your smoker with wood pellets and follow the start-up procedure. Preheat the grill, with the lid closed, to 450° F.
3. Remove chicken from marinade and season with salt and pepper.
4. Place chicken directly on the grill grate and cook for 10 minutes on each side flipping once or until internal temperature reaches 150°F.
5. Brush on remaining 1/2 cup of Traeger Sweet & Heat BBQ Sauce while chicken is still on the grill, and continue to cook 5 to 10 minutes longer or until a finished internal temperature of 165°F.
6. Remove chicken from grill and let rest 5 minutes before serving. Sprinkle with chopped parsley. Enjoy!

Easy Grilled Chicken Shawarma

Servings:
Cooking Time: 16 Minutes

Ingredients:

- 2 lbs to 2 ¼ lb chicken thighs
- Shawarma Marinade
- 2 tablespoons ground cumin
- 2 tablespoons ground coriander
- 8 garlic cloves, minced
- 2 teaspoons kosher salt
- 6 tablespoons olive oil
- 1/4 teaspoon cayenne pepper
- 2 teaspoon turmeric
- 1 teaspoon ground ginger
- 1 teaspoon ground black pepper
- 2 teaspoon allspice

Directions:

1. Supply your smoker with wood pellets and follow the start-up procedure. Preheat the grill, with the lid closed, to medium-high heat. Place all marinade ingredients in a bowl and mix, or pulse in a food processor to make a paste.
2. Rub chicken on all sides with the marinade and let sit 20 minutes.
3. Place the chicken on the grill racks, closing the lid to the BBQ, until all sides have nice grill marks, about 8 minutes each side. Move to the warming rack until cooked all the way through, about 10 minutes.
4. Enjoy the chicken shawarma over Israeli salad, or with rice and veggies, or with pita bread and tzatziki.

Cranberry Turkey Breast

Servings: 6
Cooking Time: 90 Minutes

Ingredients:

- 1 Bay Leaf
- 1/2 Tsp Black Pepper
- 3 Tbsp Butter, Divided
- 1 Celery Rib, Chopped
- To Taste, Cracked Black Pepper
- 4 Oz Cremini Mushrooms
- 1/2 Cup Dried Cranberries
- 2 Garlic Cloves, Minced
- 1 Package, Approx 2Lbs Honeysuckle White Turkey Breast, Boneless
- 1/2 Cup Marsala Wine
- 1 Tbsp Olive Oil
- 1 Rosemary Sprigs
- 1/2 Tsp Rubbed Sage
- 1/2 Tsp Salt
- To Taste, Sea Salt
- 6 Oz Stuffing Mix
- 1 1/4 Cup Turkey Stock, Divided
- 1 Yellow Onion, Chopped

Directions:

1. Supply your smoker with wood pellets and follow the start-up procedure. Preheat the grill, with the lid closed, to 325° F. If using a gas or charcoal grill, set it up for medium-low heat.

2. Melt the butter 1 tablespoon of butter and olive oil in a large skillet over medium heat. Add the onions and celery and cook, stirring frequently, until soft, 3 minutes.

3. Add the garlic and mushrooms and continue to cook for 5 minutes, until the mushrooms are slightly browned.

4. Deglaze with marsala wine, using a wooden spoon to scrape up any browned bits from the bottom of the pan.

5. Add the dried cranberries, black pepper, sage, and salt and simmer for 2 minutes, then remove from the heat.

6. Fold the stuffing into the vegetable mixture, then slowly pour over turkey stock, until stuffing is moistened.

7. Place the Honeysuckle White® Turkey Breast on a large cutting board, skin-side down, then butterfly it. Season with salt and pepper, then spoon over ⅓ of the stuffing, leaving an inch border.

8. Roll the turkey breast, starting at the side with less skin. Use butcher's twine to truss the turkey breast and secure the stuffing. Place in a cast iron skillet, top remaining butter, season with salt and pepper. Place a sprig of rosemary on top, add remaining ¼ cup of stock around the turkey, along with 1 bay leaf. Transfer to the grill.

9. Cook the turkey for 1 to 1 ½ hours, until an internal temperature of 165°F is reached.

10. Remove stuffed turkey breast from the grill, rest for 15 minutes, then slice and serve warm, with remaining stuffing.

Dry Brine Traeger Turkey

Servings: 6
Cooking Time: 360 Minutes

Ingredients:
- 1 farm fresh turkey, any size
- 1 Teaspoon kosher salt per pound of turkey
- fresh thyme
- fresh rosemary
- fresh sage
- fresh parsley

Directions:
1. Make sure to plan ahead, this recipe requires multiple days of brine time.

2. Combine desired amounts of thyme, rosemary, sage and/or parsley with kosher salt. Rub kosher salt and spice mixture over entire surface of the turkey, including the cavity.

3. Place turkey in a bag or plastic wrap and seal tight. Place turkey in the fridge for 2 days. On day 3, take the turkey out of the bag or unwrap plastic wrap. Place the turkey back in the fridge, uncovered for 24 hours.

4. Supply your smoker with wood pellets and follow the start-up procedure. Preheat the grill, with the lid closed, to 180° F.

5. Place the turkey on grill, breast up. Smoke the turkey for 3 to 4 hours. Grill: 180 °F

6. After 3 to 4 hours, increase the grill temperature to 325°F and continue to cook turkey until it reaches an internal temperature of 165°F. Enjoy!

Roasted Chicken With Wild Rice & Mushrooms

Servings: 2
Cooking Time: 120 Minutes

Ingredients:
- 1 Whole whole chicken
- salt
- pepper
- 2 Tablespoon butter
- 1 Medium onion, chopped
- 4 Strips Bacon, diced
- 1 Cup Rice, wild
- 1 mushrooms, sliced
- salt
- 2 1/4 Cup water
- 2 Tablespoon parsley, chopped

Directions:
1. Supply your smoker with wood pellets and follow the start-up procedure. Preheat the grill, with the lid closed, to 375° F.

136

2. Season inside and outside of chicken with salt and pepper.

3. In a large saucepan, melt 2 Tbsp butter over medium heat. Add onions and cook until soft, 3-5 minutes. Add bacon to onions and cook, stirring, until bacon and onions are browned. Stir in rice, mushrooms, salt, and pepper.

4. Add 2-1/4 cups of water to mixture and bring to a boil. Reduce heat to low, cover and simmer for 25 minutes, until rice has absorbed liquid. Add fresh parsley and mix.

5. Stuff cavity loosely with rice mixture. Tie chicken legs back with butcher's twine.

6. Place chicken directly on grill grate and roast for 1 hr 15 mins or until an instant-read thermometer inserted into the thickest part of the breast reads 160°F and the thigh 170°F. Grill: 375 °F Probe: 160 °F

7. Remove chicken from grill and allow to rest for 10 minutes.

8. Spoon stuffing out of chicken cavity to a platter and slice chicken. Serve immediately with chicken pieces over rice stuffing. Enjoy!

Chicken On A Throne

Servings: 6
Cooking Time: 75 Minutes

Ingredients:
- 1 can of low-carb beer or sugar-free dark-colored soda, about 12oz (350ml)
- 1 whole chicken, about 4lb (1.8kg)
- 3 tbsp barbecue rub, plus more

Directions:
1. Supply your smoker with wood pellets and follow the start-up procedure. Preheat the grill, with the lid closed, to 350° F.

2. Pour half the contents of the can into a glass for drinking. Set the half-full can aside.

3. Blot any juices off the chicken with paper towels. Sprinkle 2 teaspoons of the rub in the body and neck cavities. Sprinkle the remaining rub evenly on the outside. Tuck the wing tips behind the bird's back.

4. Carefully lower the chicken (body cavity side down) over the can. Place the chicken upright on its can on the grate. (For stability, pull the legs forward and rest them on the grate to essentially form a tripod.) Roast the chicken until the internal temperature in the thickest part of a thigh reaches 165°F (74°C), about 1 hour. (Check on your bird periodically to make sure it hasn't tipped over.) If it hasn't yet reached that temperature, continue cooking for about 15 minutes more.

5. Use heavy-duty insulated rubber gloves and tongs to carefully transfer the chicken to the kitchen. Let rest 5 minutes and then carefully ease the chicken off the can. Discard the can and its steaming liquid, being careful not to burn yourself. Carve the chicken and serve.

Cajun Spatchcock Turkey

Servings: 7
Cooking Time: 180 Minutes

Ingredients:
- 16 Oz Cajun Butter
- Sweet Heat Rub
- 1 Brined Turkey

Directions:
1. Supply your smoker with wood pellets and follow the start-up procedure. Preheat the grill, with the lid closed, to 300° F.

2. Inject the Turkey with Cajun butter and season liberally with Sweet Heat Rub.

3. Place on the grill and cook until thighs and breasts reach 165°.

4. Let rest for 30 minutes and serve.

Bbq Spatchcocked Chicken

Servings: 2
Cooking Time: 45 Minutes

Ingredients:
- 1 whole chicken
- 1/4 Cup Chicken Rub
- olive oil
- 1/2 Cup Sweet & Heat BBQ Sauce

Directions:

1. Supply your smoker with wood pellets and follow the start-up procedure. Preheat the grill, with the lid closed, to 375° F.

2. With a large knife or shears, cut the bird open along the backbone on both sides, through the ribs, and remove the backbone.

3. Brush chicken with olive oil and season both sides with Traeger Chicken rub.

4. Place the poultry on the Traeger, breast side up and cook for 35 to 40 minutes or until a thermometer inserted into the breast registers 160°F. Grill: 375 °F Probe: 160 °F

5. Remove from the grill and let rest 5 minutes before slicing. Enjoy!

Smoked Thanksgiving Turkey

Servings: 6 - 8

Cooking Time: 300 Minutes

Ingredients:

- 1 Turkey Brining Kits
- 12 – 14 Lbs Turkey
- 1 Gallon Water, Cold
- 4 Cups + 1 Gallon Water, Warm

Directions:

1. Start by defrosting the turkey overnight in the refrigerator.

2. Once turkey has been defrosted begin to make the brine by adding 4 cups of water and the brine mixture to a large stockpot.

3. Bring the mixture to a boil and add 1 gallon of cold water.

4. Place the turkey in the brine bag and pour the brine mixture over the turkey and refrigerate 1 hour per pound.

5. Once turkey has been brined rinse the turkey with cold water and set on a pan.

6. Using the seasoning in the brine box, season the turkey. Once turkey has been seasoned, supply your smoker with wood pellets and follow the start-up procedure. Preheat the grill, with the lid closed, to 275° F.

7. Place your turkey in the smoker and place the temperature probe in the deepest part of the breast.

Cook at 275 until the breast and thigh meat internal temperature has reached 165°F to 170°F.

8. Remove the turkey from the smoker, let cool, and cut the turkey into your desired pieces. Enjoy!

Bbq Pulled Turkey Sandwiches

Servings: 6

Cooking Time: 120 Minutes

Ingredients:

- 6 Whole Turkey Thighs
- Pork & Poultry Rub
- 1 1/2 Cup chicken broth
- 1 Cup 'Que BBQ Sauce
- 6 Whole Kaiser Buns, Split

Directions:

1. Season turkey thighs on both sides with the Traeger Pork & Poultry rub.

2. Supply your smoker with wood pellets and follow the start-up procedure. Preheat the grill, with the lid closed, to 180° F.

3. Arrange the turkey thighs directly on the grill grate and smoke for 30 minutes.

4. Transfer the thighs to a sturdy disposable aluminum foil or roasting pan. Pour the broth around the thighs. Cover the pan with foil or a lid.

5. Increase temperature to 325°F and preheat, lid closed. Roast the thighs until they reach an internal temperature of 180°F. Grill: 325 °F Probe: 180 °F

6. Remove pan from the grill, but leave grill on. Let the turkey thighs cool slightly until they can be comfortably handled.

7. Pour off the drippings and reserve. Remove the skin and discard.

8. Pull the turkey meat into shreds with your fingers and return the meat to the roasting pan.

9. Add 1 cup or more of your favorite Traeger BBQ Sauce along with some of the drippings.

10. Recover the pan with foil and reheat the BBQ turkey on the Traeger for 20 to 30 minutes.

11. Serve with toasted buns if desired. Enjoy!

Yucatán-spiced Chicken Thighs

Servings: 4
Cooking Time: 40 Minutes

Ingredients:

- 8 skin-on, bone-in chicken thighs, about 2½lb (1.2kg) total
- for the marinade
- 2oz (55g) achiote paste
- ¼ cup hot distilled water
- ¼ cup freshly squeezed orange juice
- 2 tbsp freshly squeezed lime juice
- 2 tbsp apple cider vinegar or distilled white vinegar
- 2 tbsp vegetable oil or extra virgin olive oil
- 2 garlic cloves, peeled and minced
- 1 tsp kosher salt, plus more
- 1 tsp dried Mexican oregano
- ½ tsp ground cumin
- ¼ tsp ground cinnamon

Directions:

1. In a small bowl, make the marinade by using a fork to crumble the achiote paste. Add the hot water and mash the paste with the fork until blended. Whisk in the orange juice, lime juice, vinegar, oil, garlic, salt, oregano, cumin, and cinnamon.
2. Place the chicken thighs in a resealable plastic bag. Pour the marinade over the chicken, turning and massaging the bag to thoroughly coat the chicken. Refrigerate for 2 hours.
3. Supply your smoker with wood pellets and follow the start-up procedure. Preheat the grill, with the lid closed, to 400° F.
4. Remove the chicken thighs from the marinade and let any excess drip off. (Discard the marinade.) Place the chicken thighs skin side down on the grate at an angle to the bars. Grill for 20 minutes and then turn. Continue to grill until the internal temperature in the thighs reaches 165°F (74°C), about 20 minutes more.
5. Transfer the thighs to a platter and serve immediately.

Lemon Rosemary Beer Can Chicken

Servings: 4
Cooking Time: 60 Minutes

Ingredients:

- 1 (3 to 3-1/2 lb) whole chicken
- 1 lemon, halved
- 1 Teaspoon kosher salt
- 1 Teaspoon ground black pepper
- 1 Teaspoon fresh finely chopped rosemary
- 1 (12 oz) can beer

Directions:

1. Supply your smoker with wood pellets and follow the start-up procedure. Preheat the grill, with the lid closed, to 400° F.
2. Coat the chicken inside and out with the juice from one lemon. In a small bowl, combine salt, pepper and rosemary, and sprinkle on the inside and outside of chicken.
3. Empty half of the beer from the can and place the can on a solid surface. Place the chicken atop the beer can, tucking the legs in the front.
4. Carefully place the chicken directly on the grill grate using the legs to support if needed. Alternatively, place the chicken atop the beer can on a sheet tray for a more stable surface, then place the sheet tray directly on the grill grate.
5. Cook the chicken until an instant-read thermometer reads 165°F when inserted in the thickest part of the breast, about 60 minutes. Grill: 400 °F Probe: 165 °F
6. Let the chicken rest 10 minutes before carving. Serve with Chardonnay or any of your favorite medium body red or white wines. Enjoy!

Chicken Tenders

Servings: 2-4
Cooking Time: 80 Minutes

Ingredients:

- 1 pound boneless, skinless chicken breast tenders
- 1 batch Chicken Rub

Directions:

1. Supply your smoker with wood pellets and follow the start-up procedure. Preheat the grill, with the lid closed, to 180°F.

2. Season the chicken tenders with the rub. Using your hands, work the rub into the meat.

3. Place the tenders directly on the grill grate and smoke for 1 hour.

4. Increase the grill's temperature to 300°F and continue to cook until the tenders' internal temperature reaches 170°F. Remove the tenders from the grill and serve immediately.

Smoked Pulled Chicken

Servings: 6
Cooking Time: 65 Minutes

Ingredients:
- To Taste, Ale House Beer Can Chicken Seasoning
- 1 Lb Chicken Breasts, Boneless, Skinless
- 1 Tbsp Cilantro, Chopped
- 1 Tsp Cumin, Ground
- 2 Jalapeños, Chopped
- 2 Tsp Olive Oil
- 1 Bag Tortilla Chips
- 1 Lb White American Cheese, Cubed
- 1 Cup Milk

Directions:
1. Supply your smoker with wood pellets and follow the start-up procedure. Preheat the grill, with the lid open, to 350° F. If using a gas or charcoal grill, preheat to medium heat.

2. Score the chicken, rub with olive oil, then season with Ale House Beer Can Chicken.

3. Transfer the chicken to the grill and cook for 8 to 10 minutes, turning occasionally.

4. Remove chicken from the grill, and reduce the temperature to 225° F. Allow the chicken to rest for 10 minutes, then pull apart with 2 forks. Set aside.

5. While the chicken is resting, heat a cast iron skillet on the grill. Partially open the sear slide, then to the skillet add the cubed cheese, jalapeño, milk, and cumin. Stir occasionally, for 5 minutes, until the cheese melts. Fold in the pulled chicken, then close the lid and allow the dip to smoke for 30 to 45 minutes.

6. Remove from grill and let rest for 5-10 minutes to thicken. Serve warm with fresh cilantro and tortilla chips.

Smoked Maple Syrup Thanksgiving Turkey

Servings: 8
Cooking Time: 375 Minutes

Ingredients:
- 1 Cup Butter, Room Temp
- 1/2 Cup Maple Syrup
- 2 Tablespoons Champion Chicken Seasoning
- 1, (Pre-Brined) Turkey, Whole

Directions:
1. Supply your smoker with wood pellets and follow the start-up procedure. Preheat the grill, with the lid closed, to 250° F.

2. Combine the melted butter and maple syrup in a bowl. With the Marinade Injector, fill with the butter and syrup mixture and pierce the meat with the needle while pushing on the plunger, injecting the flavor. You want to inject the marinade into the thickest part of the breast, thigh, and wings.

3. Next, combine the room temperature butter and Champion Chicken seasoning and spread all over the turkey, making sure that you get it under the skin as well.

4. Place the turkey in an aluminum pan to catch all the drippings (this makes incredible gravy) and place on the grill.

5. When the breast and thigh meat of the turkey reaches 165°F to 170°F, remove from grill and let rest 15 minutes before carving. Happy Thanksgiving!

Lemon Parmesan Chicken Wings

Servings: 4 -8
Cooking Time: 30 Minutes

Ingredients:
- 2 Tablespoons Unsalted Butter, Melted
- 2 Lbs Chicken Wings, Trimmed And Patted Dry
- 3 Cloves Garlic, Minced
- Juice Of 1 Lemon
- 2 Tablespoons Mustard, Dijon
- ¼ Cup Olive Oil
- ¼ Cup Shredded Parmesan Cheese
- 2 Tablespoons Parsley, Chopped

- 2 Tablespoons Champion Chicken Seasoning

Directions:

1. Supply your smoker with wood pellets and follow the start-up procedure. Preheat the grill, with the lid open, to 350° F. If you are using a charcoal or gas grill, set the temperature to medium high heat.

2. In a large resealable bag, combine the olive oil, minced garlic, lemon zest, lemon juice, Dijon mustard, Champion Chicken Seasoning, and chopped parsley. Seal the resealable bag and give it a good shake to mix the ingredients.

3. Once the chicken has finished marinating, remove the chicken from the marinade and drain. Place the chicken wings on the wing rack.

4. Place the wing rack on the grill and insert a temperature probe into the thickest part of one of the wings. Grill the wings for 5 minutes, then rotate, and grill for another 5-10 minutes, or until the internal temperature of the wings reaches 165°F.

5. Toss the wings in the large bowl with the melted butter and shredded Parmesan until well coated. Serve immediately.

County Fair Turkey Legs

Servings: 4
Cooking Time: 90 Minutes

Ingredients:

- 4 turkey legs, each about 1lb (450g)
- for the brine
- ½ gallon (1.9 liters) distilled water
- ½ cup kosher salt
- ¼ cup light brown sugar or low-carb substitute
- 2½ tsp pink curing salt #1
- 1 tsp liquid smoke (optional)

Directions:

1. In a stockpot on the stovetop over medium-high heat, make the brine by combining the ingredients. Bring the mixture to a boil. Stir until the salts and sugar dissolve. Remove the pot from the stovetop and let the brine cool to room temperature. Cover and refrigerate until cool.

2. Submerge the turkey legs in the brine. If they float, place a resealable bag of ice on top. Refrigerate for 24 hours, turning from time to time so the legs cure evenly.

3. Supply your smoker with wood pellets and follow the start-up procedure. Preheat the grill, with the lid closed, to 325° F.

4. Remove the turkey legs from the brine and discard the liquid. Rinse the legs under cold running water and pat dry with paper towels.

5. Place the turkey legs on the grate and grill for 45 minutes. Turn and continue to cook until the turkey skin is nicely browned and the internal temperature in a leg reaches 170 to 175°F (77 to 79°C), about 45 minutes. (Turkey legs have a lot of connective tissue and they seem to turn out better when cooked to a slightly higher temperature.)

6. Remove the legs from the grill and serve warm or cold.

Baked Prosciutto-wrapped Chicken Breast With Spinach And Boursin

Servings: 4
Cooking Time: 60 Minutes

Ingredients:

- 1 Tablespoon olive oil
- 10 Ounce baby spinach leaves, washed and dried
- 2 Whole packs (5.2 oz) Boursin Garlic & Fine Herbs Gournay Cheese
- 2 Pound boneless, skinless chicken breasts
- Pork & Poultry Rub
- 14 Slices prosciutto

Directions:

1. Heat olive oil in a medium sauté pan. Add spinach and sauté until wilted, about 3 to 5 minutes. Transfer to a strainer and squeeze out excess liquid. Place spinach and cheese in a medium bowl. Mix well and set aside.

2. Butterfly each chicken breast and open like a book. Cover with plastic wrap and using a meat mallet, pound out thinly. Season the chicken with Pork & Poultry Rub.

3. Lay a sheet of plastic wrap about 2 feet long down on a flat, clean surface. Lay down slices of prosciutto,

slightly overlapping and double-wide. Place the chicken on top of the prosciutto leaving a 1- 1/2 inch border.

4. Spread the spinach mixture on top of the chicken. Roll it up tightly to create a log. Tie off the ends tightly and transfer to the refrigerator. Refrigerate 2 to 3 hours or overnight.

5. Supply your smoker with wood pellets and follow the start-up procedure. Preheat the grill, with the lid closed, to 300° F.

6. Carefully remove the plastic wrap and place directly on the grill grate. Bake for an hour and a half, or until the internal temperature reaches 162°F to 165°F. Remove from Traeger and let rest for 10 minutes before slicing. Enjoy! Grill: 300 °F Probe: 162 °F

Smoked Whole Chicken

Servings: 6-8
Cooking Time: 240 Minutes

Ingredients:
- 1 whole chicken
- 2 cups Tea Injectable (using Not-Just-for-Pork Rub)
- 2 tablespoons olive oil
- 1 batch Chicken Rub
- 2 tablespoons butter, melted

Directions:
1. Supply your smoker with wood pellets and follow the start-up procedure. Preheat the grill, with the lid closed, to 180°F.
2. Inject the chicken throughout with the tea injectable.
3. Coat the chicken all over with olive oil and season it with the rub. Using your hands, work the rub into the meat.
4. Place the chicken directly on the grill grate and smoke for 3 hours.
5. Baste the chicken with the butter and increase the grill's temperature to 375°F. Continue to cook the chicken until its internal temperature reaches 170°F.
6. Remove the chicken from the grill and let it rest for 10 minutes, before carving and serving.

Roasted Stuffed Turkey Breast

Servings: 6

Cooking Time: 40 Minutes

Ingredients:
- 1 (4-5 lb) boneless turkey breast
- 5 Slices thick-cut bacon, chopped
- 3/4 Cup assorted mushrooms
- 1 Bunch scallions, chopped
- 1/8 Cup white wine
- 3 Tablespoon panko breadcrumbs
- salt
- black pepper

Directions:
1. Supply your smoker with wood pellets and follow the start-up procedure. Preheat the grill, with the lid closed, to 375° F.
2. Slice the turkey breast horizontally, making sure not to slice all the way through. Lay breast open flat.
3. Cook bacon in a skillet over medium heat until crispy. Remove bacon and set aside. Sauté mushrooms in the bacon grease until browned. Add scallions and cook for an additional two minutes. Add white wine and cook down until no wine remains. Stir in breadcrumbs and bacon, adding salt and pepper to taste.
4. Transfer filling to fridge to cool for 15 to 20 minutes. Once chilled, spread the filling onto the turkey breast, pressing lightly to make sure it adheres. Roll the turkey breast tightly and tie with butcher's twine at about 1 inch intervals. Tuck the ends of the turkey breast under and tie with twine lengthwise.
5. Season the outside of the turkey breast with salt and pepper. Place in grill for 40 minutes. Check the internal temperature, desired temperature is 165°F. Once the finished temperature is reached, remove turkey from the grill and let rest for 10 minutes. Slice and serve. Enjoy! Grill: 375 °F Probe: 165 °F

Bacon Wrapped Chicken Wings

Servings: 6
Cooking Time: 60 Minutes

Ingredients:
- 2 Pound chicken wings
- 24 Ounce beer
- 2 Teaspoon red pepper flakes

- Cajun Seasoning
- 1 Pound bacon

Directions:

1. Plan ahead, this recipe requires 12 to 24 hours to brine the wings. Trim the tips off of the wings and discard or set them aside for homemade stock.

2. Cut the skin flap between the flat and the drummette so the wing stays a little more straight and is easier to wrap.

3. Place the wings in a large bowl and cover with the beer and red pepper flakes (if desired).

4. Refrigerate for 12-24 hours before grilling.

5. Remove the wings from the brine and pat dry. Season liberally with Traeger's Cajun Shake.

6. Wrap each wing with a piece of bacon. You can secure with toothpicks, if necessary.

7. Supply your smoker with wood pellets and follow the start-up procedure. Preheat the grill, with the lid closed, to 450° F.

8. Place the wings directly on the grill grate, close the lid, and cook for 30 minutes.

9. Flip the wings and cook for an additional 30 minutes or until the bacon is crisp and the chicken is fully cooked (at least 165 degrees F). Enjoy!

Carrot Celery Chicken Drumsticks

Servings: 4
Cooking Time: 30 Minutes

Ingredients:

- Buffalo Style Dry Rub
- Carrot, Stick
- Celery, Stick
- 12 Chicken, Drumsticks

Directions:

1. Supply your smoker with wood pellets and follow the start-up procedure. Preheat the grill, with the lid closed, to 350° F.

2. Generously sprinkle the Buffalo Wing Rub all over the drumsticks. Hang each drumstick by the bone on the Wing Rack. Place in the for about 30 minutes.

3. Serve hot with celery and carrot sticks. Enjoy!

Spiced Smoked Chicken Quarters

Servings: 4
Cooking Time: 120 Minutes

Ingredients:

- 4 chicken leg quarters
- For the rub:
- 2 tbsp paprika
- 1 tbsp thyme
- 2 tbsp chili powder
- 2 tbsp cayenne pepper
- 1 tbsp garlic powder
- 1 tbsp onion powder
- 1 tbsp kosher/table salt
- 2 tbsp black pepper
- 1 tbsp olive oil

Directions:

1. Supply your smoker with wood pellets and follow the start-up procedure. Preheat the grill, with the lid closed, to 220° F.

2. Pat down chicken pieces with a paper towel to make them dry. Cut off any excess fat that's visible on the outside of the meat.

3. Apply a thin layer of oil to the chicken skin. In a small bowl, combine all the BBQ rub ingredients thoroughly. Apply BBQ rub generously to your chicken thighs, rubbing in firmly and thoroughly.

4. Transfer chicken quarters to your smoker rack.Close the lid.

5. Cook until the quarters reach an internal temperature of 165°F, about 2 hours.

6. Once cooked, increase the grill temperature to medium heat. Cook for just a few minutes, turning regularly, for a crispy skin.

Fried Chicken Sliders

Servings: 8
Cooking Time: 30 Minutes

Ingredients:

- 8 Slider Buns
- ½ Cup Buttermilk
- 4 Horizontally Cut Chicken Breasts
- 2 Cups Flour, All-Purpose

- 1 Tablespoon Hot Sauce
- ¼ Cup Mayonnaise
- 2 Quarts Cooking Canola Or Soybean Oil
- ½ Cup Spicy Bread And Butter Pickle Slices
- ½ Tablespoon Champion Chicken Seasoning

Directions:

1. Supply your smoker with wood pellets and follow the start-up procedure. Preheat the grill, with the lid open, to 350° F. If you're using a gas or charcoal grill, set it up for medium heat.

2. Place a deep cast iron pan on the grill and fill it with about 3 inches of cooking oil. Place a temperature probe into the oil.

3. While the oil heats, combine the buttermilk, hot sauce and Champion Chicken seasoning in a resealable plastic bag. Seal and shake to mix, then place the chicken in the bag and turn to coat.

4. Place the flour on a plate and dip the chicken in the flour to coat. Place the chicken on a wire rack set on a baking sheet and allow the coated chicken to set for 10 minutes, then dip again in the flour.

5. Once the oil in the cast iron pan reaches 350°F, place a temperature probe in a piece of chicken and fry the chicken, 2-3 pieces at a time. The oil temperature in the pan will drop by 25-30 degrees, so make sure not to put more than 3 pieces of chicken in the pan or your chicken will be greasy.

6. Fry the chicken until golden brown, crispy, and the internal temperature of the chicken is 170°F. Remove the chicken and place on a plate lined with paper towels. Allow the chicken to drain and rest for 5 minutes. Fry the remaining chicken pieces, reinserting the temperature probe.

7. Once the chicken is all fried, place the chicken on the slider buns, top with spicy bread and butter pickles, and a swoop of mayo, serve immediately.

Kansas City Hot Fried Chicken

Servings: 4
Cooking Time: 25 Minutes

Ingredients:

- 1 Whole Chicken, cut into pieces

- 1 1/2 Cup buttermilk
- 2 Tablespoon hot sauce
- 4 Cup all-purpose flour
- 1 Teaspoon salt
- 1/2 Teaspoon black pepper
- 1/2 Tablespoon red pepper flakes
- 12 Ounce Bacon, Uncooked, Chopped
- vegetable oil

Directions:

1. Supply your smoker with wood pellets and follow the start-up procedure. Preheat the grill, with the lid closed, to 180° F.

2. Smoke the 4 pieces of chicken for about 10 min. Grill: 180 °F

3. Mix buttermilk and hot sauce together in a large bowl, keep mixture ultra chilled.

4. In a separate bowl, mix the dry ingredients and bacon together, set aside.

5. Remove chicken and place in ice-cold buttermilk mixture for about an hour in the refrigerator.

6. Heat Vegetable Oil in a frying pan to 370°F (195 C).

7. Remove chicken from the liquid and batter it in dry ingredient mixture, drop into frying oil for about 10-15 minutes.

8. Serve with pickled hot peppers. Enjoy!

Bacon Weaved Stuffed Turkey Breast

Servings: 8
Cooking Time: 60 Minutes

Ingredients:

- 1/2 Cup celery, diced
- 14 Ounce Stuffing Mix
- 2 Tablespoon chopped sage
- 4 Tablespoon Chicken Rub
- 1/2 Cup dried sweetened cranberries
- 2 Cup apple cider
- 20 Strips thick-cut bacon

Directions:

1. Prepare the stuffing: Add all stuffing ingredients into a large bowl and toss to mix together.

2. Create a bacon weave and lay it out in a 5x5 pattern on cutting board.

3. Using a long, thin knife, butterfly each of the turkey breasts. Stuff each breast with a generous amount of stuffing and close.

4. Place turkey breast on prepared bacon weave, carefully wrap turkey, and secure with tooth picks. Repeat for the second breast.

5. Supply your smoker with wood pellets and follow the start-up procedure. Preheat the grill, with the lid closed, to 375° F.

6. Place the breasts seam side down on a rimmed baking sheet. Transfer directly to grill.

7. Place the bacon wrapped turkey breasts directly to the Traeger and cook for approximately 45 mins to 1 hour or until an instant read thermometer inserted into the center of the stuffing reaches 165 degrees F. Grill: 375 ˚F Probe: 165 ˚F

8. If the bacon gets too dark, cover with foil. Slice and enjoy!

Smoked Avocado Turkey Tamale Pie

Servings: 6
Cooking Time: 240 Minutes

Ingredients:
- 1 Avocado, Diced (For Topping)
- 15 Oz Black Beans, Drained (For Filling)
- To Taste, Blackened Sriracha Rub Seasoning
- 2 Tsp Blackened Sriracha Rub Seasoning (For Filling)
- To Taste, Blackened Sriracha Rub Seasoning (For Polenta)
- 2 Tbsp Butter (For Polenta)
- 2 Tbsp Cilantro, Chopped (For Topping)
- 1 Cup Corn Kernels (For Filling)
- 2 Cups Enchilada Sauce (For Filling)
- 1/2 Jalapeño, Minced (For Topping)
- 2 Cups Milk Or Water (For Polenta)
- 1 Cup Polenta, Or Fine Cornmeal (For Polenta)
- 2 Scallions, Sliced (For Topping)
- 2 Cups Smoked Turkey Breast, Shredded (For Filling)
- 2 1/2 Lbs Split Turkey Breast , Bone-In
- 2 Cups Turkey Stock (For Polenta)

- 4 Oz White Cheddar, Shredded (For Polenta)
- 4 Oz White Cheddar, Shredded (For Topping)

Directions:
1. Supply your smoker with wood pellets and follow the start-up procedure. Preheat the grill, with the lid closed, to 225° F. If using a gas or charcoal grill, set it up for low, indirect heat.

2. Season the turkey breast with Blackened Sriracha, then transfer to the grill, on a rack, over indirect heat.

3. Smoke the turkey breast for 2 ½ to 3 hours, until an internal temperature of 160° F. Remove the turkey from the grill, allow to rest for 20 minutes, then shred with 2 forks.

4. While the turkey is resting, prepare the polenta:

5. Place a deep, cast iron skillet on the grill, then increase the temperature to 375° F. Add chicken broth and milk to a skillet and bring to a boil.

6. Whisk in the polenta, then reduce the heat to a simmer, stirring often for 5 minutes. Season with Blackened Sriracha, then stir in cheese and butter. Remove the skillet from the grill and smooth out the polenta in an even layer.

7. In a large glass measuring cup or mixing bowl, combine the turkey, enchilada sauce, black beans, corn and Blackened Sriracha.

8. Spoon the turkey mixture over the polenta, then top with 4 ounces of shredded cheese. Place on the grill, over indirect heat and bake for 20 to 25 minutes, until the filling is bubbling along the edge and the cheese is melted.

9. Remove the skillet from the grill and allow it to rest for 10 minutes. Serve warm, garnished with avocado, scallions, jalapeño, and fresh cilantro.

Savory Cajun Bbq Chicken

Servings: 4
Cooking Time: 25 Minutes

Ingredients:
- ½ Cup Barbecue Sauce
- ¼ Cup Beer, Any Brand
- 1 Tablespoon Butter
- 1 Pound Boneless, Skinless Chicken Breasts

- 2 Cloves Garlic Clove, Minced
- ¼ Teaspoon Ground Thyme
- 1 Teaspoon Hot Sauce
- Juice Of 1 Lime
- 1 Tablespoon Olive Oil
- ½ Teaspoon Oregano
- 2 Tablespoons Sweet Heat Rub
- 1 Tablespoon Worcestershire Sauce

Directions:

1. In a small mixing bowl, mix together the Sweet Heat Rub, oregano, and ground thyme.

2. Rub the chicken breasts all over with olive oil, making sure to completely coat the meat. Generously season the chicken breasts on all sides with the Sweet Heat mixture.

3. Supply your smoker with wood pellets and follow the start-up procedure. Preheat the grill, with the lid closed, to 350° F. If you're using a gas or charcoal grill, set it up for medium heat. Insert a temperature probe into the thickest part of one of the chicken breasts and place the meat on the grill. Grill the meat on one side for 10-12 minutes, then flip and grill for another 5-7 minutes, or until the chicken breasts are golden brown and juicy and reaches an internal temperature of 165°F.

4. Remove the chicken from the grill and allow to rest for 10 minutes.

5. While the chicken rests, make the sauce. Combine the butter, barbecue sauce, beer, Worcestershire sauce, lime juice, and minced garlic in a heat proof saucepan and place on the grill. Bring the sauce to a boil. Once it boils, remove it from the heat, whisk it and serve with the chicken.

Cajun Brined Maple Smoked Turkey Breast

Servings: 4
Cooking Time: 180 Minutes

Ingredients:
- 1 Gallon water
- 3/4 Cup canning and pickling salt
- 3 Tablespoon minced garlic
- 3 Tablespoon dark brown sugar

- 2 Tablespoon Worcestershire sauce
- 2 Tablespoon Cajun seasoning
- 1 (5-6 lb) bone-in turkey breast
- 3 Tablespoon extra-virgin olive oil
- 2 Tablespoon Cajun seasoning

Directions:

1. In a large food safe container or bucket, combine all of the ingredients for the brine with 1 gallon water. Stir until the salt is dissolved.

2. Place the turkey breast in the brine and weigh it down to ensure it is fully submerged. Cover and brine in a refrigerator for 1 to 2 days.

3. Remove the turkey breast from the brine and pat dry. Drizzle with the olive oil using your hands to cover all areas of the bird. Season liberally with Cajun seasoning. Probe: 165 °F

4. Supply your smoker with wood pellets and follow the start-up procedure. Preheat the grill, with the lid closed, to 225° F.

5. Place the turkey breast directly on the grill grate, close the lid and cook for 3 hours. After 3 hours, increase the temperature to 425°F and continue to cook for another 30 minutes or until the internal temperature reads 165°F when a thermometer is inserted into the thickest part of the breast. Grill: 225 °F Probe: 165 °F

6. Remove the turkey breast from the grill and allow to rest for at least 15 minutes before slicing. Slice and serve. Enjoy!

Grilled Cheesy Chicken

Servings: 4
Cooking Time: 45 Minutes

Ingredients:
- 4 Aged Chedder Cheese, Sliced
- 32 Oz Chicken Broth
- 1 Tsp Extra-Virgin Olive Oil
- Sweet Heat Rub And Grill
- 4 Plump Chicken, Boneless/Skinless

Directions:

1. Supply your smoker with wood pellets and follow the start-up procedure. Preheat the grill, with the lid open, to 350° F.

2. Remove the chicken from the brine. Pat the breasts dry and lightly brush olive oil on both sides of the chicken. Take your knife and slice diagonally across the top of each breast. Sprinkle a lit amount of Sweet Heat Rub and Grill on each side.

3. Barbecue your chicken breasts for 30 minutes. Next, place a slice of cheddar cheese on top of each breast.

4. Heat for another 5-10 minutes or until the cheese has fully melted into the incisions you made earlier. Remove and serve for a tender chicken breast with a spicy kick and hot cheesy center. You'll receive too much credit for a recipe this easy.

Turkey & Bacon Kebabs With Ranch-style Dressing

Servings: 8
Cooking Time: 25 Minutes

Ingredients:
- 1½lb (680g) skinless turkey tenders or boneless, skinless turkey breasts, cut into 1-inch (2.5cm) chunks
- 8 strips of thick-cut bacon
- 12 fresh bay leaves (optional)
- for the dressing
- 1 cup reduced-fat mayo
- 1 cup light sour cream
- ½ cup buttermilk or whole milk, plus more
- 2 tbsp minced fresh parsley
- 2 tbsp minced fresh chives
- 1 tbsp minced fresh dill
- 2 tsp freshly squeezed lemon juice
- 1 tsp Worcestershire sauce
- 1 tsp garlic salt
- 1 tsp onion powder
- ½ tsp coarse salt, plus more
- ½ tsp freshly ground black pepper, plus more

Directions:
1. In a large bowl, make the dressing by whisking together the mayo, sour cream, and buttermilk until smooth. Whisk in the remaining ingredients. Pour half the mixture into a small bowl. Cover and refrigerate.

2. Add the turkey to the mixture remaining in the bowl and toss to coat thoroughly. If the dressing seems too thick (dip-like), add more buttermilk 1 tablespoon at a time. Cover and refrigerate for 2 to 4 hours.

3. Supply your smoker with wood pellets and follow the start-up procedure. Preheat the grill, with the lid closed, to 375° F.

4. Place the bacon on the grate and cook until some of the fat has rendered and the bacon begins to brown, about 15 minutes. Remove the bacon from the grill to cool. Cut the bacon into 1-inch (2.5cm) squares. Set aside.

5. Drain the tenders and discard any excess dressing. Alternate threading the turkey, bacon pieces, and 3 bay leaves on a bamboo skewer. Repeat the threading with 3 more skewers.

6. Place the kebabs on the grate and grill until the turkey is cooked through, about 4 to 5 minutes per side, turning as needed.

7. Transfer the skewers to a platter. Serve with the reserved dressing.

Mini Turducken Roulade

Servings: 6
Cooking Time: 120 Minutes

Ingredients:
- 1 (16-ounce) boneless turkey breast
- 1 (8-to 10-ounce) boneless duck breast
- 1 (8-ounce) boneless, skinless chicken breast
- Salt
- Freshly ground black pepper
- 2 cups Italian dressing
- 2 tablespoons Cajun seasoning
- 1 cup prepared seasoned stuffing mix
- 8 slices bacon
- Butcher's string

Directions:
1. Butterfly the turkey, duck, and chicken breasts, cover with plastic wrap and, using a mallet, flatten each ½ inch thick.

2. Season all the meat on both sides with a little salt and pepper.

3. In a medium bowl, combine the Italian dressing and Cajun seasoning. Spread one-fourth of the mixture on top of the flattened turkey breast.

4. Place the duck breast on top of the turkey, spread it with one-fourth of the dressing mixture, and top with the stuffing mix.

5. Place the chicken breast on top of the duck and spread with one-fourth of the dressing mixture.

6. Supply your smoker with wood pellets and follow the start-up procedure. Preheat, with the lid closed, to 275°F.

7. Tightly roll up the stack, tie with butcher's string, and slather the whole thing with the remaining dressing mixture.

8. Wrap the bacon slices around the turducken and secure with toothpicks, or try making a bacon weave (see the technique for this in the Jalapeño-Bacon Pork Tenderloin recipe).

9. Place the turducken roulade in a roasting pan. Transfer to the grill, close the lid, and roast for 2 hours, or until a meat thermometer inserted in the turducken reads 165°F. Tent with aluminum foil in the last 30 minutes, if necessary, to keep from overbrowning.

10. Let the turducken rest for 15 to 20 minutes before carving. Serve warm.

Skinny Smoked Chicken Breasts

Servings: 4-6
Cooking Time: 85 Minutes

Ingredients:
- 2½ pounds boneless, skinless chicken breasts
- Salt
- Freshly ground black pepper

Directions:
1. Supply your smoker with wood pellets and follow the start-up procedure. Preheat the grill, with the lid closed, to 180°F.
2. Season the chicken breasts all over with salt and pepper.
3. Place the breasts directly on the grill grate and smoke for 1 hour.

4. Increase the grill's temperature to 325°F and continue to cook until the chicken's internal temperature reaches 170°F. Remove the breasts from the grill and serve immediately.

Italian Grilled Barbecue Chicken Wings

Servings: 4
Cooking Time: 18 Minutes

Ingredients:
- 1 cup KRAFT Zesty Italian Dressing
- 2 pounds chicken wings/drummettes
- 1/2 cup barbecue sauce

Directions:
1. Pour dressing over chicken in large bowl; toss to coat.
2. Refrigerate at least 30 minutes to marinate.
3. Supply your smoker with wood pellets and follow the start-up procedure. Preheat the grill, with the lid closed, to 400° F. Drain chicken; discard marinade.
4. Grill chicken 8 minutes on each side or until done.
5. Brush with barbecue sauce; grill for another 2 minutes.
6. Remove from grill and serve.

Sweet Cajun Wings

Servings: 4
Cooking Time: 30 Minutes

Ingredients:
- 2 Pound chicken wings
- Pork & Poultry Rub
- Cajun Shake

Directions:
1. Coat wings in Traeger Sweet rub and Traeger Cajun shake.
2. Supply your smoker with wood pellets and follow the start-up procedure. Preheat the grill, with the lid closed, to 350° F.
3. Cook for 30 minutes or until skin is brown and center is juicy and an instant-read thermometer reads at least 165°F. Serve, enjoy! Grill: 350 °F Probe: 165 °F

Bbq Breakfast Sausage

Servings: 4 - 6
Cooking Time: 35 Minutes

Ingredients:

- 1/4 Cup Bbq Sauce
- 1 Tbsp Brown Sugar
- 4 Oz Cheddar Cheese, Cut Into Sticks
- To Taste, Cracked Black Pepper
- 6 Eggs, Scrambled
- 4 Oz Ham, Diced
- 1 Package, Approx 1 Lb Shady Brook Farms Ground Turkey Sausage
- 10 Oz Turkey Bacon

Directions:

1. Supply your smoker with wood pellets and follow the start-up procedure. Preheat the grill, with the lid closed, to 375° F. If using a gas or charcoal grill, set it up for medium-high heat.

2. Lay out a piece of plastic wrap then make a bacon weave using your favorite turkey bacon. Top with the Shady Brooks Farms Turkey Sausage and spread out into an even layer with your fingers.

3. Spoon the scrambled eggs into the center of the sausage, then place half of the cheese sticks in the middle, followed by ham, then remaining cheese.

4. Gently lift up one end of the plastic wrap and begin rolling the "not so fatty." Once the roll is completed, remove the plastic wrap and secure the ends of the bacon together with toothpicks, if needed.

5. Set in a cast iron skillet, sprinkle with brown sugar, and season with cracked pepper. Transfer to the grill and cook for 30 minutes, until an internal temperature of 155°F.

6. Baste with BBQ sauce and cook for an additional 5 minutes until the sauce is set and the internal temperature increased to 165°F.

7. Remove from the grill and rest for 5 minutes before slicing and serving warm.

Smoke Roasted Chicken With Herb Butter

Servings: 4

Cooking Time: 60 Minutes

Ingredients:

- 8 Tablespoon butter, room temperature
- 1 Scallions, minced
- 1 Clove garlic, minced
- 2 Tablespoon Fresh Herbs (Thyme, Rosemary, Oregano, Basil, Sage or Parsley, Minced)
- 1 1/2 Tablespoon Chicken Rub
- 1/2 Tablespoon fresh lemon juice
- 1 (4 to 4-1/2 lb) chicken
- Chicken Rub

Directions:

1. In a small bowl, combine butter, scallions, garlic, minced fresh herbs, Traeger Chicken Rub and lemon juice. Blend well with a wooden spoon.

2. Remove any giblets from the cavity of the chicken. Wash the chicken inside and out with cold running water. Dry thoroughly with paper towels.

3. Sprinkle a generous amount of Traeger Chicken Rub into the cavity of the chicken.

4. Gently loosen the skin around the chicken breast and slide in a few tablespoons of the herb butter and cover evenly. Smear the outside of the chicken with the remaining herb butter.

5. Tuck the chicken wings behind the back. Tie the legs together with butcher's twine.

6. Sprinkle the outside of the chicken with more Traeger Chicken Rub and insert sprigs of fresh herbs into the cavity of the chicken if desired.

7. Supply your smoker with wood pellets and follow the start-up procedure. Preheat the grill, with the lid closed, to 400° F.

8. When grill is hot, place chicken directly on the grill grate, breast side up. Cook for 1 to 1-1/4 hours or until the internal temperature registers 165°F. If the chicken is browning too quickly, loosely cover the breast and legs with foil and continue to cook. Grill: 400 °F Probe: 165 °F

9. Remove from the grill and let rest 15 minutes at room temperature before carving. Serve. Enjoy!

Chicken Parmesan Sliders With Pesto Mayonnaise

Servings: 4
Cooking Time: 30 Minutes

Ingredients:

- 2 Pound Chicken, ground
- 1 Cup Parmesan cheese
- 1 Tablespoon Worcestershire sauce
- black pepper
- 1 Cup mayonnaise
- 2 Tablespoon Pesto Sauce
- 3 Roma tomatoes
- 1 red onion, sliced
- Baby Spinach

Directions:

1. Line a baking sheet with plastic wrap. In a large mixing bowl, combine the ground chicken, the Parmesan, the Worcestershire, and a few grinds of black pepper. Wet your hands with cold water, and use them to mix the ingredients.

2. Divide the meat mixture in half, then form six 2-inch patties out of each half. Place the patties on the baking sheet, cover with another sheet of plastic wrap, and refrigerate for at least 1 hour.

3. Combine the mayonnaise and pesto in a small bowl and whisk together. Cover and refrigerate until serving time.

4. Supply your smoker with wood pellets and follow the start-up procedure. Preheat the grill, with the lid closed, to 300° F.

5. Arrange the chicken patties on the grill grate and grill, turning once, until the patties are cooked through (165F), about 30 minutes. Grill: 300 °F Probe: 165 °F

6. To serve, put a chicken patty on the bottom of a slider bun and top with a dollop of the pesto mayonnaise. Add tomato, onion, and spinach as desired. Replace the top of the bun and skewer with a frilled toothpick, if desired.

Spatchcocked Chicken With Toasted Fennel & Garlic

Servings: 6
Cooking Time: 45 Minutes

Ingredients:

- 6 Pound whole chicken
- 1 Tablespoon toasted fennel seed
- 2 Clove garlic, minced
- 1 Tablespoon salt
- 1/2 Tablespoon pepper

Directions:

1. To Spatchcock the chicken, remove the backbone by cutting down both sides of the backbone.

2. Next turn the bird over and make a cut down the keel bone, which is right in the center. This will allow the chicken to lay flat.

3. Supply your smoker with wood pellets and follow the start-up procedure. Preheat the grill, with the lid closed, to 450° F.

4. While the grill is preheating, rub the chicken with the fennel, garlic, salt, and pepper, and let it come almost to room temperature (this will help it cook faster).

5. Place the chicken, skin-side down on the grill. Cook 8 to 10 minutes, or until there are good grill marks. Grill: 450 °F

6. Turn the chicken over and cook until the meat reaches an internal temperature of 160 degrees. Enjoy! Grill: 450 °F Probe: 160 °F

Smoked Wings

Servings: 6
Cooking Time: 50 Minutes

Ingredients:

- 24 chicken wings, flats and drumettes separated
- 12 Ounce Italian dressing
- 3 Ounce Chicken Rub
- 5 Ounce 'Que BBQ Sauce
- 3 Ounce chili sauce

Directions:

1. Wash all wings and place into resealable bag. Add Italian dressing to the resealable bag containing the

wings. Place in refrigerator and allow to marinate for 6 to 12 hours.

2. Supply your smoker with wood pellets and follow the start-up procedure. Preheat the grill, with the lid closed, to 225° F.

3. Remove wings from marinade and shake off excess marinade. Season all sides of the wings with Traeger Chicken Rub and let sit for 15 minutes before putting wings on the Traeger.

4. In a small bowl, combine the BBQ and chili sauces. Set aside.

5. Cook wings to an internal temperature of 160°F. Remove the wings and toss in chili barbecue sauce. Grill: 225 °F Probe: 160 °F

6. Increase the grill temperature to 375°F and preheat. Once at temperature, place the wings on the Traeger and sear both sides until the internal temperature reaches 165°F. Grill: 375 °F Probe: 165 °F

7. Remove the wings from grill and let rest for 5 minutes. Serve with your favorite side wing dressing or sauce. Enjoy!

Bourbon-brined Turkey Thighs

Servings: 4
Cooking Time: 135 Minutes

Ingredients:
- 4 skin-on, bone-in turkey thighs, about 2lb (1kg) total
- 6 tbsp unsalted butter, at room temperature
- 4 large fresh sage leaves
- coarse salt
- freshly ground black pepper
- for the brine
- 1 quart (1 liter) distilled water
- ¼ cup coarse salt, plus more
- ¼ cup light brown sugar or low-carb substitute
- ¼ cup bourbon (optional)

Directions:
1. In a saucepan on the stovetop over medium-high heat, make the brine by combining the water, salt, brown sugar, and bourbon (if using). Bring to a boil. Stir until the salt and sugar dissolve. Remove the saucepan from the stovetop and let the brine cool to room temperature.

2. Place the turkey in a resealable plastic bag and pour the brine over the thighs. Refrigerate for 4 hours.

3. Supply your smoker with wood pellets and follow the start-up procedure. Preheat the grill, with the lid closed, to 250° F.

4. Drain the turkey thighs and discard the brine. Rinse under cold running water and pat dry with paper towels. Gently lift the skin of each thigh and push 2 teaspoons of butter underneath. Top the butter with a sage leaf, smoothing it out so it lays flat under the skin. Rub the outside of the skin with more butter. Lightly season with salt and pepper.

5. Place the turkey thighs on the grate at an angle to the bars. Smoke for 1½ hours. Raise the temperature to 375°F (191°C) and roast until the skin is golden brown and the internal temperature in the thickest part of the meat reaches 170°F (77°C), about 30 to 45 minutes.

6. Transfer the thighs to a platter. Let rest for 3 minutes before serving.

Traeger Bbq Half Chickens

Servings: 2
Cooking Time: 60 Minutes

Ingredients:
- 1 (3 to 3-1/2 lb) fresh young chicken
- Leinenkugel's Summer Shandy Rub
- Apricot BBQ Sauce

Directions:
1. Place the chicken breast side down, on a cutting board with the neck pointing away from you. Cut along one side of the backbone, staying as close to the bone as possible, from the neck to the tail. Repeat on the other side of the backbone then remove it.

2. Open the chicken and slice through the white cartilage at the tip of the breastbone to pop it open. Cut down either side of the breast bone then use your fingers to pull it out. Flip the chicken over so it is skin side up and cut down the center splitting the chicken in half. Tuck the wings back on each chicken half.

151

3. Season on both sides with Traeger Leinenkugel's Summer Shandy Rub.

4. Supply your smoker with wood pellets and follow the start-up procedure. Preheat the grill, with the lid closed, to 375° F.

5. Place chicken directly on the grill grate skin side up and cook until the internal temperature reaches 160°F, about 60-90 minutes. Grill: 375 °F Probe: 160 °F

6. Brush the BBQ sauce all over the chicken skin and cook for an additional 10 minutes. Remove from grill and let rest 5 minutes before serving. Enjoy! Grill: 375 °F

Teriyaki Apple Cider Turkey

Servings: 8-10
Cooking Time: 180 Minutes

Ingredients:
- 1/2 Cup Apple Cider
- 1/4 Cup Melted Butter, Unsalted
- 1 Teaspoon Cornstarch
- 2 Finely Chopped Garlic, Cloves
- 1/2 Teaspoon Ginger, Ground
- 2 Tablespoon Honey
- 2 Tablespoon Champion Chicken Seasoning
- 1 Shady Brook Farms® Whole Turkey, Thawed
- 2 Tablespoon Soy Sauce
- 1 Tablespoon Water, Cold

Directions:
1. Supply your smoker with wood pellets and follow the start-up procedure. Preheat the grill, with the lid closed, to 300° F.

2. In a saucepan, whisk together melted butter, garlic, soy sauce, apple cider, ground ginger, and honey. Bring to a boil then reduce to a simmer.

3. Place the turkey in an aluminum roasting pan.

4. With a marinade injector, fill with the mixture and pierce the meat with the needle while pushing on the plunger, injecting the flavor. You want to inject into the thickest part of the breast, thigh, and wings.

5. Next, rub entire turkey with your favorite poultry seasoning or the Champion Chicken seasoning. For added flavor, throw some extra garlic gloves into the cavity and apple cider in the aluminum pan.

6. Place the turkey in the grill and cook until the internal temperature reaches 165-170°F.

7. In a separate bowl, mix cornstarch and cold water together and add to the leftover original mixture to create a glaze. Glaze the turkey with the remaining mixture with approximately 15-20 minutes left. Skin will darken because of the sugar in the glaze.

8. Let the turkey rest 20-25 minutes before carving and enjoy!

Spatchcocked Chicken With White Barbecue Sauce

Servings: 4
Cooking Time: 60 Minutes

Ingredients:
- 1 whole chicken, about 4 to 4½lb (1.8 to 2kg), preferably organic or farm raised
- extra virgin olive oil
- White Barbecue Sauce
- chopped fresh chives (optional)
- for the brine
- ½ gallon (1.9 liters) distilled water
- ½ cup kosher salt
- 2 tbsp light brown sugar or low-carb substitute
- for the rub
- ¼ cup coarse salt
- ¼ cup granulated light brown sugar or low-carb substitute
- ¼ cup sweet or smoked paprika
- 2 tbsp freshly ground black pepper
- 1 tbsp granulated garlic
- 2 tsp dried thyme
- ½ tsp ground cayenne

Directions:
1. In a large stockpot on the stovetop over medium-high heat, make the brine by combining the ingredients. Bring the mixture to a boil. Stir until the salt and sugar dissolve. Remove the pot from the stovetop and let the brine cool to room temperature. Cover and refrigerate until cool.

2. Remove the backbone of the chicken by using a sharp knife, starting at the tail and cutting through the

rib bones. Repeat on the other side of the backbone. Fold the two halves backward to release the cartilaginous breastbone. (You might have to use a knife to slice through the thin skin on either side.) Remove the breastbone. Turn the chicken over and gently flatten it with the palm of your hand. Submerge the chicken in the brine. If it floats, place a resealable bag of ice on top. Refrigerate for 4 to 6 hours.

3. Supply your smoker with wood pellets and follow the start-up procedure. Preheat the grill, with the lid closed, to 325° F.

4. In a small bowl, make the rub by combining the ingredients.

5. Rinse the chicken with cold running water and dry with paper towels. (Discard the brine.) Coat the skin with olive oil. Lightly dust the chicken on both sides with the rub. (Save the remainder for another grill session.) Tuck the wingtips behind the chicken's back.

6. Place the chicken ribs side down on the grate and grill until the skin is nicely browned and the internal temperature in a thigh reaches 170°F (77°C), about 1 hour.

7. Transfer the chicken to a platter. Spoon the white barbecue sauce over the chicken. Spread the sauce with a basting brush, letting it pool in places. Lightly scatter the chives over the top. Carve the chicken and serve with extra sauce on the side.

Spicy Bbq Whole Chicken

Servings: 4
Cooking Time: 180 Minutes

Ingredients:
- 6 Thai chiles
- 2 Tablespoon sweet paprika
- 1 Scotch bonnet pepper
- 2 Tablespoon sugar
- 3 Tablespoon salt
- 1 white onion
- 5 Clove garlic
- 4 Cup grapeseed oil
- 1 whole chicken

Directions:

1. In a food processor or blender, puree the Thai chiles, paprika, Scotch bonnet pepper, sugar, salt, onion, garlic and grapeseed oil together until smooth.

2. Smother the chicken with mixture and let rest in fridge overnight.

3. Supply your smoker with wood pellets and follow the start-up procedure. Preheat the grill, with the lid closed, to 300° F.

4. Place chicken on grill, breast side up and smoke for 3 hours, or until it reaches an internal temperature of 165°F in the breast. Grill: 300 °F Probe: 165 °F

5. Remove from grill and allow to rest for 10 to 15 minutes before slicing. Serve with sides of choice. Enjoy!

Green Chile Chicken Enchiladas

Servings: 6
Cooking Time: 45 Minutes

Ingredients:
- 2 Cups Chicken, Shredded
- 1 (12 Oz) Package Colby Jack Cheese, Shredded
- 1 Enchilada Sauce, Can
- 1 Can Green Chile, Drained
- 1 Onion, Diced
- 1 Tablespoon Sweet Rib Rub
- 1 Cup Sour Cream
- 1 Package Flour Tortilla

Directions:

1. Supply your smoker with wood pellets and follow the start-up procedure. Preheat the grill, with the lid open, to 300° F.

2. In a bowl, mix - the chicken, green chiles, Sweet Heat seasoning, sour cream, diced onion, and half the bag of shredded cheese.

3. Place a large spoonful of the chicken mixture in the center of a tortilla and roll it up. Repeat with the remaining tortillas, then place in the baking pan, and pour the enchilada sauce over the tortilla pans. Top with the remainder of the shredded cheese.

4. Wrap the top of the pan tightly in aluminum foil and grill for 45 minutes or until the enchilada sauce is bubbly. Remove from the grill and serve.

Bacon-wrapped Chicken Breasts

Servings: 4 - 6
Cooking Time: 270 Minutes

Ingredients:

- 5 Oz Frozen Spinach, Thawed, Strained
- 8 Bacon Slices
- 1 Tbsp Butter
- 4 Chicken Breasts, Boneless, Skinless, Butterflied
- 2 Garlic Clove, Minced
- 1 Cup Italian Cheese Blend, Shredded
- 8 Oz Mushrooms, Sliced Thin
- 1 Tbsp Olive Oil
- 1 Tbsp Hickory Bacon Rub
- 1 Yellow Onion, Chopped

Directions:

1. Supply your smoker with wood pellets and follow the start-up procedure. Preheat the grill, with the lid open, to 375° F. If using a gas or charcoal grill, set heat to medium heat. For all other grills, preheat cast iron skillet on grill grates.

2. Heat olive oil and butter on griddle, then add mushrooms and cook for about 3 minutes, stirring frequently. Add chopped onion and garlic and cook for 2 minutes. Add spinach and sauté another minute, then transfer vegetables to a heat-safe bowl to cool slightly.

3. Season the butterflied chicken breasts with Hickory Bacon, coating both sides. Sprinkle half of cheese over each butterflied chicken breast, followed by the sautéed vegetables, and the remaining half of the cheese.

4. On a metal sheet tray, lay out two bacon slices. Gently fold chicken breast halves together and place on top of bacon slices, then wrap tightly with bacon. To secure, tuck ends of bacon underneath, or insert a toothpick to hold it together. Repeat with remaining breasts.

5. Arrange the chicken breasts, bacon seam down, directly on the grill grate and grill, turning once or twice, until the bacon is crisp and golden brown, about 25 to 30 minutes, or until internal temperature reaches 165°F.

6. Remove from grill, allow to rest for 5 minutes, remove any toothpicks, then serve hot.

Nashville Spiced Smoked Chicken

Servings: 6
Cooking Time: 40 Minutes

Ingredients:

- 6 drumsticks
- 1 quart Butter Milk
- 1 tbsp Louisiana Hot Sauce
- 1 tbsp Ground Cumin
- 1/2 tbsp Chili powder
- 1 tbsp Onion Powder
- 1 tbsp Garlic Powder
- 1/2 tbsp White Pepper
- 1 tbsp Red Cayenne Pepper
- 1 tbsp Black Pepper
- 2 tbsp Brown Sugar

Directions:

1. Soak wings overnight in marinade.
2. Remove chicken from marinade.Dry off chicken and wash off buttermilk.
3. Drizzle chicken with olive oil.
4. Apply dry rub to drumsticks by rubbing thoroughly.
5. Let drumsticks rest in dry rub for at least 30 minutes.
6. Supply your smoker with wood pellets and follow the start-up procedure. Preheat the grill, with the lid closed, to 325° F, using Apple Wood Pellets.
7. Cook chicken on 325 degrees for 30-40 minutes or until internal temperature reach 160 degrees F.
8. Let chicken rest for 10 minutes before serving.

Smoked Cheesy Chicken Quesadilla

Servings: 4-8
Cooking Time: 180 Minutes

Ingredients:

- 2-3 Boneless, Skinless Chicken Breasts
- 1 Jalapeno, Chopped
- 1 Onion, Chopped
- Sweet Heat Rub
- 1, Chopped Red Bell Pepper
- 1-2 Cups Salsa
- 3 Cups Shredded Cheddar Cheese
- 3 Cups Shredded Monterey Or Pepper Jack Cheese
- Taco Sauce

- 20 Taco-Size Tortilla

Directions:

1. Supply your smoker with wood pellets and follow the start-up procedure. Preheat the grill, with the lid closed, to 350° F. If you're using a gas or charcoal grill, set it up for medium heat. Preheat with lid closed for 10-15 minutes.

2. Sprinkle chicken breasts generously in Sweet Heat Rub and rub to coat evenly. Place chicken breasts directly on preheated grill grates and cook for 45 minutes, or until the chicken is completely cooked (165°F internal temperature), tender, and falling apart. Remove from the grill and let cool slightly. Shred with meat claws and set aside. Turn grill up to 375°F.

3. In a large bowl, add the shredded chicken, onion, red bell pepper, jalapeno, and taco sauce. Mix to combine then set aside.

4. Cut each tortilla in half. Add about 2 tablespoons each of the cheddar cheese, Monterey Jack cheese, and chicken mixture to each tortilla half. Roll the tortillas into cones, starting from the cut edge, making sure not to push the ingredients out of the tortilla.

5. Place the small bowl in the center of the pizza plan and begin to stack quesadilla cones in a ring around the bowl. The points of each cone should be in the center just touching the bowl. Sprinkle cheese over the layer and repeat another layer with the remaining cones, finishing with a final sprinkle of cheese.

6. Remove bowl from the center of the ring and place the pizza pan directly on the grill grates. Cook with the lid closed for 15-20 minutes, or until the cheese is melted and the edges are browned and crispy.

7. Fill small bowl with salsa and return to the center of the ring. Serve immediately and enjoy!

Cider-brined Turkey

Servings: 8
Cooking Time: 180 Minutes

Ingredients:

- 1 whole turkey, about 12 to 14lb (4.5 to 5.4kg), thawed if frozen
- 1 white onion, peeled and sliced into quarters
- 1 apple, cut into wedges
- 2 celery stalks, sliced into 2-inch (5cm) pieces
- sprigs of fresh sage, rosemary, parsley, or thyme
- 8 tbsp unsalted butter, at room temperature
- coarse salt
- freshly ground black pepper
- for the brine
- 1 quart (1 liter) apple cider or apple juice
- 3 quarts (3 liters) cold distilled water
- ¾ cup coarse salt
- ½ cup light brown sugar or low-carb substitute
- 3 garlic cloves, peeled and smashed with a chef's knife
- 3 bay leaves

Directions:

1. In a large food-safe bucket, make the brine by combining the apple cider, water, salt, and brown sugar. Stir until the salt and sugar dissolve. Add the garlic and bay leaves. Submerge the turkey in the brine. If it floats, place a resealable bag of ice on top. Refrigerate for at least 8 hours and up to 16 hours.

2. Supply your smoker with wood pellets and follow the start-up procedure. Preheat the grill, with the lid closed, to 350° F.

3. Remove the turkey from the brine and pat dry with paper towels. Discard the brine. Place the onion, apple, celery, and herbs in the main cavity. Tie the legs together with butcher's twine. Fold the wings behind the back. Rub the outside with butter. Lightly season with salt and pepper.

4. Place the turkey breast side up on a wire rack in a shallow roasting pan. Place the pan on the grate and roast the turkey until the internal temperature in the thickest part of a thigh reaches 165°F (74°C), about 2½ to 3 hours.

5. Transfer the turkey to a cutting board and let rest for 20 minutes. (Save the drippings to make from-scratch turkey gravy.) Carve the turkey and arrange the meat on a large platter before serving.

Bbq Chicken Tostada

Servings: 4
Cooking Time: 50 Minutes

Ingredients:
- 4 Whole boneless, skinless chicken thighs
- salt and pepper
- 8 Whole Corn Tostada
- Refried Beans
- lettuce
- green onion, coarsely chopped
- cilantro, chopped
- guacamole

Directions:
1. Supply your smoker with wood pellets and follow the start-up procedure. Preheat the grill, with the lid closed, to 350° F.
2. While grill heats, trim excess fat and skin from chicken thighs.
3. Season with a light layer of salt and pepper.
4. Place chicken thighs on the grill grate and cook for 35 minutes.
5. Check internal temperature; chicken is done when a thermometer inserted reads 175 degrees F. Remove from the grill and let rest for 10 minutes before shredding.
6. Place tostadas on grill while chicken is resting for 5 minutes.
7. Build tostadas starting with refried beans, sliced lettuce, shredded chicken, tomatoes, green onions, cilantro, guacamole. Enjoy!

Smoked Quarters

Servings: 2-4
Cooking Time: 120 Minutes

Ingredients:
- 4 chicken quarters
- 2 tablespoons olive oil
- 1 batch Chicken Rub
- 2 tablespoons butter

Directions:

1. Supply your smoker with wood pellets and follow the start-up procedure. Preheat the grill, with the lid closed, to 180°F.
2. Coat the chicken quarters all over with olive oil and season them with the rub. Using your hands, work the rub into the meat.
3. Place the quarters directly on the grill grate and smoke for 1½ hours.
4. Baste the quarters with the butter and increase the grill's temperature to 375°F. Continue to cook until the chicken's internal temperature reaches 170°F.
5. Remove the quarters from the grill and let them rest for 10 minutes before serving.

Hot Turkey Sandwich With Gravy

Servings: 4
Cooking Time: 10 Minutes

Ingredients:
- 8 Slices Bread, Sliced
- 1 Cup Gravy, Prepared
- 2 Cups Leftover Turkey, Shredded

Directions:
1. Supply your smoker with wood pellets and follow the start-up procedure. Preheat the grill, with the lid closed, to 400° F.
2. Place the BBQ Grill Mat on the grates of your preheated grill and lay the shredded turkey evenly across the mat to reheat for about 10 minutes.
3. Prepare or reheat the gravy. You"ll want to have the gravy warmed and ready as soon as the turkey is reheated and the bread is toasted.
4. Hold each slice of bread over the flame broiler to toast to your liking.
5. When all of your ingredients are hot, scoop 1/2 cup of the shredded turkey onto a piece of bread, generously cover with gravy and top with another piece of toasted bread. Serve immediately.

Chicken Breast Calzones

Servings: 4
Cooking Time: 24 Minutes

Ingredients:

- 4 boneless, skinless chicken breasts, each about 6 to 8oz (170 to 225g)
- coarse salt
- freshly ground black pepper
- 1 cup good-quality Italian tomato sauce or marinara
- 4oz (110g) thinly sliced pepperoni or diced smoked ham
- 4oz (110g) provolone, fontina, or mozzarella cheese
- 8 fresh basil leaves
- 4 thin slices of prosciutto
- extra virgin olive oil
- freshly grated Parmesan cheese

Directions:

1. Supply your smoker with wood pellets and follow the start-up procedure. Preheat the grill, with the lid closed, to 425° F.
2. Use a sharp, thin-bladed knife to cut a deep pocket in the side of each breast, angling the knife toward the opposite side. (Don't cut all the way through.) Season the inside of each breast with salt and pepper. Add a couple spoonfuls of tomato sauce to each pocket. Add 1 ounce (25g) of pepperoni, 1 ounce (25g) of provolone, and 2 basil leaves.
3. Wrap each breast crosswise with a slice of prosciutto and then pin each breast closed with two toothpicks. Lightly brush the breasts with olive oil and season the outside with salt and pepper.
4. Place the breasts on the grate at an angle to the bars. Grill for 10 to 12 minutes and then turn with a thin-bladed spatula. Dust the tops with grated Parmesan. Continue to cook until the chicken is cooked through and the cheese has melted, about 10 to 12 minutes more.
5. Transfer the chicken to a platter. Let rest for 3 minutes and then remove the toothpicks. Serve immediately.

Bacon Wrapped Turkey Legs

Servings: 8

Cooking Time: 180 Minutes

Ingredients:

- 1 Gallon water
- 1/4 Cup Rub
- 3 Cup Morton Tender Quick Home Meat Cure
- 1/2 Cup brown sugar
- 6 Whole black peppercorns
- 2 Whole bay leaves
- 8 (1-1/2 lb each) turkey legs
- 8 Slices bacon

Directions:

1. Plan ahead, these turkey legs brine overnight. In a large stockpot, combine one gallon of water, Traeger Rub, curing salt, brown sugar, peppercorns and bay leaves.
2. Bring to a boil over high heat to dissolve the salt and sugar granules. Take off of the heat and add in 1/2 gallon of water and ice. Make sure the brine is at least to room temperature, if not colder. (You may need to refrigerate the brine for an hour or so.)
3. Add the turkey legs making sure they are completely submerged in the brine.
4. After 24 hours, drain the turkey legs and discard the brine. Rinse the brine off the legs with cold water, then dry thoroughly with paper towels.
5. Supply your smoker with wood pellets and follow the start-up procedure. Preheat the grill, with the lid closed, to 250° F.
6. Lay the turkey legs directly on the grill grate.
7. After 2-1/2 hours, wrap a piece of bacon around each leg and finish cooking them for the last 30 to 40 minutes. Grill: 250 ˚F
8. The total cooking time for the legs will be 3 hours, or until the internal temperature reaches 165°F on an instant-read meat thermometer. Serve and enjoy! Grill: 250 ˚F Probe: 165 ˚F

Whole Smoked Honey Chicken

Servings: 4
Cooking Time: 40 Minutes

Ingredients:

- 1 Tablespoon Honey
- 1 ½ Lemon
- 4 Tablespoons Champion Chicken Seasoning
- 4 Tablespoons Unsalted Butter
- 1, 4 Pound Chicken, Giblets Removed And Patted Dry

Directions:

1. Supply your smoker with wood pellets and follow the start-up procedure. Preheat the grill, with the lid open, to 225° F.
2. In a small saucepan, melt together the butter and honey over low heat. Squeeze ½ lemon into the honey mixture and remove from the heat.
3. Smoke the chicken, skin side down until the chicken is lightly browned and the skin releases from the grate without ripping, about 6-8 minutes.
4. Turn the chicken over and baste with the honey butter mixture.
5. Continue to smoke the chicken, basting every 45 minutes, until the thickest part of the chicken reaches 160°F.

Grilled Honey Chicken Wings

Servings: 4 - 8
Cooking Time: 30 Minutes

Ingredients:

- 2 Chipotles Chopped In Adobo
- 1 Apple Cider Vinegar
- 2 Tablespoons Balsamic Vinegar
- ¼ Cup Brown Sugar
- 2 ½ Lbs Chicken Wings, Trimmed And Patted Dry
- ¼ Cup Honey
- ½ Cup Ketchup
- ¼ Cup Adobo Sauce
- 2 Tablespoons Sweet Rib Rub
- 2 Teaspoons Worcestershire Sauce

Directions:

1. Supply your smoker with wood pellets and follow the start-up procedure. Preheat the grill, with the lid open, to 350° F. If you're using a charcoal or gas grill, set up the grill for medium high heat.
2. In a large bowl, whisk together the apple cider vinegar, ketchup, brown sugar, honey, chopped chipotle peppers with adobo sauce, balsamic vinegar, Worcestershire sauce, and Sweet Rib Rub. Whisk the glaze until it's well combined.
3. Add the wings to the glaze and place the bowl in the refrigerator. Marinade the chicken wings for up to 12 hours. Once the wings have finished marinating, remove the chicken wings from the marinade and place the chicken wings onto the wing rack.
4. Once all the wings have been placed on the wing rack, place the wing rack on the grill. Insert a temperature probe into the thickest part into one of the wings and grill the wings for 5 minutes, and then rotate the rack 180° and grill for another 5 minutes. Remove the wings once they have an internal temperature of 165°F and the juice from the chicken runs clear.
5. Remove the wings from the grill and serve immediately.

Apricot Glazed Ham

Servings: 8
Cooking Time: 60 Minutes

Ingredients:

- 1 Cup Apricot Preserves
- 1/2 Cup apricot brandy
- 1/4 Cup honey
- 1/4 Cup brown sugar, firmly packed
- 1/4 Teaspoon ground cloves
- 6 Ounce Apricot Nectar, bottled or ginger ale
- 1 Large ham
- fresh parsley
- apricot, halved

Directions:

1. Supply your smoker with wood pellets and follow the start-up procedure. Preheat the grill, with the lid closed, to 325° F.

2. In a saucepan, stir together the apricot preserves, apricot brandy, honey, brown sugar, cloves, and apricot nectar and simmer over medium heat until the preserves, honey, and brown sugar have melted. Set aside and keep warm.

3. Place ham in large roasting pan lined with aluminum foil. Place pan on grill and cook for 1.5 hours.

4. Open Grill and glaze ham with reserved mixture. Continue cooking for another 30 minutes or until a thermometer is inserted into the thickest part of the meat and reaches an internal temperatures of 135 degrees F. Probe: 135 °F

5. Garnish the platter with the parsley and apricots, if desired. Enjoy!

Smoked Honey Chicken Drumsticks

Servings: 4
Cooking Time: 30 Minutes

Ingredients:

- 1/2 Cup Apple Cider Vinegar
- 12 Chicken Drumsticks
- 2 Tablespoons Dijon Mustard
- 1/4 Cup Honey
- 1/4 Cup Ketchup
- 1 Tablespoon Sweet Heat Rub
- 1/2 Cup Soy Sauce

Directions:

1. Supply your smoker with wood pellets and follow the start-up procedure. Preheat the grill, with the lid open, to 225° F. Remove the wings from the marinade and place the drumsticks into the Buffalo Wing Rack.

2. Smoke for 60 minutes, or until a thermometer inserted into the thickest part of the drumstick registers at 170°F.

3. Turn the heat up to 350°F and cook for 5 to 10 minutes to make the skin crisp.

4. Remove from the smoker, serve immediately and enjoy!

Smoke-roasted Chicken Thighs

Servings: 12-15
Cooking Time: 120 Minutes

Ingredients:

- 3 pounds chicken thighs
- 2 teaspoons salt
- 2 teaspoons freshly ground black pepper
- 2 teaspoons garlic powder
- 2 teaspoons onion powder
- 2 cups prepared Italian dressing

Directions:

1. Place the chicken thighs in a shallow dish and sprinkle with the salt, pepper, garlic powder, and onion powder, being sure to get under the skin.

2. Cover with the Italian dressing, coating all sides, and refrigerate for 1 hour.

3. Supply your smoker with wood pellets and follow the start-up procedure. Preheat, with the lid closed, to 250°F.

4. Remove the chicken thighs from the marinade and place directly on the grill, skin-side down. Discard the marinade.

5. Close the lid and roast the chicken for 1 hour 30 minutes to 2 hours, or until a meat thermometer inserted in the thickest part of the thighs reads 165°F. Do not turn the thighs during the smoking process.

COCKTAILS RECIPES

Smoked Berry Cocktail

Servings: 2
Cooking Time: 15 Minutes

Ingredients:

- 1/2 Cup strawberries, stemmed
- 1/2 Cup blackberries
- 1/2 Cup blueberries
- 8 Ounce bourbon or iced tea
- 2 Ounce lime juice
- 3 Ounce simple syrup
- soda water
- fresh mint, for garnish

Directions:

1. Supply your smoker with wood pellets and follow the start-up procedure. Preheat the grill, with the lid closed, to 180° F.
2. Wash berries well, spread them on a clean cookie sheet and place on the grill. Smoke berries for 15 minutes. Grill: 180 °F
3. Remove berries from grill and transfer to a blender. Puree berries until smooth then pass through a fine mesh strainer to remove seeds.
4. To create a layered cocktail, pour 2 ounces of berry puree in the bottom of a glass. Next, pour 2 ounces of bourbon or iced tea over the back of a spoon into the glass, then 1/2 ounce lime juice and 1/2 ounce simple syrup, top with soda water and ice. Finish with mint or extra berries for garnish.
5. Repeat the same process for 3 more servings. Enjoy!

Smoking Gun Cocktail

Servings: 2
Cooking Time: 45 Minutes

Ingredients:

- 2 Jar vermouth soaked cocktail onions
- 3 Ounce vodka
- 1 Ounce dry vermouth

Directions:

1. Supply your smoker with wood pellets and follow the start-up procedure. Preheat the grill, with the lid closed, to 180° F.
2. To make the smoked onion vermouth: Pour jar of vermouth soaked cocktail onions onto a shallow sheet pan. Smoke for 45 minutes. Remove from grill and set aside to chill. Grill: 180 °F
3. To make the cocktail: Add vodka, 1 teaspoon liquid from the smoked onions and dry vermouth to a mixing glass. Shake and strain into a chilled martini glass.
4. Garnish with smoked cocktail onions on a skewer. Enjoy!

Traeger Smoked Daiquiri

Servings: 2
Cooking Time: 25 Minutes

Ingredients:

- 2 limes, sliced
- 2 Tablespoon granulated sugar
- 3 Ounce Rum
- 1 Ounce Smoked Simple Syrup
- 1 1/2 Ounce lime juice

Directions:

1. Supply your smoker with wood pellets and follow the start-up procedure. Preheat the grill, with the lid closed, to 350° F.
2. Toss the lime slices with granulated sugar and place directly on the grill grate. Cook 20-25 minutes or until grill marks form. Remove from grill and cool. Grill: 350 °F
3. In a mixing glass add rum, Traeger Simple Syrup, and fresh lime juice. Add ice to the mixing glass and shake. Strain contents into a chilled glass.
4. Garnish with a grilled lime wheel. Enjoy!

In Traeger Fashion Cocktail

Servings: 2
Cooking Time: 20 Minutes

Ingredients:

- 2 Whole orange peel
- 2 Whole lemon peel
- 3 Ounce bourbon
- 1 Ounce Smoked Simple Syrup
- 6 Dash Bitters Lab Charred Cedar & Currant Bitters

Directions:

1. Supply your smoker with wood pellets and follow the start-up procedure. Preheat the grill, with the lid closed, to 350° F.
2. Place the lemon and orange peel directly on the grill grate and cook 20 to 25 minutes or until lightly browned. Grill: 350 °F
3. Add bourbon, Traeger Smoked Simple Syrup and bitters to a mixing glass and stir over ice. Stir until glass is chilled and contents are well diluted.
4. Strain into a new glass over fresh ice and garnish with grilled lemon and orange peel. Enjoy!

Smoked Apple Cider

Servings: 2
Cooking Time: 30 Minutes

Ingredients:

- 32 Ounce apple cider
- 2 cinnamon sticks
- 4 whole cloves
- 3 star anise
- 2 Pieces orange peel
- 2 Pieces lemon peel

Directions:

1. Supply your smoker with wood pellets and follow the start-up procedure. Preheat the grill, with the lid closed, to 225° F.
2. Combine the cider, cinnamon stick, star anise, clove, lemon and orange peel in a shallow baking dish.

3. Place directly on the grill grate and smoke for 30 minutes. Remove from grill, strain and transfer to four mugs. Grill: 225 °F
4. Finish with a slice of apple and a cinnamon stick to serve. Enjoy!

Grilled Blood Orange Mimosa

Servings: 4
Cooking Time: 15 Minutes

Ingredients:

- 3 blood orange, halved
- 2 Tablespoon granulated sugar
- 1 Bottle sparkling wine
- thyme sprigs, for garnish

Directions:

1. Supply your smoker with wood pellets and follow the start-up procedure. Preheat the grill, with the lid closed, to 375° F.
2. When the grill is hot, dip the cut side of the orange halves in sugar and place cut side down directly on the grill grate. Grill: 375 °F
3. Grill the oranges for 10-15 minutes or until grill marks develop. Grill: 375 °F
4. Remove from the grill and let cool at room temperature.
5. When cool enough to handle, juice the oranges and strain through a fine strainer removing any pulp.
6. Pour 5 oz of sparkling wine into each glass and top with 1 oz blood orange juice.
7. Garnish with a sprig of thyme. Enjoy!

Sunset Margarita

Servings: 2
Cooking Time: 55 Minutes

Ingredients:

- 4 oranges
- 2 Cup plus 1 teaspoon agave
- 1/2 Cup water
- 1 Ounce burnt orange agave
- 3 Ounce reposado tequila
- 1 1/2 Ounce fresh squeezed lime juice
- Jacobsen Salt Co. Cherrywood Smoked Salt

Directions:

1. Supply your smoker with wood pellets and follow the start-up procedure. Preheat the grill, with the lid closed, to 350° F.

2. For the Burnt Orange Agave Syrup: Cut one orange in half and brush cut side with agave. Place cut side down directly on the grill grate and grill for 15 minutes or until grill marks develop. Grill: 350 °F

3. While the orange halves are grilling, slice the other orange and brush both sides of the slices with agave. Place slices directly on the grill grate next to the halves and cook for 15 minutes or until grill marks develop. Grill: 350 °F

4. Remove orange halves from grill grate and let cool. After they have cooled, juice halves and strain. Set aside.

5. Combine 1/4 cup water and agave in a shallow dish and mix well. Remove orange slices from the grill and place in the agave mixture, reserving a few for garnish.

6. Reduce the grill temperature to 180 degrees F and place the shallow dish with agave and oranges directly on the grill grate. Smoke for 40 minutes. Remove from heat and strain. Set aside. Grill: 180 °F

7. To Mix Drink: Rim glass with Jacobsen Smoked Salt. Combine tequila, fresh lime juice, grilled orange juice and burnt orange agave syrup in a glass. Add ice and shake well.

8. Strain into a rimmed glass over clean ice. Garnish with a grilled orange slice. Enjoy!

Ryes And Shine Cocktail

Servings: 2
Cooking Time: 30 Minutes

Ingredients:

- 2 lemon, cut into wheels for garnish
- 6 Tablespoon granulated sugar
- 2 Ounce rye
- 1 Ounce bourbon
- 3 Ounce lemon juice
- 1 Ounce Smoked Simple Syrup
- 6 Dash Fernet-Branca

Directions:

1. Supply your smoker with wood pellets and follow the start-up procedure. Preheat the grill, with the lid closed, to 325° F.

2. Toss lemon wheels with granulated sugar to coat on both sides. Place wheels directly on the grill grate and cook for 15 minutes on each side or until grill marks form. Grill: 325 °F

3. Add rye, bourbon, lemon juice, Traeger Smoked Simple Syrup and Fernet-Branca to a shaker and shake until slightly diluted (about 10 to 15 seconds).

4. Pour into a fresh glass, serve neat and garnish with a grilled lemon wheel. Enjoy!

Grilled Peach Sour Cocktail

Servings: 2
Cooking Time: 15 Minutes

Ingredients:

- 2 peach, sliced
- 2 Tablespoon sugar
- 1 1/2 Ounce Smoked Simple Syrup
- 4 Ounce bourbon
- 6 Dash Bitters Lab Apricot Vanilla Bitters
- 2 Sprig fresh thyme, for garnish

Directions:

1. Supply your smoker with wood pellets and follow the start-up procedure. Preheat the grill, with the lid closed, to 325° F.

2. Toss peach slices with granulated sugar and place directly on grill grate. Cook for 20 minutes or until grill marks form. Remove from grill and let cool. Grill: 325 °F

3. Place peaches and Traeger Smoked Simple Syrup into tin and muddle. Peaches should form about an ounce of juice during the muddling. Once completed, add remaining ingredients and shake.

4. Pour contents into glass over fresh ice and garnish with fresh thyme. Enjoy!

Zombie Cocktail Recipe

Servings: 2
Cooking Time: 45 Minutes

Ingredients:

- fresh squeezed orange juice
- pineapple juice
- 2 Ounce light rum
- 2 Ounce dark rum
- 2 Ounce lime juice
- 1 Ounce Smoked Simple Syrup
- 6 Ounce smoked orange and pineapple juice
- 2 grilled orange peel, for garnish
- 2 grilled pineapple chunks, for garnish

Directions:

1. Supply your smoker with wood pellets and follow the start-up procedure. Preheat the grill, with the lid closed, to 180° F.
2. Smoked Orange and Pineapple Juice: Pour equal parts fresh squeezed orange juice and pineapple juice into a shallow sheet pan and smoke for 45 minutes. Remove and let cool. Measure out 3 ounces of juice and reserve any remaining juice in the refrigerator for future use. Grill: 180 ˚F
3. Add dark and light rums, 3 ounces smoked orange and pineapple juice, lime juice and Traeger Smoked Simple Syrup to a mixing glass.
4. Add ice, shake and strain over clean ice into a Tiki glass.
5. Garnish with a grilled orange peel and grilled pineapple. Enjoy!

Smoked Hot Buttered Rum

Servings: 4
Cooking Time: 30 Minutes

Ingredients:

- 2 Cup water
- 1/4 Cup brown sugar
- 1/2 Stick butter, melted
- 1 Teaspoon ground cinnamon
- 1/4 Teaspoon ground nutmeg
- ground cloves
- salt

- 6 Ounce Rum

Directions:

1. Supply your smoker with wood pellets and follow the start-up procedure. Preheat the grill, with the lid closed, to 180° F.
2. In a shallow baking dish, combine 2 cups water with all ingredients except for the rum and place directly on the grill grate. Smoke for 30 minutes. Grill: 180 ˚F
3. Remove from the grill and pour into the pitcher of a blender. Process until somewhat frothy.
4. Pour 1.5 ounces of rum each into 4 glasses. Split hot butter mixture evenly between the four glasses.
5. Garnish with a cinnamon stick and freshly grated nutmeg. Enjoy!

Strawberry Mule Cocktail

Servings: 2
Cooking Time: 15 Minutes

Ingredients:

- 8 grilled strawberries, plus more for serving
- 3 Ounce vodka
- 1 Ounce Smoked Simple Syrup
- 1 Ounce lemon juice
- 6 Ounce ginger beer
- fresh mint leaves

Directions:

1. Supply your smoker with wood pellets and follow the start-up procedure. Preheat the grill, with the lid closed, to 400° F.
2. Place strawberries directly on the grill grate and cook 15 minutes or until grill marks appear. Grill: 400 ˚F
3. For the cocktail: Add vodka, grilled strawberries, Traeger Smoked Simple Syrup and lemon juice to a shaker. Shake vigorously.
4. Double strain into a fresh glass or copper mug with crushed ice.
5. Top with ginger beer and garnish with extra grilled strawberries and fresh mint. Enjoy!

Garden Gimlet Cocktail

Servings: 2
Cooking Time: 45 Minutes

Ingredients:

- 2 Cup honey
- 4 lemons, zested
- 4 Sprig rosemary, plus more for garnish
- 1/2 Cup water
- 4 Slices cucumber
- 1 1/2 Ounce lime juice
- 3 Ounce vodka

Directions:

1. Supply your smoker with wood pellets and follow the start-up procedure. Preheat the grill, with the lid closed, to 180° F.
2. To make smoked lemon and rosemary honey syrup, thin 1 cup honey by adding 1/4 cup water to a shallow pan. Add lemon zest and 2 sprigs rosemary.
3. Place the pan directly on the grill grate and smoke 45 minutes to an hour. Remove from heat, strain and cool. Grill: 180 °F
4. In a cocktail shaker, muddle the cucumbers and 1oz of the smoked lemon and rosemary honey syrup.
5. After muddling, add lime juice, vodka, and ice. Shake and double strain into a coup glass.
6. Garnish with a sprig of rosemary. Enjoy!

Grilled Hawaiian Sour

Servings: 2
Cooking Time: 15 Minutes

Ingredients:

- 2 Whole pineapple, trimmed and sliced
- 1/2 Cup palm sugar
- 3 Ounce bourbon
- 2 Ounce grilled pineapple juice
- 2 Ounce Smoked Simple Syrup
- 10 Ounce lemon juice
- 2 grilled pineapple chunk, for garnish
- 2 pineapple leaf, for garnish

Directions:

1. Supply your smoker with wood pellets and follow the start-up procedure. Preheat the grill, with the lid closed, to 350° F.
2. For the Grilled Pineapple Juice: Dust pineapple slices with palm sugar. Place directly on the grill grate and cook for 8 minutes per side. Grill: 350 °F
3. Remove from grill and let cool. Reserve a few pieces for garnish. Run remaining pineapple pieces through centrifugal juicer to extract juice.
4. To Make the Drink: Add bourbon, grilled pineapple juice, simple syrup and lemon juice to a cocktail strainer with ice. Shake vigorously. Double strain into a chilled coupe glass. Garnish with grilled pineapple chunk and pineapple leaf. Enjoy!

Smoked Pomegranate Lemonade Cocktail

Servings: 2
Cooking Time: 45 Minutes

Ingredients:

- 32 Ounce POM Juice
- 2 Cup pomegranate seeds
- 3 Ounce vodka
- 8 Ounce lemonade
- lemon wheel, for garnish
- fresh mint, for garnish

Directions:

1. Supply your smoker with wood pellets and follow the start-up procedure. Preheat the grill, with the lid closed, to 225° F.
2. For the Smoked Pomegranate Ice Cubes: Pour one small container of POM juice and 1 cup of pomegranate seeds into a shallow sheet pan. Smoke on the Traeger for 45 minutes. Pull off grill and let sit until cooled. Grill: 180 °F
3. Pour smoked POM juice into ice molds of your choice and put into freezer.
4. When ready to serve, place the frozen pomegranate cubes into a mason jar. Pour vodka and lemonade over the ice cubes.
5. Garnish with a lemon wheel and fresh mint. Enjoy!

Smoked Mulled Wine

Servings: 10
Cooking Time: 60 Minutes

Ingredients:

- 2 Bottle red wine
- 1/2 Cup whiskey
- 1/2 Cup white rum
- 1/2 Cup honey
- 1 cinnamon stick
- 2 pods star anise
- 4 whole cloves
- 1 (3 in) orange peel

Directions:

1. Supply your smoker with wood pellets and follow the start-up procedure. Preheat the grill, with the lid closed, to 180° F.
2. In a shallow baking dish, combine wine, whiskey, rum, honey, cinnamon stick, star anise, cloves and orange peel. Stir well until combined.
3. Place the dish directly on the grill grate and smoke for one hour until the mixture is warm. Grill: 180 °F
4. Remove from grill and ladle into mugs leaving the mulling spices behind. Garnish with fresh cinnamon sticks, anise, orange zest or a combination. Enjoy!

Batter Up Cocktail

Servings: 2
Cooking Time: 60 Minutes

Ingredients:

- 2 whole nutmeg
- 4 Ounce Michter's Bourbon
- 3 Teaspoon pumpkin puree
- 1 Ounce Smoked Simple Syrup
- 2 Large egg

Directions:

1. Supply your smoker with wood pellets and follow the start-up procedure. Preheat the grill, with the lid closed, to 180° F.
2. Place whole nutmeg on a sheet tray and place in the grill. Smoke 1 hour. Remove from grill and let cool. Grill: 180 °F

3. Add everything to a shaker and shake without ice. Add ice, then shake and strain into a chilled highball glass.
4. Garnish with grated, smoked nutmeg. Enjoy!

Smoked Ice Mojito Slurpee

Servings: 2
Cooking Time: 30 Minutes

Ingredients:

- water
- 1 Cup white rum
- 1/2 Cup lime juice
- 1/4 Cup Smoked Simple Syrup
- 12 Whole fresh mint leaves
- 4 Sprig mint
- 4 Whole lime wedge, for garnish

Directions:

1. Supply your smoker with wood pellets and follow the start-up procedure. Preheat the grill, with the lid closed, to 180° F.
2. For optimal flavor, use Super Smoke if available. Grill: 180 °F
3. Remove water from grill and pour smoked water into ice cube trays. Place in freezer until frozen.
4. Add rum, lime juice, Traeger Smoked Simple Syrup, mint and smoked ice to a blender.
5. Blend until a slushy consistency and pour into glasses.
6. Garnish with a mint sprig and lime wedge. Enjoy!

Grilled Frozen Strawberry Lemonade

Servings: 4
Cooking Time: 15 Minutes

Ingredients:

- 1 Pound fresh strawberries
- 1/2 Cup turbinado sugar
- 8 lemon, halved
- 1/4 Cup Cointreau
- 1/4 Cup simple syrup
- 2 Cup ice
- 1 Cup Titos Vodka

Directions:

1. Supply your smoker with wood pellets and follow the start-up procedure. Preheat the grill, with the lid closed, to High heat.
2. Dip the lemon halves in turbinado sugar and place directly on the grill grate. Toss the strawberries with remaining sugar and place next to the lemons.
3. Cook until grill marks develop on both, about 15 min for lemons and 10 min for strawberries.
4. Remove from heat and let cool.
5. Juice grilled lemons straining out any seeds or pulp. Pour into a blender pitcher.
6. Remove stems from grilled strawberries and place in blender pitcher with lemon juice. Add simple syrup, vodka, cointreau, and 2 cups of ice.
7. Puree until smooth and transfer to 4-6 glasses. Garnish with grilled strawberries and grilled lemon slices if desired. Enjoy!

Smoked Sangria

Servings: 6
Cooking Time: 45 Minutes

Ingredients:
- 1 (750 ml) medium-bodied red wine
- 1/4 Cup Grand Marnier
- 1/4 Cup Smoked Simple Syrup
- 1 Cup fresh cranberries
- 1 Whole apple, sliced
- 2 Whole limes, sliced
- 4 cinnamon stick
- soda water

Directions:
1. Supply your smoker with wood pellets and follow the start-up procedure. Preheat the grill, with the lid closed, to 180° F.
2. In a shallow dish, combine red wine, Grand Marnier, Traeger Smoked Simple Syrup and cranberries, and place directly on the grill grate.
3. Smoke for 30 to 45 minutes or until the liquid picks up desired amount of smoke. Remove from grill and place in the fridge to cool. Grill: 180 °F

4. When the mixture has cooled, place in a large pitcher. Add sliced apples, limes, cinnamon sticks and ice to pitcher.
5. Top with soda water, if desired. Enjoy!

Smoked Pumpkin Spice Latte

Servings: 4
Cooking Time: 45 Minutes

Ingredients:
- 1 Small sugar pumpkin
- olive oil
- 1 Can sweetened condensed milk
- 1 Cup whole milk
- 2 Tablespoon Smoked Simple Syrup
- 1 Teaspoon pumpkin pie spice
- pinch of salt
- cinnamon
- whipped cream
- shaved nutmeg
- 8 Ounce smoked cold brew coffee

Directions:
1. Supply your smoker with wood pellets and follow the start-up procedure. Preheat the grill, with the lid closed, to 325° F.
2. Cut the sugar pumpkin in half, scoop out the seeds and discard. Place the pumpkin halves cut side up on a baking sheet and brush lightly with olive oil.
3. Place the sheet tray directly on the grill grate and cook 45 minutes or until the flesh is tender. Remove from heat and place on the counter to cool. Grill: 325 °F
4. When the pumpkin is cool enough to handle, scoop out the flesh and mash until smooth.
5. Place 3 Tbsp of the pumpkin puree in a separate bowl and reserve the remaining for another use.
6. Add the sweetened condensed milk, whole milk, Traeger Smoked Simple Syrup, pumpkin pie seasoning and salt to the pumpkin puree. Whisk to combine.
7. Pour the cold brew over ice, add desired amount of pumpkin spice creamer and top with whipped cream, cinnamon, and shaved nutmeg if desired. Enjoy!

Fig Slider Cocktail

Servings: 2

Cooking Time: 15 Minutes

Ingredients:

- 2 peach, halved
- 4 oranges
- honey
- sugar
- 2 Teaspoon orange fig spread
- 1 Ounce fresh lemon juice
- 4 Ounce bourbon
- 3 Ounce honey glazed grilled orange juice

Directions:

1. Supply your smoker with wood pellets and follow the start-up procedure. Preheat the grill, with the lid closed, to 325° F.

2. Pit the peach and cut in half. Cut one of the oranges in half. Glaze the peach and orange cut sides with honey and set directly on the grill grate until the honey caramelizes and fruit has grill marks. Grill: 325 °F

3. Cut the second orange into wheels and coat with granulated sugar on both sides. Place directly on the grill grate and cook 15 minutes each side or until grill marks form. Grill: 325 °F

4. In a mixing tin, add grilled peaches, bourbon, orange fig spread, fresh lemon juice and honey glazed orange juice.

5. Shake vigorously to blend the juices and fig spread. Strain over clean ice. Garnish with grilled orange wheel. Enjoy!

Bacon Old-fashioned Cocktail

Servings: 2

Cooking Time: 20 Minutes

Ingredients:

- 16 Slices bacon
- 1/2 Cup warm water (110°F to 115°F)
- 1500 mL bourbon
- 1/2 Fluid Ounce maple syrup
- 4 Dash Angostura bitters
- 2 fresh orange peel

Directions:

1. Smoke bacon prior to making Old Fashioned using this recipe for Applewood Smoked Bacon.

2. To Make Bacon: Supply your smoker with wood pellets and follow the start-up procedure. Preheat the grill, with the lid closed, to 325° F.

3. Place bacon in a single layer on a cooling rack that fits inside a baking sheet pan. Cook in Traeger for 15-20 minutes or until bacon is browned and crispy. Reserve bacon for later. Let the fat cool slightly; you'll use the fat to infuse the bourbon. Grill: 325 °F

4. Combine 1/4 cup of warm (not hot) liquid bacon fat with the entire contents of a 750ml bottle of bourbon in a glass or heavy plastic container.

5. Use a fork to stir well. Let it sit on the counter for a few hours, stirring every so often.

6. After about four hours, put bourbon fat mixture into the freezer. After about an hour, the fat will congeal and you can simply scoop it out with a spoon. You can fine-strain the mixture through a sieve to remove all fat if desired.

7. Combine ingredients with ice and stir until cold. Strain over fresh ice in an Old Fashioned glass and garnish with reserved bacon and orange peel. Enjoy!

Smoked Salted Caramel White Russian

Servings: 4

Cooking Time: 20 Minutes

Ingredients:

- 16 Ounce half-and-half
- salted caramel sauce
- 6 Ounce vodka
- 6 Ounce Kahlúa

Directions:

1. Supply your smoker with wood pellets and follow the start-up procedure. Preheat the grill, with the lid closed, to 180° F.

2. Pour the half-and-half in a shallow baking dish and place directly on the grill grate. In another shallow baking dish, pour 2 to 3 cups of water and place on the grill next to the half-and-half.

3. Smoke both the half-and-half and water for 20 minutes. Remove from the grill and let cool. Grill: 180 °F

4. Place the half-and-half in the fridge until ready to use. Pour the smoked water into ice cube trays and transfer to the freezer until completely frozen.

5. Separate the smoked ice cubes into four glasses. Drizzle the salted caramel sauce around the inside of the glass.

6. Pour 1-1/2 ounce vodka and 1-1/2 ounce Kahlúa into each of the glasses and top with the smoked half-and-half. Enjoy!

Smoky Scotch & Ginger Cocktail

Servings: 2
Cooking Time: 60 Minutes

Ingredients:
- 1 Ounce ginger syrup
- 1/2 Ounce brandied cherry juice
- 1/2 Ounce agave nectar
- 4 Ounce scotch
- 1 1/2 Ounce lemon juice
- 2 Slices grilled lemon, for garnish
- 2 cherry, for garnish

Directions:
1. Supply your smoker with wood pellets and follow the start-up procedure. Preheat the grill, with the lid closed, to 180° F.

2. For the smoked ginger cherry syrup: Place ginger syrup, cherry juice and agave nectar in a shallow dish and place the dish directly on the grill grate.

3. Smoke for 60 minutes, or until the mixture has picked up the smoke flavor. Remove from grill and allow to cool for 30 minutes. Grill: 180 °F

4. Place smoked ginger cherry syrup, scotch and lemon juice into a shaker tin and shake with ice. Strain into a glass over fresh ice and garnish with a grilled lemon wheel and cherry. Enjoy!

A Smoking Classic Cocktail

Servings: 2
Cooking Time: 60 Minutes

Ingredients:
- 2 Bottle Angostura orange bitters
- 10 sugar cubes
- 8 Ounce Champagne
- lemon twist

Directions:
1. Supply your smoker with wood pellets and follow the start-up procedure. Preheat the grill, with the lid closed, to 180° F.

2. For the Smoked Orange Bitters: In a small skillet, combine 1 bottle of Angostura orange bitters with a splash of water and 4 sugar cubes.

3. Place skillet on the grill grate and smoke for 60 minutes. Cool the smoked bitters and put back into the bottle. Grill: 180 °F

4. Add a sugar cube to each Champagne flute and soak the sugar cubes with the smoked bitters.

5. Add champagne and a lemon twist in a flute glass. Enjoy!

Cran-apple Tequila Punch With Smoked Oranges

Servings: 2
Cooking Time: 15 Minutes

Ingredients:
- 6 Cup apple juice, chilled
- 6 Cup light cranberry cocktail
- 1 Cup cranberries, fresh or thawed
- 3 Large oranges, halved
- 1 Cup sugar, for rimming glasses
- 2 Tablespoon lemon juice
- 2 Cup reposado tequila
- 1 Cup orange-flavored liqueur, such as Grand Marnier or Cointreau
- 2 Bottle sparkling wine (such as prosecco) or sparkling water

Directions:
1. Combine 1 cup each of the apple and cranberry juices, then pour into ice cube trays. If the cube molds are big enough, place a few cranberries into each cube. Freeze for 6 hours to overnight.

2. Supply your smoker with wood pellets and follow the start-up procedure. Preheat the grill, with the lid closed, to 180° F.

3. Place the orange halves cut-side down on the grill and smoke for 15 minutes. Remove from the grill and juice oranges. Reserve smoked orange juice. Grill: 180 ˚F

4. When ready to serve, place the sugar on a flat plate. Pour the lemon juice into a bowl that will fit the rim of each glass.

5. Carefully dip the rim of each glass in the lemon juice, then dip in the sugar to create a 1/8" sugar rim. Turn the glass right-side up and allow to dry for a few minutes before using.

6. Just before serving, mix the remaining apple juice, cranberry cocktail and smoked orange juice with the tequila, orange liqueur, and sparkling wine in a large bowl or pitcher. Taste, adding more of any ingredient to meet your preference.

7. When ready to serve, place a few ice cubes in each glass, then pour a cup of the punch over the top. Alternatively, place all of the ice cubes in the punch bowl and allow guests to help themselves. Enjoy!

Smoked Cold Brew Coffee

Servings: 8
Cooking Time: 120 Minutes

Ingredients:
- 12 Ounce coarse ground coffee
- heavy cream or milk
- sugar

Directions:

1. Place half the coffee grounds in a plastic container and slowly pour 3-1/2 cups water over the top of the grounds. Add remaining grounds and pour another 3-1/2 cups water over the top in a circular motion.

2. Press the grounds down into the water using the back of a spoon. Cover and transfer to the refrigerator and let sit for 18 to 24 hours.

3. Remove from refrigerator and strain into a clean container through a fine mesh strainer or double layer of cheese cloth.

4. Supply your smoker with wood pellets and follow the start-up procedure. Preheat the grill, with the lid closed, to 180° F.

5. Pour cold brew into a shallow baking dish and place directly on the grill grate. Smoke for 1 to 2 hours depending on desired level of smoke. Grill: 180 ˚F

6. Remove from grill and place over an ice bath to cool. Drink as is over ice, with cream or sugar or use in your favorite coffee recipes. Enjoy!

Smoked Hibiscus Sparkler

Servings: 4
Cooking Time: 30 Minutes

Ingredients:
- 1/2 Cup sugar
- 2 Tablespoon dried hibiscus flowers
- 1 Bottle sparkling wine
- crystallized ginger, for garnish

Directions:

1. Supply your smoker with wood pellets and follow the start-up procedure. Preheat the grill, with the lid closed, to 180° F.

2. Place water in a shallow baking dish and place directly on the grill grate. Smoke the water for 30 minutes or until desired smoke flavor is achieved. Grill: 180 ˚F

3. Pour water into a small saucepan and add sugar and hibiscus flowers. Bring to a simmer over medium heat and cook until sugar is dissolved.

4. Strain out the hibiscus flowers and transfer your simple syrup to a small container and refrigerate until chilled.

5. Pour 1/2 ounce smoked hibiscus simple syrup in the bottom of a champagne glass and top with sparkling wine.

6. Drop in a few pieces of crystallized ginger to garnish. Enjoy!

Smoked Jacobsen Salt Margarita

Servings: 2
Cooking Time: 1 Day

Ingredients:

- kosher sea salt
- 3 Cup Jacobsen Co. Honey
- 6 Ounce tequila
- 4 Ounce fresh squeezed lime juice
- 1/2 Cup Jacobsen Salt Co. Cherrywood Smoked Salt or smoked kosher salt
- 2 Ounce simple syrup
- 2 Teaspoon orange liqueur

Directions:

1. If making your own smoked salt, take kosher sea salt (however much you want to smoke) and spread it out on a tray.
2. Supply your smoker with wood pellets and follow the start-up procedure. Preheat the grill, with the lid closed, to 165° F.
3. Place tray of salt directly on the grill grate and smoke for about 24 hours, stirring the salt every 8 hours. Once it has smoked for 24 hours, take off grill and use in all your favorite dishes. Note: If you want to skip the long smoke session, use Jacobsen Salt Co. Cherrywood Smoked Salt. Grill: 165 °F
4. Simple Syrup: Put the honey and 1 cup water in a small saucepan. Cook over low heat, stirring, for about 20 min.
5. Fill a cocktail shaker with ice. Add tequila, lime juice, simple syrup and orange liqueur. Cover and shake until mixed and chilled, about 30 seconds.
6. Place smoked salt on a plate. Press the rim of a chilled rocks glass into the salt to rim the edge. Strain margarita into the glass. Enjoy!

Smoked Barnburner Cocktail

Servings: 2
Cooking Time: 45 Minutes

Ingredients:

- 16 Ounce fresh raspberries
- 1/2 Cup Smoked Simple Syrup
- 1 1/2 Ounce smoked raspberry syrup

- 3 Ounce reposado tequila
- 1 Ounce lime juice
- 1 Ounce lemon juice
- 2 grilled lime wheel, for garnish

Directions:

1. Supply your smoker with wood pellets and follow the start-up procedure. Preheat the grill, with the lid closed, to 180° F.
2. For Smoked Raspberry Syrup: Place fresh raspberries on a grill mat and smoke for 30 minutes. After the raspberries have been smoked, reserve a few for garnish and place the remainder into a shallow sheet pan with Traeger Smoked Simple Syrup. Grill: 180 °F
3. Place sheet pan on the grill grate and smoke for 45 minutes. Remove from grill and let cool. Strain through a fine mesh sieve discarding solids. Transfer the syrup to the refrigerator until ready to use. Makes about 1/2 cup of smoked raspberry syrup. Grill: 180 °F
4. For cocktail: Add 3/4 ounce smoked raspberry syrup, tequila, lime juice and lemon juice with ice into a mixing glass. Shake and pour over clean ice. Garnish with smoked raspberries and a grilled lime wheel. Enjoy!

Smoked Pineapple Hotel Nacional Cocktail

Servings: 2
Cooking Time: 20 Minutes

Ingredients:

- 2 pineapple
- 1/2 Cup water
- 1/2 Cup sugar
- 3 Fluid Ounce white rum
- 1 1/2 Fluid Ounce lime juice
- 1 1/2 Fluid Ounce Pineapple Syrup
- 1 Fluid Ounce apricot brandy
- 2 Dash Angostura bitters

Directions:

1. For the Syrup: Supply your smoker with wood pellets and follow the start-up procedure. Preheat the grill, with the lid closed, to 180° F.
2. Trim both ends of the pineapple, discard the ends. Cut the pineapple into slices about 3/4" thick. Don't

worry about the skin, it doesn't hurt to leave it on. Place the pineapple slices on the grill and smoke for about 15 minutes on each sideTrim both ends of the pineapple and discard the ends. Cut the pineapple into slices about 3/4 inch thick. Don't worry about the skin, it doesn't hurt to leave it on. Place the pineapple slices on the grill and smoke for about 15 minutes per side. Grill: 180 ℉

3. While the pineapple is smoking, combine 1/4 cup water and sugar in a saucepan over low heat, stirring constantly, until sugar is dissolved. Pour syrup into a large bowl and set aside.

4. When the pineapple is done cooking, cut each slice into eight or so wedges and add the wedges to the bowl with the simple syrup, tossing to coat and cover.

5. Leave the mixture to macerate for at least 4 hours (or up to 24) in the refrigerator, stirring from time to time.

6. Strain the syrup into a clean bowl through a fine-mesh strainer and press on the pineapple with a ladle to extract as much liquid as possible. You can bottle and refrigerate the syrup for up to 4 days.

7. To make the cocktail: Combine the rum, lime juice, pineapple syrup, apricot brandy, and bitters in a cocktail shaker or mixing glass. Fill with ice cubes and shake until cold.

8. Strain into a chilled cocktail glass. Garnish with a lime wheel and serve. Enjoy!

Dublin Delight Cocktail

Servings: 2
Cooking Time: 20 Minutes

Ingredients:
- 2 orange, sliced
- 3 Fluid Ounce Teeling Whiskey
- 1 1/2 Fluid Ounce Smoked Simple Syrup
- 6 Dash aromatic bitters
- 6 Fluid Ounce Guinness beer
- 2 Amarena cherry, for garnish

Directions:
1. Supply your smoker with wood pellets and follow the start-up procedure. Preheat the grill, with the lid closed, to 450° F.

2. Place orange slices directly on the grill grate and cook 20 to 25 minutes. Remove from grill and let cool. Grill: 450 ℉

3. In a mixing glass, add whiskey, Traeger Smoked Simple Syrup and bitters. Add ice and shake. Pour over a beer glass filled with ice and top off with cold Guinness.

4. Garnish with a grilled orange slice and Amarena cherry. Enjoy!

Grilled Peach Mint Julep

Servings: 2
Cooking Time: 45 Minutes

Ingredients:
- 2 Whole peach
- 4 Ounce whiskey
- 2 Cup sugar
- 4 Tablespoon pink peppercorns
- 20 Whole fresh mint leaves, plus more for garnish
- 2 lime wedge, for garnish
- 4 Ounce bourbon

Directions:
1. For the Grilled Whiskey Peaches: cut peach into slices, then soak peach slices in whiskey in the refrigerator for 4 to 6 hours.

2. For the Pink Peppercorn Simple Syrup: In a shallow pan, combine sugar, 1 cup water and pink peppercorns.

3. Supply your smoker with wood pellets and follow the start-up procedure. Preheat the grill, with the lid closed, to 180° F.

4. Cook syrup down on the grill for 30 minutes, or until desired smoke flavor has been reached. Remove from the grill. Grill: 180 ℉

5. Increase Traeger temperature to 350℉ and preheat. Place the whiskey peach slices directly on the grill grate and cook 10 to 12 minutes or until peaches soften and get grill marks. Grill: 350 ℉

6. To make the Julep: Muddle 1/2 ounce Pink Peppercorn Simple Syrup with 10 fresh mint leaves and 4 slices of grilled whiskey peaches.

7. Add crushed ice over the rim of the glass. Pour bourbon over the crushed ice and stir. Garnish with 1 large sprig of mint and fresh lime. Enjoy!

Smoked Irish Coffee

Servings: 2
Cooking Time: 15 Minutes

Ingredients:

- 10 Ounce hot coffee
- 1/2 Cup heavy cream
- 1 Tablespoon sugar
- 2 Ounce Irish whiskey
- freshly grated nutmeg, for garnish (optional)

Directions:

1. Supply your smoker with wood pellets and follow the start-up procedure. Preheat the grill, with the lid closed, to 180° F.
2. Place the coffee and cream in separate shallow baking dishes and place both directly on the grill grate. Smoke for 10 to 15 minutes until the liquids pick up a slight smoke flavor. Grill: 180 °F
3. Remove from the grill and cool the cream. When the cream is cool, add sugar and whip in a stand mixer or by hand to soft peaks.
4. Pour the hot coffee into two mugs then add 2 ounces of whiskey to each.
5. Top with smoked whipped cream and finish with freshly grated nutmeg, if desired. Enjoy!

Smoked Texas Ranch Water

Servings: 4
Cooking Time: 60 Minutes

Ingredients:

- 3 Whole limes
- 1 Tablespoon Blackened Saskatchewan Rub
- 12 Ounce blanco tequila
- 24 Ounce Topo Chico or other sparkling mineral water
- 8 Slices jalapeño, optional

Directions:

1. Supply your smoker with wood pellets and follow the start-up procedure. Preheat the grill, with the lid closed, to 225° F.
2. Cut two of the limes in half and sprinkle with Traeger Blackened Saskatchewan Rub. Place the four lime halves on the edge of the grill grate and smoke for 1 hour. Remove from grill and set aside to cool. Grill: 225 °F
3. Pour some of the rub onto a small plate. Cut the third lime into 1/4 wedges and use the lime to rub the rim of 4 cocktail glasses, turn the glasses upside down, and into the rub to salt the rim.
4. Place several ice cubes into your rimmed glasses and pour 3 ounces tequila, 6 ounces Topo Chico, squeeze the juice of one smoked lime (discard after squeezing), and add one fresh lime wedge to each. If using the jalapeño, add one or two slices to each glass (muddle if desired).
5. Stir to combine and enjoy!

Traeger Old Fashioned

Servings: 2
Cooking Time: 60 Minutes

Ingredients:

- 2 orange
- 2 Cup cherries
- 3 Ounce bourbon
- 1 Ounce Smoked Simple Syrup
- 8 Dash Bitters Lab Apricot Vanilla Bitters

Directions:

1. Supply your smoker with wood pellets and follow the start-up procedure. Preheat the grill, with the lid closed, to 180° F.
2. While Traeger preheats, slice whole orange into wheels.
3. Place cherries on a small sheet pan and place in the Traeger. Place orange slices directly on the grill grate.
4. Smoke cherries for 1 hour and oranges for 25 minutes, depending on taste, before removing from the grill. Let oranges and cherries cool. Grill: 180 °F
5. Pour bourbon into glass, followed by Traeger Smoked Simple Syrup and bitters. Add ice and stir for 45 seconds or until drink is well-diluted.
6. Strain contents into new glass over fresh ice. Skewer orange wheel and add cherry for garnish. Enjoy!

Traeger Boulevardier Cocktail

Servings: 2
Cooking Time: 60 Minutes

Ingredients:

- 4 oranges
- 1/2 Cup honey
- 1500 mL rye whiskey
- 1 1/2 Ounce Campari
- 1 1/2 Ounce sweet vermouth
- 2 Tablespoon granulated sugar
- 3 Ounce grilled orange infused rye

Directions:

1. Supply your smoker with wood pellets and follow the start-up procedure. Preheat the grill, with the lid closed, to 350° F.
2. Slice 2 oranges in half and coat cut side with honey. Peel remaining orange and place peels on the grill. Cook 20 to 25 minutes. Grill: 350 °F
3. Remove from grill and let cool. Place orange halves cut side down directly on the grill grate and cook 20 to 30 minutes or until dark grill marks appear. Remove orange halves and allow to cool. Grill: 350 °F
4. Place orange halves into a bottle of rye whiskey and let steep for 10 to 12 hours. The longer they steep, the sweeter and more pronounced the orange flavor will be.
5. Add all ingredients into a mixing glass and stir until diluted. Strain into a fresh coupe glass and serve neat.
6. Garnish with grilled orange peel. Enjoy!

Grilled Rabbit Tail Cocktail

Servings: 2
Cooking Time: 25 Minutes

Ingredients:

- 1 1/2 Ounce lemon juice
- 4 Ounce Apple Brandy
- 1 Ounce orange juice
- 1 Ounce Smoked Simple Syrup

Directions:

1. Supply your smoker with wood pellets and follow the start-up procedure. Preheat the grill, with the lid closed, to 350° F.

2. Place lemon halves directly on the grill grate and cook for 20-25 minutes or until grill marks appear. Remove from grill and let cool. Once cool enough to handle, juice the lemons then chill and reserve the juice. Grill: 350 °F
3. Using the proportions listed above and considering the size and consumption rate of your tailgate crew or party, mix all the above ingredients in a large thermos and top with a bit of ice.
4. Using 6-8 oz glasses or cups, guests can serve themselves from the thermos and garnish each drink with a grilled apple slice. Enjoy!

Traeger Paloma Cocktail

Servings: 2
Cooking Time: 25 Minutes

Ingredients:

- 4 grapefruit, halved
- Smoked Simple Syrup
- 10 Stick cinnamon
- 3 Ounce reposado tequila
- 1 Ounce lime juice
- 1 Ounce Smoked Simple Syrup
- grilled lime, for garnish
- cinnamon stick, for garnish

Directions:

1. Supply your smoker with wood pellets and follow the start-up procedure. Preheat the grill, with the lid closed, to 350° F.
2. Grilled Grapefruit Juice: Cut 2 grapefruits in half. Place a cinnamon stick in each grapefruit half and glaze with Traeger Smoked Simple Syrup. Place on grill grate and cook for 20 minutes or until edges start to burn and it acquires grill marks. Remove from heat and let cool. Grill: 350 °F
3. After grapefruits have cooled, squeeze and strain juice. It should yield 10 to 12 ounces of juice.
4. In a mixing glass, add tequila, lime juice, Traeger Smoked Simple Syrup and 2 ounces of the grilled grapefruit juice.
5. Add ice and shake. Strain over ice in an old fashioned glass.
6. Add a grilled lime slice and cinnamon stick to garnish. Enjoy!

Smoked Grape Lime Rickey

Servings: 4
Cooking Time: 45 Minutes

Ingredients:

- 1/2 Pound red grapes
- 1/2 Cup plus 1 tablespoon sugar
- 1/2 Cup water
- 1 limes, sliced
- 2 limes, halved
- 1 Tablespoon sugar
- 1 L lemon lime soda

Directions:

1. Supply your smoker with wood pellets and follow the start-up procedure. Preheat the grill, with the lid closed, to 180° F.
2. Rinse grapes well and place in a shallow baking dish. Combine 1/2 cup sugar and water and stir until sugar dissolves. Pour over grapes.
3. Place the baking dish directly on the grill grate and smoke for 30 to 40 minutes until grapes are tender. Grill: 180 °F
4. Remove from the grill and pour entire contents of the baking dish in a blender. Puree on high until smooth then pass the mixture through a fine mesh strainer.
5. Increase Traeger temperature to 350°F . Grill: 350 °F
6. Toss the lime slices and lime halves with 1 tablespoon sugar and place directly on the grill grate. Cook for 15 to 20 minutes or until grill marks develop. Remove from grill and set slices aside. When cool enough to handle, juice grilled lime halves. Grill: 350 °F
7. To build the drink, fill a pint glass with ice. Pour in 1-1/2 ounce grilled lime juice, 1-1/2 ounce smoked grape syrup and top off with soda. Garnish with grilled lime slice. Enjoy!

Honey Glazed Grapefruit Shandy Cocktail

Servings: 2
Cooking Time: 20 Minutes

Ingredients:

- 4 grapefruits
- 4 Tablespoon honey
- granulated sugar
- 2 Ounce bourbon
- 1 Ounce Smoked Simple Syrup
- 4 Ounce honey glazed grilled grapefruit, juiced
- 2 Bottle Ballast Point Grapefruit Sculpin

Directions:

1. Supply your smoker with wood pellets and follow the start-up procedure. Preheat the grill, with the lid closed, to 375° F.
2. For the honey glazed grapefruit: Slice one grapefruit in half and coat with 2 tablespoons honey.
3. Take the other grapefruit and slice into wheels. Toss the wheels in granulated sugar until well coated.
4. Place the grapefruit halves and wheels directly on the grill grate, cut side down, and cook for 20 to 30 minutes. Remove from grill and set the wheels aside. Grill: 375 °F
5. Squeeze the grapefruit halves into a measuring cup. It should yield about 2 oz juice.
6. Pour the grapefruit juice into a shaker and add bourbon and Traeger Smoked Simple Syrup then top with ice. Shake for 10-15 seconds.
7. Strain into glass, add ice and fill with beer. Garnish with the grilled grapefruit wheel. Enjoy!

Smoked Plum And Thyme Fizz Cocktail

Servings: 2
Cooking Time: 60 Minutes

Ingredients:

- 6 fresh plums
- 4 Fluid Ounce vodka
- 1 1/2 Fluid Ounce fresh lemon juice
- 2 Ounce smoked plum and thyme simple syrup
- 4 Fluid Ounce club soda
- 2 Slices smoked plum, for garnish
- 2 Sprig fresh thyme, for garnish
- 8 Sprig thyme
- 2 Cup Smoked Simple Syrup

Directions:

1. Supply your smoker with wood pellets and follow the start-up procedure. Preheat the grill, with the lid closed, to 180° F.

2. Cut plums in half and remove the pit. Place the plum halves directly on the grill grate and smoke for 25 minutes. Grill: 180 °F

3. For the Plum and Thyme Simple Syrup: After 25 minutes, remove plums from the grill and cut into quarters. Add plums and thyme sprigs to 1 cup of Traeger Smoked Simple Syrup. Smoke the mixture for 45 minutes. Remove from grill, strain and let cool. Grill: 180 °F

4. Add vodka, fresh lemon juice and smoked plum and thyme simple syrup to a mixing glass.

5. Add ice and shake. Strain over clean ice, top off with club soda and garnish with a piece of thyme and slice of smoked plum. Enjoy!

Grilled Peach Smash Cocktail

Servings: 2
Cooking Time: 10 Minutes

Ingredients:
- 2 peach, sliced and grilled
- 10 fresh mint leaves
- 1 1/2 Ounce Smoked Simple Syrup
- 4 Ounce bourbon
- 2 mint sprig, for garnish

Directions:
1. Supply your smoker with wood pellets and follow the start-up procedure. Preheat the grill, with the lid closed, to 375° F.

2. Cut the peach into 6 slices and brush with Traeger Smoked Simple Syrup. Place directly on the grill grate and cook 10 to 12 minutes or until peaches soften and get grill marks. Grill: 375 °F

3. In a mixing glass, add 3 slices of grilled peaches, 5 mint leaves and Traeger Smoked Simple Syrup.

4. Muddle ingredients to release oils of the mint and juices from the grilled peaches. Add bourbon and crushed ice.

5. Shake and pour into a stemless wine glass. Top off with more crushed ice. Garnish with a grilled peach and mint sprig. Enjoy!

Smoked Eggnog

Servings: 4
Cooking Time: 60 Minutes

Ingredients:
- 2 Cup whole milk
- 1 Cup heavy cream
- 4 egg yolk
- Cup sugar
- 3 Ounce bourbon
- 1 Teaspoon vanilla extract
- 1 Teaspoon nutmeg
- 4 egg white
- whipped cream

Directions:
1. Plan ahead, this recipe requires chill time.

2. Supply your smoker with wood pellets and follow the start-up procedure. Preheat the grill, with the lid closed, to 180° F.

3. Pour the milk and the cream into a baking pan and smoke on the Traeger for 60 minutes. Grill: 180 °F

4. Meanwhile, in the bowl of a stand mixer, beat the egg yolks until they lighten in color. Gradually add 1/3 cup sugar and continue to beat until sugar completely dissolves.

5. After the milk and cream have smoked, add them along with the bourbon, vanilla and nutmeg into the egg mixture and stir to combine.

6. Place the egg whites in the bowl of a stand mixer and beat to soft peaks. When you lift the beaters the whites will make a peak that slightly curls down.

7. With the mixer still running, gradually add 1 tablespoon of sugar and beat until stiff peaks form.

8. Gently fold the egg whites into the cream mixture and then whisk to thoroughly combine.

9. Chill eggnog for a couple hours to let the flavors meld. Garnish with a dash of nutmeg and whipped cream on top. Enjoy!

Traeger Gin & Tonic

Servings: 2

Cooking Time: 45 Minutes

Ingredients:

- 1/2 Cup berries
- 2 orange, sliced
- 4 Tablespoon granulated sugar
- 3 Ounce gin
- 1 Cup tonic water
- 2 Sprig fresh mint, for garnish

Directions:

1. Supply your smoker with wood pellets and follow the start-up procedure. Preheat the grill, with the lid closed, to 180° F.

2. For the Smoked Berries: Spread mixed fresh berries on a sheet pan and place directly on the grill grate. Smoke for 30 minutes then remove from grill. Grill: 180 °F

3. For the Orange Slices: Increase the grill temperature to 450°F and preheat, lid closed for 15 minutes. Grill: 450 °F

4. Toss the orange slices with granulated sugar and place directly on grill grate. Cook for about 5 minutes, turning once or until the slices have developed grill marks. Grill: 450 °F

5. Pour gin into a glass, add ice and berries, then top with tonic water. Garnish with a fresh mint sprig and grilled orange wheel. Enjoy!

Smoke And Bubz Cocktail

Servings: 2

Cooking Time: 45 Minutes

Ingredients:

- 16 Ounce POM Juice
- 2 Cup pomegranate seeds
- 6 Ounce sparkling white wine
- 2 lemon twist, for garnish
- 2 Teaspoon pomegranate seeds

Directions:

1. Supply your smoker with wood pellets and follow the start-up procedure. Preheat the grill, with the lid closed, to 180° F.

2. For the Smoked Pomegranate Juice: Pour POM juice and a cup of pomegranate seeds into a shallow sheet pan. Smoke on the Traeger for 45 minutes. Pull off grill, strain, discard seeds and let sit until chilled. Grill: 180 °F

3. Add 1-1/2 ounces of the smoked pomegranate juice to the bottom of a champagne flute.

4. Add sparkling white wine, a few fresh pomegranate seeds and a lemon twist to garnish. Enjoy!

Smoked Raspberry Bubbler Cocktail

Servings: 2

Cooking Time: 45 Minutes

Ingredients:

- 2 Cup fresh raspberries
- Smoked Simple Syrup
- 8 Ounce sparkling wine

Directions:

1. Supply your smoker with wood pellets and follow the start-up procedure. Preheat the grill, with the lid closed, to 180° F.

2. Smoked Raspberry Syrup: Place 1 cup fresh raspberries on a grill mat and smoke for 30 minutes. Grill: 180 °F

3. After the raspberries have been smoked, set a few aside for garnish. Place the remainder into a shallow sheet pan with Traeger Smoked Simple Syrup. Place back on the grill grate and let smoke for 45 minutes. Remove from heat and allow to cool. Strain and refrigerate until ready to use. Grill: 180 °F

4. Place 1 ounce of the smoked raspberry syrup in the bottom of a champagne flute and top off with sparkling white wine or champagne.

5. Garnish with smoked raspberries. Enjoy!

Smoky Mountain Bramble Cocktail

Servings: 2

Cooking Time: 15 Minutes

Ingredients:

- 16 Ounce blackberries

- 2 Cup sugar
- 10 smoked blackberries
- 3 Ounce vodka
- 1 1/2 Ounce Alpine Distilling Preserve Liqueur
- 1 1/2 Ounce lemon juice
- 1 Ounce smoked blackberry syrup

Directions:

1. Supply your smoker with wood pellets and follow the start-up procedure. Preheat the grill, with the lid closed, to 180° F.

2. To make Smoked Blackberry Simple Syrup: Place blackberries on a grill mat and smoke for 15 to 20 minutes. Grill: 180 °F

3. Combine 1 cup water and sugar in a small sauce pan and warm over medium heat until sugar dissolves. Remove from heat and place 2/3 of blackberries in the simple syrup and macerate.

4. Strain through a fine mesh strainer and store for up to 14 days.

5. To make the cocktail: Muddle 4 to 5 smoked blackberries in a cocktail shaker. Add vodka, Preserve Liqueur, lemon and smoked blackberry syrup. Add ice and shake vigorously. Double strain into an old fashioned glass.

6. Garnish with a smoked blackberry and lemon twist. Enjoy!

VEGETABLES RECIPES

Smoked & Loaded Baked Potato

Servings: 4
Cooking Time: 60 Minutes

Ingredients:

- 6 Yukon Gold or russet potatoes
- 8 Slices bacon
- 1/2 Cup butter, melted
- 1 Cup sour cream
- 1 1/2 Cup shredded cheddar cheese, divided
- salt and pepper
- 1 Bunch green onions, thinly sliced

Directions:

1. Supply your smoker with wood pellets and follow the start-up procedure. Preheat the grill, with the lid closed, to 375° F.
2. Poke potatoes with a fork, then place straight onto the grill. Cook for 1 hour. Grill: 375 °F
3. At the same time, cook bacon on a baking sheet on the grill for about 20 minutes; remove, cool and crumble. Grill: 375 °F
4. Once potatoes are done, remove and allow to cool for 15 minutes.
5. Cut each potato lengthwise, creating long halves. Use a small spoon to scoop out about 70% of the potato to make a boat, keeping a thick layer of potato near skin.
6. Place excess potato in a bowl and reserve. Lightly mash extra potato with a fork; add butter, sour cream, 1/2 cup cheese and season with salt and pepper.
7. Take the potato skins and fill with potato mixture, then sprinkle with extra cheese and bacon.
8. Place back on grill for about 10 minutes or until warm and cheese has melted. Garnish with green onions and extra sour cream. Enjoy! Grill: 375 °F

Grilled Cabbage Steaks With Warm Bacon Vinaigrette

Servings: 4
Cooking Time: 10 Minutes

Ingredients:

- 3 Strips thick-cut lean bacon, cut into 1/4 inch strips
- 1 Large shallot, minced
- 2 Tablespoon sherry vinegar
- 1 Tablespoon whole grain mustard
- 1 Teaspoon chopped thyme
- 2 Tablespoon olive oil, plus more as needed
- 1 Head green cabbage, cut into 3/4 inch thick slices (about 6 steaks)
- salt and pepper

Directions:

1. Supply your smoker with wood pellets and follow the start-up procedure. Preheat the grill, with the lid closed, to 450° F.
2. For the Vinaigrette: In a large skillet, cook the bacon in 2 tablespoons olive oil over medium-high heat until browned and crisp. Remove bacon from heat and stir in the shallot, vinegar, mustard and thyme then set aside.
3. Brush cabbage steaks with olive oil and season with salt and pepper. Place cabbage steaks directly on grill grate and grill for 5 minutes per side. Grill: 450 °F
4. Remove cabbage steaks from grill and drizzle with bacon vinaigrette. Enjoy!

Braised Creamed Green Beans

Servings: 4
Cooking Time: 25 Minutes

Ingredients:

- 6 Tablespoon butter
- 2 Clove garlic, pressed or minced
- 1 shallot, thinly sliced
- 1 Cup heavy cream
- 1 Pinch ground nutmeg
- salt
- 3 Pound mixed greens such as kale, chard or collards; washed, stems removed and torn into bite sized pieces

Directions:

1. Supply your smoker with wood pellets and follow the start-up procedure. Preheat the grill, with the lid closed, to 325° F.

2. In a saucepan, heat 2 tablespoons of the butter over high heat until it foams. Add the garlic and shallot and cook over medium-low heat, stirring, until softened and golden, about 5 minutes.

3. Add the cream, bring to a simmer and cook until slightly thickened, about 10 minutes.

4. Add the nutmeg and salt to taste. Using a hand blender, purée until smooth.

5. In a cast iron pan, heat the remaining 4 tablespoons butter over high heat until it foams.

6. Add the greens and cook until tender but still bright green, about 5 minutes.

7. Sprinkle with salt and add the cream mixture. Cover and transfer to the grill.

8. Braise greens for 15-20 minutes until the cream is bubbling and greens are tender. Grill: 325 ˚F

9. Season to taste with nutmeg and salt. Serve hot. Enjoy!

Carolina Baked Beans

Servings: 12-15
Cooking Time: 180 Minutes

Ingredients:

- 3 (28-ounce) cans baked beans (I like Bush's brand)
- 1 large onion, finely chopped
- 1 cup The Ultimate BBQ Sauce
- ½ cup light brown sugar
- ¼ cup Worcestershire sauce
- 3 tablespoons yellow mustard
- Nonstick cooking spray or butter, for greasing
- 1 large bell pepper, cut into thin rings
- ½ pound thick-cut bacon, partially cooked and cut into quarters

Directions:

1. Supply your smoker with wood pellets and follow the start-up procedure. Preheat, with the lid closed, to 300°F.

2. In a large mixing bowl, stir together the beans, onion, barbecue sauce, brown sugar, Worcestershire sauce, and mustard until well combined

3. Coat a 9-by-13-inch aluminum pan with cooking spray or butter.

4. Pour the beans into the pan and top with the bell pepper rings and bacon pieces, pressing them down slightly into the sauce.

5. Place a layer of heavy-duty foil on the grill grate to catch drips, and place the pan on top of the foil. Close the lid and cook for 2 hours 30 minutes to 3 hours, or until the beans are hot, thick, and bubbly.

6. Let the beans rest for 5 minutes before serving.

Stuffed Jalapenos

Servings: 8
Cooking Time: 60 Minutes

Ingredients:

- 40 Whole jalapeño
- 8 Ounce cream cheese, room temperature
- 1 Cup Sharp Cheddar Grated
- 1 1/2 Teaspoon Pork & Poultry Rub
- 2 Tablespoon sour cream
- 1 Whole (14 oz) cocktail sausages
- 20 Whole Slices of Smoked Bacon, Cut in Half

Directions:

1. Wash and dry the peppers. Cut the stem ends off with a paring knife, and using the same knife or a small metal spoon, carefully scrape the seeds and ribs out of each pepper. Set aside.

2. In a small bowl, combine the cream cheese, grated cheese, Traeger Pork and Poultry Rub, and the sour cream.

3. Transfer the mixture to a sturdy resealable plastic bag and trim 1/2-inch off one of the lower corners with a scissors. Squeeze the cream cheese mixture into each pepper, filling each a little over the halfway point.

4. Stuff one sausage into each pepper. Wrap the outside of each with a piece of bacon, securing with 1 or 2 toothpicks.

5. Arrange the peppers on a foil-lined baking sheet. Supply your smoker with wood pellets and follow the start-up procedure. Preheat the grill, with the lid closed, to 180° F, and smoke the peppers for 1 to 1-1/2 hours.

6. Increase the heat to 350 degrees F and continue to cook for 20 to 30 minutes, or until the bacon begins to render its fat and crisp. Enjoy! Grill: 350 ˚F

Roasted Jalapeno Cheddar Deviled Eggs

Servings: 6
Cooking Time: 30 Minutes

Ingredients:
- 7 Eggs, hard boiled
- 3 Tablespoon mayonnaise
- 1 Teaspoon brown mustard
- 1 Teaspoon apple cider vinegar
- 1 Dash hot sauce
- 1 jalapeño pepper, seeded and minced
- salt and pepper
- 1/2 Cup shredded cheddar cheese
- paprika

Directions:
1. Supply your smoker with wood pellets and follow the start-up procedure. Preheat the grill, with the lid closed, to 180° F.
2. Place your eggs directly on the grill grate and smoke for 30 minutes.
3. Remove from the grill and allow the eggs to cool. Smoking the eggs will give them a slightly yellowed color, but an intense smoky flavor. If a classic white egg is your preference, then skip this step.
4. Slice the eggs lengthwise and scoop the egg yolks directly into a gallon zip top bag.
5. Add the mayo, mustard, vinegar, hot sauce, roasted jalapeños and salt and pepper to the bag.
6. Zip the bag closed and, using your hands, knead all of the ingredients together in the bag until completely smooth.
7. Squeeze the yolk mixture into one corner of the bag and then cut the corner off. Pipe the yolk mixture into the whites.
8. Sprinkle with the finely shredded cheddar or paprika and chill until you are ready to serve. Enjoy!

Roasted Green Beans With Bacon

Servings: 4
Cooking Time: 20 Minutes

Ingredients:
- 1 1/2 Pound green beans, ends trimmed
- 4 Strips bacon, cut into small pieces
- 4 Tablespoon extra-virgin olive oil
- 2 Clove garlic, minced
- 1 Teaspoon kosher salt

Directions:
1. Supply your smoker with wood pellets and follow the start-up procedure. Preheat the grill, with the lid closed, to 350° F.
2. Toss all ingredients together and spread out evenly on a sheet tray.
3. Place the tray directly on the grill grate and roast until the bacon is crispy and beans are lightly browned, about 20 minutes. Enjoy! Grill: 450 °F

Butternut Squash

Servings: 4
Cooking Time: 45 Minutes

Ingredients:
- 1 Whole butternut squash
- Veggie Rub
- Blackened Saskatchewan Rub
- olive oil

Directions:
1. Cut squash in half and lightly coat with mixture of olive oil, Traeger Veggie Shake, and Traeger Blackened Saskatchewan.
2. Wrap in foil with 1/2 cup (120mL) of water.
3. Supply your smoker with wood pellets and follow the start-up procedure. Preheat the grill, with the lid closed, to 450° F.
4. Place squash on grill for 45 minutes. Remove from grill and unwrap. Enjoy!

Roasted New Potatoes With Compound Butter

Servings: 4
Cooking Time: 45 Minutes

Ingredients:
- 2 Pound Small Red, White or Purple Potatoes (or Combination of All Three)

- 3 Tablespoon olive oil
- salt and pepper
- 2 Stick Butter, unsalted
- 1 Tablespoon shallot, minced
- 3 Tablespoon Finely Chopped Herbs, Such As Tarragon, Parsley, Basil or Combination
- 2 Teaspoon kosher salt

Directions:

1. Supply your smoker with wood pellets and follow the start-up procedure. Preheat the grill, with the lid closed, to 400° F. Cut the potatoes in half and place in a large mixing bowl. Cover with the olive oil, a teaspoon of salt and generous grinding of pepper.

2. Place on a large baking sheet so there is space between the potatoes. Place on the grill and roast for 45 minutes to 1 hour, until crispy skinned. Toss once during cooking. Grill: 400 °F

3. To make the butter: Place it in a medium sized shallow mixing bowl. Use a wooden spoon or strong spatula to break it up and soften it even more. Sprinkle the shallot, herbs, and salt over the butter, then use the spoon to combine the ingredients. Taste, adding more salt or herbs if necessary. Reserve a few tablespoons of the butter to serve on the potatoes.

4. To freeze the butter for future use, place a foot long piece of plastic wrap on the counter. Spread the butter out into a 6" log across the long direction of the plastic wrap towards the bottom. Begin to roll the plastic wrap away from you to roll it into a log, twisting the sides of the plastic wrap like a candy wrapper to secure.

5. Using your hands, shape the log into an even cylinder. Once it's wrapped tightly, place in the freezer. Then when more is needed, simply slice off coins of it to serve over grilled steak, chicken, veggies, or roasted potatoes. The butter holds well in the freezer for up to one month. Enjoy! *Cook times will vary depending on set and ambient temperatures.

Baked Sweet Potato Casserole With Marshmallow Fluff

Servings: 6
Cooking Time: 60 Minutes

Ingredients:

- 3 Pound sweet potatoes
- 1/2 Cup milk
- 1 Cup brown sugar
- 3 eggs
- 4 Tablespoon butter
- 1/2 Teaspoon salt
- 3 egg white
- 1 Pinch salt
- 1 Pinch ground cinnamon

Directions:

1. Supply your smoker with wood pellets and follow the start-up procedure. Preheat the grill, with the lid closed, to 375° F.

2. Rinse, dry and pierce the sweet potatoes and place in grill whole. Cook for 45 minutes or until fork tender. Remove from grill and peel. Grill: 375 °F

3. Once peeled, mash the sweet potatoes in a large bowl with the milk, brown sugar, eggs, butter and salt. Place mashed potatoes in a baking dish and cook for 35 minutes. Grill: 375 °F

4. While the potatoes bake, make the fluff. Make a double boiler by bringing a small pot of water to a simmer, then placing the bowl of your stand mixer or another large stainless steel bowl atop the water.

5. Add the 3 egg whites, 2/3 cup brown sugar, a pinch of salt and a pinch of cinnamon to the bowl and whisk continuously until the sugar dissolves and the liquid is warm to the touch.

6. Transfer the bowl from the stovetop to your stand mixer and use the whisk attachment to whip the whites on medium-high speed until it turns glossy with stiff peaks, about 5-8 minutes.

7. Once the casserole has finished baking, use a rubber spatula to cover the sweet potato mixture with the fluff. Use the back of the spatula to create dramatic peaks.

8. Return to the grill for 5-7 minutes, or until the fluff starts to turn golden and the peaks are just shy of burnt. Remove from grill and enjoy!

Whole Roasted Cauliflower With Garlic Parmesan Butter

Servings: 4
Cooking Time: 45 Minutes

Ingredients:
- 1 Whole head cauliflower
- 1/4 Cup olive oil
- salt and pepper
- 1/2 Cup butter, melted
- 1/4 Cup shredded Parmesan cheese
- 2 Clove garlic, minced
- 1/2 Tablespoon chopped parsley

Directions:

1. Supply your smoker with wood pellets and follow the start-up procedure. Preheat the grill, with the lid closed, to 450° F.
2. Brush the cauliflower with olive oil and season liberally with salt and pepper.
3. Put cauliflower in a cast iron skillet, place directly on the grill grate and cook for 45 minutes until golden brown and the center is tender.
4. While the cauliflower is cooking, combine the melted butter, parmesan, garlic and parsley in a small bowl.
5. During the last 20 minutes of cooking, baste the cauliflower with the melted butter mixture.
6. Remove the cauliflower from the grill and top with extra parmesan and parsley if desired. Enjoy!

Roasted Sheet Pan Vegetables

Servings: 4
Cooking Time: 25 Minutes

Ingredients:
- 1 Small head purple cauliflower, stemmed and cut into 2 inch florets
- 1 Small head yellow cauliflower, stemmed and cut into 2 inch florets
- 4 Cup butternut squash
- 2 Cup oyster or shiitake mushrooms, rinsed and sliced
- 3 Tablespoon olive oil
- 2 Teaspoon kosher salt
- freshly ground black pepper
- 1/4 Cup chopped flat-leaf parsley

Directions:

1. Supply your smoker with wood pellets and follow the start-up procedure. Preheat the grill, with the lid closed, to 450° F.
2. In a large mixing bowl, combine all of the vegetables. Drizzle olive oil over the top, along with kosher salt and a generous grinding of black pepper.
3. Using your hands, toss the vegetables until they are evenly coated.
4. Spread out onto 1 or 2 half sheet pans or baking sheets, ensuring there is a little space between the veggies. (If they are too crowded, the vegetables will steam instead of roast and you won't get that crispy texture.)
5. Place the sheet pans on the grill and cook for 15 minutes. Open and stir, then close the lid and continue to cook until the vegetables are brown around the edges, about 5 to 15 minutes longer. Grill: 450 °F
6. Toss with parsley and serve immediately. The vegetables are also delicious at room temperature. Enjoy!

Smoked Macaroni Salad

Servings: 4
Cooking Time: 20 Minutes

Ingredients:
- 1 Pound macaroni, uncooked
- 1/2 Small red onion, diced
- 1 green bell pepper, diced
- 1/2 Cup shredded carrot
- 1 Cup mayonnaise
- 3 Tablespoon white wine vinegar
- 2 Tablespoon sugar
- salt
- black pepper

Directions:

1. Bring a large stock pot of salted water to a boil over medium heat and cook pasta according to package directions. Make sure to cook to al dente, strain, and rinse under cold water.

2. Supply your smoker with wood pellets and follow the start-up procedure. Preheat the grill, with the lid closed, to 225° F.

3. Spread cooked pasta out on a sheet tray and place sheet tray directly on the grill grate. Smoke for 20 minutes, remove from heat, and transfer directly to the refrigerator to cool. Grill: 225 °F

4. While the pasta is cooling mix the dressing. Place all ingredients in a medium bowl and whisk to combine.

5. When pasta is cool combine chopped veggies, smoked pasta and dressing in a large bowl.

6. Cover with plastic wrap and place in the fridge for 20 minutes before serving. Enjoy!

Baked Heirloom Tomato Tart

Servings: 4
Cooking Time: 45 Minutes

Ingredients:
- 1 Whole Puff Pastry Sheet
- 2 Pound heirloom tomatoes, various shapes and sizes
- 1/2 Tablespoon kosher salt
- 1/2 Cup Ricotta Cheese
- 5 Whole eggs
- 1 To Taste salt and pepper
- 1/2 Teaspoon thyme leaves
- 1/2 Teaspoon red pepper flakes
- 4 Sprig thyme

Directions:
1. Supply your smoker with wood pellets and follow the start-up procedure. Preheat the grill, with the lid closed, to 350° F.

2. Place the puff pastry on a parchment lined sheet tray, and make a cut ¾ of the way through the pastry, ½" from the edge.

3. Slice the tomatoes and season with salt. Place on a sheet tray lined with paper towels.

4. In a small bowl combine the ricotta, 4 of the eggs, salt, thyme leaves, red pepper flakes and black pepper. Whisk together until combined. Spread the ricotta mixture over the puff pastry, staying within ½" from the edge.

5. In a small bowl whisk the last egg. Brush the egg wash onto the exposed edges of the pastry.

6. Place the sheet tray directly on the grill grate and bake for 45 minutes, rotating half-way through. Grill: 350 °F

7. When the edges are browned and the moisture from the tomatoes has evaporated, remove from the grill and let cool 5-7 minutes before serving. Enjoy!

Baked Kale Chips

Servings: 4
Cooking Time: 20 Minutes

Ingredients:
- 2 Bunch kale, leaves washed and stems removed
- 1 As Needed extra-virgin olive oil
- 1 To Taste sea salt

Directions:
1. Dry the kale leaves well and lay them out on a sheet tray. Drizzle lightly with olive oil and sprinkle with sea salt.

2. Supply your smoker with wood pellets and follow the start-up procedure. Preheat the grill, with the lid closed, to 250° F.

3. Place the sheet tray directly on the grill grate and cook until kale is lightly browned and crispy, about 20 minutes. Enjoy! Grill: 250 °F

Grilled Broccoli Rabe

Servings: 4
Cooking Time: 10 Minutes

Ingredients:
- 4 Tablespoon extra-virgin olive oil
- 4 Bunch broccoli rabe or broccolini
- kosher salt
- 1 lemon, halved

Directions:
1. Supply your smoker with wood pellets and follow the start-up procedure. Preheat the grill, with the lid closed, to 450° F.

2. On a platter or in a mixing bowl, drizzle the olive oil over the broccoli rabe. Use your hands to mix thoroughly,

coating the vegetables evenly with the oil. Season with sea salt.

3. Place the broccoli rabe in one layer directly on the lowest grill grate. Close the lid and cook for 5 to 10 minutes. You want there to be some color and slight char on the first side. Flip and cook for a few more minutes. Grill: 450 °F

4. Transfer the broccoli rabe to a serving platter and squeeze the juice of half a lemon evenly over the top.

5. Serve with more lemon wedges on the side. Enjoy!

Roasted New Potatoes

Servings: 4
Cooking Time: 25 Minutes

Ingredients:

- 2 Pound small new potatoes
- 3 Tablespoon butter, melted
- 2 Tablespoon olive oil
- 2 Tablespoon whole mustard seeds
- salt and pepper
- 2 Tablespoon freshly minced chives
- 2 Tablespoon freshly minced parsley

Directions:

1. Place potatoes in a colander and rinse with cold water. Dry on paper towels and transfer to a rimmed baking sheet large enough to hold them in a single layer.

2. Drizzle the potatoes with butter and olive oil, then sprinkle them with the mustard seeds. Season with salt and pepper.

3. Supply your smoker with wood pellets and follow the start-up procedure. Preheat the grill, with the lid closed, to 400° F.

4. Place the baking sheet with the potatoes on the grill grate. Roast for about 25 minutes shaking the pan once or twice, until potatoes are tender and the skins are slightly wrinkled. Grill: 400 °F

5. Transfer potatoes to a bowl or platter. Top with fresh chives and parsley. Enjoy!

Steak Fries With Horseradish Creme

Servings: 6
Cooking Time: 25 Minutes

Ingredients:

- 5 Potatoes, Baking
- 2 Tablespoon extra-virgin olive oil
- 1 Teaspoon butter
- 3 Clove garlic, crushed
- 1 Teaspoon onion powder
- 2 Teaspoon Jacobsen Salt Co. Pure Kosher Sea Salt
- 1 Teaspoon black pepper

Directions:

1. Wash the potatoes thoroughly, and cut them in eighths, then toss them in the olive oil, butter, crushed garlic, onion powder, salt, and pepper.

2. Supply your smoker with wood pellets and follow the start-up procedure. Preheat the grill, with the lid closed, to 450° F.

3. In order to get great grill marks, line up the wedges on the front of the grill and the back of the grill, turning to get grill marks on all sides.

4. Once they have been seared, move them to the center of the grill and finish cooking about ten more minutes, serve hot with the horseradish mayo. Enjoy!

Baked Bacon Green Bean Casserole

Servings: 6
Cooking Time: 50 Minutes

Ingredients:

- 1 1/2 Pound Green Beans, fresh
- 1 Can cream of mushroom soup
- 1/2 Cup milk
- 1/2 Teaspoon Worcestershire sauce
- 1/2 Teaspoon black pepper
- 2/3 Cup French's Original Crispy Fried Onions
- 8 Slices bacon
- 1/4 Cup red bell pepper, diced
- 2/3 French's Original Crispy Fried Onions

Directions:

1. In a mixing bowl, combine beans, soup, milk, Worcestershire sauce, black pepper, 2/3 cup of the onions, 6 of the slices of crumbled bacon, and red bell pepper. Transfer to a 1-1/2 quart casserole dish.

2. Supply your smoker with wood pellets and follow the start-up procedure. Preheat the grill, with the lid closed, to 350° F.

3. Cook casserole until the filling is hot and bubbling, 35 to 40 minutes. Grill: 350 ℉

4. Top with remaining onions and the last 2 slices of crumbled bacon and cook for 5 to 10 minutes more, or until the onions are crisp and beginning to brown. Serve, enjoy! Grill: 350 ℉

Baked Stuffed Avocados

Servings: 6
Cooking Time: 15 Minutes

Ingredients:
- 4 avocados, halved and pit removed
- 8 eggs
- 2 Cup shredded cheddar cheese
- 1/4 Cup cherry tomatoes, halved
- 4 Slices Bacon, cooked & chopped
- salt and pepper
- 1 scallion, thinly sliced

Directions:
1. Supply your smoker with wood pellets and follow the start-up procedure. Preheat the grill, with the lid closed, to 450° F.

2. After removing the pit from the avocado, scoop out a little of the flesh to make enough room to fit 1 egg per half.

3. Fill the bottom of a cast iron pan with kosher salt and nestle the avocado halves into the salt, cut side up. The salt helps to keep them in place while cooking, like ice with oysters.

4. Crack one egg into each half, top with shredded cheddar cheese, cherry tomatoes and bacon. Season with salt and pepper to taste.

5. Place the cast iron pan directly on the grill grate and bake the avocados for 12 to 15 minutes until the cheese is melted and the egg is just set. Grill: 450 ℉

6. Remove from the grill and let rest 5 to 10 minutes. Top with sliced scallions and enjoy!

Roasted Sweet Potato Steak Fries

Servings: 4
Cooking Time: 40 Minutes

Ingredients:
- 3 Whole sweet potatoes
- 4 Tablespoon extra-virgin olive oil
- salt and pepper
- 2 Tablespoon fresh chopped rosemary

Directions:
1. Supply your smoker with wood pellets and follow the start-up procedure. Preheat the grill, with the lid closed, to 450° F.

2. Cut sweet potatoes into wedges and toss with olive oil, salt, pepper and rosemary. Spread on a parchment lined baking sheet and put in the grill. Cook for 15 minutes then flip and continue to cook until lightly browned and cooked through, about 40 to 45 minutes total. Grill: 450 ℉

3. Serve with your favorite dipping sauce. Enjoy! Grill: 450 ℉

Grilled Chili-lime Corn

Servings: 8
Cooking Time: 45 Minutes

Ingredients:
- 12 Corn, ears
- 1 Teaspoon chili powder
- 1/2 Teaspoon onion powder
- 1 Teaspoon Leinenkugel's Summer Shandy Rub
- 2 lime, juiced
- 1 Tablespoon lime zest

Directions:
1. Soak the ears of corn, still in their husk, in water for 4 to 8 hours.

2. Supply your smoker with wood pellets and follow the start-up procedure. Preheat the grill, with the lid closed, to 350° F.

3. Place corn directly on grill grates. Turn corn every 15 minutes for 45 minutes total cooking time. Grill: 350 ℉

4. Combine chili powder, onion powder, Summer Shandy rub, lime juice, lime zest and butter in an oven safe dish and place in grill for 10 minutes. Remove corn and butter from the grill.

5. Pull corn husk back, but not off and remove corn silk. Using the corn husk as a handle, brush the corn with the melted chili-lime butter. Enjoy!

Roasted Vegetable Napoleon

Servings: 4
Cooking Time: 30 Minutes

Ingredients:
- 2 Whole sweet potatoes
- 2 Whole zucchini
- 2 Whole Squash
- 1 Whole red onion
- 2 Whole Bell Pepper, Red
- salt and pepper

Directions:
1. Supply your smoker with wood pellets and follow the start-up procedure. Preheat the grill, with the lid closed, to High heat.

2. Salt and pepper all vegetables and grill them on both sides. Begin with the peppers and onions as they will take a little longer to cook. Grill: 450 °F

Spicy Asian Brussels Sprouts

Servings: 4
Cooking Time: 10 Minutes

Ingredients:
- 2 Cup fresh Brussels sprouts
- 2 Tablespoon vegetable oil
- 1 Tablespoon Asian BBQ Rub
- 1/4 Cup Thai sweet chile sauce

Directions:
1. Supply your smoker with wood pellets and follow the start-up procedure. Preheat the grill, with the lid closed, to 350° F.

2. Spread the halved brussel sprouts in a single layer on a lined cookie sheet. Drizzle with the oil and toss to coat.

3. Sprinkle the brussel sprouts evenly with an Asian BBQ rub and put the cookie sheet on the grill. Close the lid and cook for 7-8 minutes. Grill: 350 °F

4. Toss the brussels sprouts in the Thai Chili Sauce and return to the grill for an additional 3-4 minutes, or until the sprouts are crisp-tender. Grill: 350 °F

5. Serve immediately. Enjoy!

Parmesan Roasted Cauliflower

Servings: 4
Cooking Time: 40 Minutes

Ingredients:
- 1 Head cauliflower, cut into florets
- 1 Medium onion, sliced
- 4 Clove garlic, unpeeled
- 4 Tablespoon olive oil
- salt
- black pepper
- 1 Teaspoon fresh thyme
- 1/2 Cup Parmesan cheese, grated

Directions:
1. Supply your smoker with wood pellets and follow the start-up procedure. Preheat the grill, with the lid closed, to 400° F.

2. On a baking tray, mix together cauliflower, onion, thyme, garlic, olive oil, salt and pepper.

3. Place tray on preheated grill and cook until cauliflower is firm and almost tender (about 25 minutes). Grill: 400 °F

4. Sprinkle cauliflower with Parmesan cheese and continue to cook on the Traeger for another 10 to 15 minutes. Cauliflower should be tender and the Parmesan crisp. Serve immediately, enjoy!

Baked Winter Squash Au Gratin

Servings: 8
Cooking Time: 45 Minutes

Ingredients:
- 2 Cup heavy cream
- salt and pepper
- 3 Cup shredded Gruyere cheese
- 4 Clove garlic, diced

- 2 Tablespoon butter
- 3 yellow potatoes, peeled and cubed
- 1 butternut squash seeded, peeled and cubed
- 1 acorn squash seeded, peeled and cubed

Directions:

1. Supply your smoker with wood pellets and follow the start-up procedure. Preheat the grill, with the lid closed, to 375° F.

2. In a medium saucepan, cook the cream, stirring constantly, until it comes to a low boil. Add salt, pepper, garlic and shredded Gruyere cheese. Stir until cheese is melted.

3. Grease a 9x13 inch baking dish with 2 tablespoons of butter. In a large mixing bowl, combine potatoes, butternut and acorn squash. Stir in the cheese sauce. Place mixture in the prepared baking dish and place in grill.

4. Cook for 45 minutes or until potatoes and squash are fork tender. Remove from grill and let cool for 10 minutes before serving. Enjoy! Grill: 375 °F

Roasted Beet & Bacon Salad

Servings: 4
Cooking Time: 45 Minutes

Ingredients:

- 2 Medium raw beets, peeled and thinly sliced
- 8 Slices bacon
- 1/4 Cup raw pecans or walnuts
- 2 Medium ripe pears, sliced
- 2 Large avocados, diced
- 1 Head red leaf lettuce or baby spinach, torn into bite-size pieces
- 1/4 Cup champagne vinaigrette

Directions:

1. Supply your smoker with wood pellets and follow the start-up procedure. Preheat the grill, with the lid closed, to 400° F.

2. Place beets on a foil-lined baking sheet and top with bacon. Place baking sheet directly on the grill grate (while preheating) and cook for 25 minutes. Grill: 400 °F

3. Toss to coat beets in rendered bacon fat.

4. Spread everything out in a single layer and continue to cook for another 15 minutes, or until beets are tender and bacon is crispy. Grill: 400 °F

5. Add pecans or walnuts and roast for 5 more minutes. Spoon out nuts and place on paper towels to drain and cool.

6. Once bacon is cool to the touch, roughly chop into medium pieces.

7. Place bacon, beets, nuts, pears, avocado and lettuce in a large salad bowl. Drizzle with champagne vinaigrette, toss to coat, and serve. Enjoy!

Grilled Corn On The Cob With Parmesan And Garlic

Servings: 6
Cooking Time: 30 Minutes

Ingredients:

- 4 Tablespoon butter, melted
- 2 Clove garlic, minced
- salt and pepper
- 8 ears fresh corn
- 1/2 Cup shaved Parmesan
- 1 Tablespoon chopped parsley

Directions:

1. Supply your smoker with wood pellets and follow the start-up procedure. Preheat the grill, with the lid closed, to 450° F.

2. Place butter, garlic, salt and pepper in a medium bowl and mix well.

3. Peel back corn husks and remove the silk. Rub corn with half of the garlic butter mixture.

4. Close husks and place directly on the grill grate. Cook for 25 to 30 minutes, turning occasionally until corn is tender. Grill: 450 °F

5. Remove from grill, peel and discard husks. Place corn on serving tray, drizzle with remaining butter and top with Parmesan and parsley.

Chef Curtis' Famous Chimichurri Sauce

Servings: 4
Cooking Time: 5 Minutes

Ingredients:

- 2 Whole lemon, halved
- 2 Medium flat-leaf Italian parsley, washed and chopped with the majority of stems cut off
- 4 Clove garlic, diced
- 1/4 Cup red wine vinegar
- 1/2 Teaspoon black pepper
- 1/4 Cup extra-virgin olive oil
- 1 Teaspoon salt

Directions:

1. Supply your smoker with wood pellets and follow the start-up procedure. Preheat the grill, with the lid closed, to 450° F.
2. Place lemon halves directly on the grill grate and cook for 5 minutes or until grill marks appear. Grill: 450 °F
3. Take lemons off grill and juice. Combine all of the ingredients in a food processor or blender and purée until smooth, or leave slightly chunky for some texture.
4. Add additional olive oil to taste for a milder flavor if preferred. Serve on protein or as a dip. Enjoy!

Roasted Mashed Potatoes

Servings: 8
Cooking Time: 40 Minutes

Ingredients:

- 5 Pound Yukon Gold potatoes
- 1 1/2 Stick butter, softened
- 1 1/2 Cup heavy whipping cream, room temperature
- kosher salt
- white pepper

Directions:

1. Supply your smoker with wood pellets and follow the start-up procedure. Preheat the grill, with the lid closed, to 300° F.

2. Peel and cut potatoes into 1/2 inch cubes. Place the potatoes in a shallow baking dish with 1/2 cup water and cover. Bake until tender, about 40 minutes. Grill: 300 °F
3. In a medium saucepan, combine cream and butter. Cook over medium heat until butter is melted.
4. Remove potatoes from the grill and drain water.
5. Transfer potatoes to a bowl and mash using a potato masher. Gradually add in cream and butter mixture and mix using the masher. Be careful not to overwork or the potatoes will becomes gluey. Season with salt and pepper to taste. Enjoy!

Broccoli-cauliflower Salad

Servings: 4
Cooking Time: 25 Minutes

Ingredients:

- 1½ cups mayonnaise
- ½ cup sour cream
- ¼ cup sugar
- 1 bunch broccoli, cut into small pieces
- 1 head cauliflower, cut into small pieces
- 1 small red onion, chopped
- 6 slices bacon, cooked and crumbled (precooked bacon works well)
- 1 cup shredded Cheddar cheese

Directions:

1. In a small bowl, whisk together the mayonnaise, sour cream, and sugar to make a dressing.
2. In a large bowl, combine the broccoli, cauliflower, onion, bacon, and Cheddar cheese.
3. Pour the dressing over the vegetable mixture and toss well to coat.
4. Serve the salad chilled.

Roasted Do-ahead Mashed Potatoes

Servings: 6
Cooking Time: 50 Minutes

Ingredients:

- 5 Pound Yukon Gold or russet potatoes
- 9 Tablespoon butter
- 8 Ounce cream cheese
- 1/2 Cup milk

- salt and pepper

Directions:

1. Peel the potatoes and cut into chunks that are roughly the same size. Cover with cold water and add a teaspoon of salt. Bring to a boil over high heat, then reduce the heat to medium and simmer the potatoes until they are tender.

2. Drain the potatoes and return them to the pot. Stir over low heat for 2 to 3 minutes to evaporate any excess moisture.

3. Mash the potatoes with a hand-held potato masher. (Alternative, rice the potatoes using a ricer.) Incorporate 8 tbsp butter and cream cheese. Add milk until the potatoes are of a good consistency. Stir in salt and pepper to taste.

4. Butter the inside of a casserole dish. Spread the potatoes out in an even layer in the casserole dish, smoothing the top with a spatula. Cool, cover, and refrigerate if not cooking right away. Before cooking, let the potatoes warm to room temperature (about an hour).

5. Supply your smoker with wood pellets and follow the start-up procedure. Preheat the grill, with the lid closed, to 350° F.

6. Bake the potatoes for 45 to 50 minutes, or until hot through. Grill: 350 °F

Grilled Asparagus And Hollandaise Sauce

Servings: 4
Cooking Time: 10 Minutes

Ingredients:

- 1 Pound asparagus
- 2 Teaspoon red pepper flakes
- 2 Tablespoon olive oil
- salt and pepper
- 4 egg yolk
- 1 Tablespoon lemon juice
- 1/2 Cup butter, melted
- cayenne pepper
- salt

Directions:

1. Supply your smoker with wood pellets and follow the start-up procedure. Preheat the grill, with the lid closed, to 375° F.

2. In a large bowl, mix asparagus with olive oil, red pepper flakes and salt. Arrange asparagus on a cooking sheet and take to the grill. Cook for approximately 10 to 15 minutes. Grill: 375 °F

3. In an aluminum bowl, whisk the egg yolks well. Add the lemon juice and whisk until creamy.

4. Place bowl over a double boiler, over low heat, making sure that it does not touches the water.

5. While whisking, add the melted butter slowly. Whisk until it doubles the volume. Take off the heat, still whisking and add the cayenne pepper and salt.

6. Arrange asparagus over a serving plater. Pour hollandaise sauce over asparagus and serve. Enjoy!

Green Bean Casserole

Servings: 6
Cooking Time: 25 Minutes

Ingredients:

- 1/2 Stick butter
- 1 Small onion
- 1/2 Cup sliced button mushrooms
- 4 Can green beans, drained
- 2 Can cream of mushroom soup
- 1 Teaspoon Lawry's Seasoned Salt
- pepper
- 1 Can French's Original Crispy Fried Onions
- 1 Cup grated sharp cheddar cheese

Directions:

1. Supply your smoker with wood pellets and follow the start-up procedure. Preheat the grill, with the lid closed, to 375° F.

2. Melt butter in a cast iron skillet and add onions and mushrooms, stirring occasionally until softened.

3. Add drained green beans and cream of mushroom soup and stir gently to combine.

4. Season with seasoned salt and pepper and sprinkle the top with grated cheddar cheese and fried onions.

5. Bake for 25 minutes. Serve warm, enjoy! Grill: 375 °F

Smoked Beet-pickled Eggs

Servings: 4
Cooking Time: 30 Minutes

Ingredients:

- 6 Eggs, hard boiled
- 1 Red Beets, scrubbed and trimmed
- 1 Cup apple cider vinegar
- 1 Cup Beet, juice
- 1/4 Onion, Sliced
- 1/3 Cup granulated sugar
- 3 Cardamom
- 1 star anise

Directions:

1. Supply your smoker with wood pellets and follow the start-up procedure. Preheat the grill, with the lid closed, to 275° F.
2. Place the peeled hard boiled eggs directly on the grill and smoke for 30 minutes. Grill: 275 °F
3. Put the smoked eggs in a quart size glass jar with the cooked/chopped beets in the bottom.
4. In a medium sauce pan, add the vinegar, beet juice, onion, sugar, cardamom and anise.
5. Bring to a boil and cook, uncovered, until sugar has dissolved and the onions are translucent (about 5 minutes).
6. Remove from the heat and let cool for a few minutes.
7. Pour the vinegar and onions mixture over the eggs and beets in the jar, covering the eggs completely.
8. Securely close with the jar lid. Refrigerate up to a month. Enjoy!

Double-smoked Cheese Potatoes

Servings: 12
Cooking Time: 35 Minutes

Ingredients:

- 4 large baking potatoes (12 to 14 ounces each—preferably organic)
- 1 1/2 tablespoons bacon fat or butter, melted, or extra virgin olive oil
- Coarse salt (sea or kosher) and freshly ground black pepper
- 4 strips artisanal bacon (like Nueske's), cut crosswise into 1/4-inch slivers
- 6 tablespoons (3/4 stick) cold unsalted butter, thinly sliced
- 2 scallions, trimmed, white and green parts finely chopped (about 4 tablespoons)
- 2 cups coarsely grated smoked or regular white cheddar cheese (about 8 ounces)
- 1/2 cup sour cream
- Spanish smoked paprika (pimentón) or sweet paprika, for sprinkling

Directions:

1. Supply your smoker with wood pellets and follow the start-up procedure. Preheat the grill, with the lid closed, to 400° F. Add enough wood for 1 hour of smoking as specified by the manufacturer.
2. Scrub the potatoes on all sides with a vegetable brush. Rinse well under cold running water and blot dry with paper towels. Prick each potato several times with a fork (this keeps the spud from exploding and facilitates the smoke absorption). Brush or rub the potato on all sides with the bacon fat and season generously with salt and pepper.
3. Place the potatoes on the smoker rack. Smoke until the skins are crisp and the potatoes are tender in the center (they'll be easy to pierce with a slender metal skewer), about 1 hour.
4. Meanwhile, place the bacon in a cold skillet and fry over medium heat until browned and crisp, 3 to 4 minutes. Drain off the bacon fat (save the fat for future potatoes).
5. Transfer the potatoes to a cutting board and let cool slightly. Cut each potato in half lengthwise. Using a spoon, scrape out most of the potato flesh, leaving a 1/4-inch-thick shell. (It's easier to scoop the potatoes when warm.) Cut the potato flesh into 1/2-inch dice and place in a bowl.
6. Add the bacon, 4 tablespoons of the butter, the scallions, and cheese to the potato flesh and gently stir to mix. Stir in the sour cream and salt and pepper to taste; the mixture should be highly seasoned. Stir as little and as gently as possible so as to leave some texture to the potatoes.

7. Spoon the potato mixture back into the potato shells, mounding it in the center. Top each potato half with a thin slice of the remaining butter and sprinkle with paprika. The potatoes can be prepared up to 24 hours ahead to this stage, covered, and refrigerated.

8. Just before serving, preheat your smoker to 400 °F. Add enough wood for 30 minutes of smoking. Place the potatoes in a shallow aluminum foil pan and re-smoke them until browned and bubbling, 15 to 20 minutes.

Grilled Fingerling Potato Salad

Servings: 6
Cooking Time: 15 Minutes

Ingredients:

- 10 Whole scallions
- 2/3 Cup extra-virgin olive oil, divided
- 1 1/2 Pound fingerling potatoes, cut in half lengthwise
- pepper
- 2 Teaspoon kosher salt, divided, plus more as needed
- 2 Tablespoon rice vinegar
- 2 Teaspoon lemon juice
- 1 Small jalapeño, sliced

Directions:

1. Supply your smoker with wood pellets and follow the start-up procedure. Preheat the grill, with the lid closed, to 450° F.

2. Brush the scallions with oil and place on the grill.

3. Cook until lightly charred, about 2 to 3 minutes. Remove and let cool. Grill: 450 °F

4. Once the scallions have cooled, slice and set aside.

5. Brush the fingerling potatoes with oil (reserving 1/3 cup for later use), then salt and pepper. Place cut-side down on the grill until cooked through, about 4 to 5 minutes. Grill: 450 °F

6. In a bowl, whisk the remaining 1/3 cup olive oil, 1 teaspoon salt, rice vinegar and lemon juice. Next mix in the scallions, potatoes and sliced jalapeño.

7. Season with salt and pepper, and serve. Enjoy!

Traeger Smoked Coleslaw

Servings: 8
Cooking Time: 20 Minutes

Ingredients:

- 1 Head purple cabbage, shredded
- 1 Head green cabbage, shredded
- 1 Cup shredded carrots
- 2 scallions, thinly sliced
- 1 1/2 Cup mayonnaise
- 1/8 Cup white wine vinegar
- 1 Teaspoon celery seed
- 1 Teaspoon sugar
- salt and pepper

Directions:

1. Supply your smoker with wood pellets and follow the start-up procedure. Preheat the grill, with the lid closed, to 180° F.

2. Spread cabbage and carrots out on a sheet tray and place directly on the grill grates. Smoke for 20 to 25 minutes or until cabbage picks up desired amount of smoke. Grill: 180 °F

3. Remove from grill and transfer to the refrigerator immediately to cool. While cabbage is cooling, make the dressing.

4. For the dressing, combine all ingredients in a small bowl and mix well.

5. Place smoked cabbage and carrots in a large bowl and pour dressing over them. Stir to coat well.

6. Transfer to a serving dish and sprinkle with scallions. Enjoy!

Grilled Asparagus And Spinach Salad

Servings: 8
Cooking Time: 10 Minutes

Ingredients:

- 4 Fluid Ounce apple cider vinegar
- 8 Fluid Ounce Honey Bourbon BBQ Sauce
- 2 Bunch asparagus, ends trimmed
- 3 Fluid Ounce extra-virgin olive oil
- 2 Ounce Beef Rub
- 24 Ounce Spinach, fresh
- 4 Ounce candied pecans

- 4 Ounce feta cheese

Directions:

1. Combine apple cider vinegar and Traeger Apricot BBQ Sauce to create salad dressing.

2. Supply your smoker with wood pellets and follow the start-up procedure. Preheat the grill, with the lid closed, to High heat.

3. Toss the asparagus with Olive Oil and the Beef Shake. Put asparagus in the Traeger Grilling Basket and move the basket to the grill grate.

4. Grill for about 10 minutes. Remove the asparagus once it is cooked. Grill: 350 ˚F

5. Place the hot asparagus right on top of the bowl of spinach.

6. Add candied pecans, feta cheese & salad dressing then toss and serve. Enjoy!

Portobello Marinated Mushroom

Servings: 2
Cooking Time: 15 Minutes

Ingredients:

- 1 Teaspoon chopped thyme
- 1 Teaspoon rosemary, chopped
- 1 Teaspoon Oregano, chopped
- 3 Tablespoon extra-virgin olive oil
- 1 To Taste Jacobsen Salt Co. Pure Kosher Sea Salt
- 1 To Taste pepper
- 6 Whole Portobello Mushroom
- 2 Whole russet potatoes

Directions:

1. Supply your smoker with wood pellets and follow the start-up procedure. Preheat the grill, with the lid closed, to 450° F.

2. Mix fresh herbs, olive oil, salt, and pepper together in a bowl. Rub over mushrooms. Grill both sides of mushrooms for approximately 2-3 minutes on each side. Grill: 450 ˚F

3. Clean the potatoes and slice into long strips.

4. Heat the oil on the Traeger in a sauce pan; drop the potatoes in the hot oil and fry for 7-8 minutes. Let the potatoes cool slightly on a sheet pan. Enjoy! Grill: 450 ˚F

Smoked Mushrooms

Servings: 4
Cooking Time: 45 Minutes

Ingredients:

- Pound Mushrooms, fresh
- 1/2 Cup apple cider vinegar
- 1/2 Cup soy sauce
- 1 Teaspoon Blackened Saskatchewan Rub

Directions:

1. Clean mushrooms and place in a large Ziploc bag. Add apple cider vinegar, soy sauce and rub.

2. Mix well and allow to marinate in the refrigerator for at least 2 hours.

3. Supply your smoker with wood pellets and follow the start-up procedure. Preheat the grill, with the lid closed, to 350° F.

4. Place cast iron skillet inside grill for 20 minutes to warm up.

5. Add the mushrooms and marinade slowly into the cast iron skillet.

6. Cook uncovered for 15 minutes, then cover the skillet and cook another 30 minutes until mushrooms are tender. Grill: 350 ˚F

7. Remove skillet from grill and let mushrooms cool down for 5 minutes before serving. Enjoy!

Smoked Pickled Green Beans

Servings: 4
Cooking Time: 45 Minutes

Ingredients:

- 1 Pound Green Beans, blanched
- 1/2 Cup salt
- 1/2 Cup sugar
- 1 Tablespoon red pepper flakes
- 2 Cup white wine vinegar
- 2 Cup ice water

Directions:

1. Supply your smoker with wood pellets and follow the start-up procedure. Preheat the grill, with the lid closed, to 180° F.

2. Place the blanched green beans on a mesh grill mat and place mat directly on the grill grate. Smoke the green beans for 30-45 minutes until they've picked up the desired amount of smoke. Remove from grill and set aside until the brine is ready. Grill: 180 ˚F

3. In a medium sized saucepan, bring all remaining ingredients, except ice water, to a boil over medium high heat on the stove. Simmer for 5-10 minutes then remove from heat and steep 20 minutes more. Pour brine over ice water to cool.

4. Once brine has cooled, pour over the green beans and weigh them down with a few plates to ensure they are completely submerged. Let sit 24 hours before use. Enjoy!

Baked Loaded Tater Tots

Servings: 6
Cooking Time: 35 Minutes

Ingredients:
- 2 Pound frozen tater tots
- 1 Can Black Beans
- 1 1/2 Cup leftover chili
- 1 Cup leftover queso
- 1 red onion, finely diced
- 1/2 Cup chopped cilantro
- 1/2 Cup sour cream
- 1 jalapeños, sliced

Directions:
1. Supply your smoker with wood pellets and follow the start-up procedure. Preheat the grill, with the lid closed, to 375° F.
2. Spread frozen tots out on a sheet tray and place directly on the grill grate.
3. Cook for 20 to 25 minutes or until tots are crispy. Grill: 375 ˚F
4. Top with warmed chili, queso and beans. Place back on the grill for 15 minutes. Grill: 375 ˚F
5. Remove from grill and top with red onion, cilantro, sour cream and jalapeño. Enjoy!

Grilled Zucchini Squash Spears

Servings: 4

Cooking Time: 10 Minutes

Ingredients:
- 4 Medium zucchini
- 2 Tablespoon olive oil
- 1 Tablespoon sherry vinegar
- 2 thyme, leaves pulled
- salt and pepper

Directions:
1. Clean the zucchini and cut the ends off. Cut each in half lengthwise, then each half into thirds.
2. Combine remaining ingredients in a medium Ziplock bag and add the spears. Toss and mix well to coat the zucchini.
3. Supply your smoker with wood pellets and follow the start-up procedure. Preheat the grill, with the lid closed, to 350° F.
4. Remove the spears from the bag and place directly on the grill grate cut side down.
5. Cook for 3-4 minutes per side, until grill marks appear and zucchini is tender. Grill: 350 ˚F
6. Remove from grill and finish with more thyme leaves if desired. Enjoy!

Christmas Brussel Sprouts

Servings: 6
Cooking Time: 50 Minutes

Ingredients:
- 1/2 Pound thick-cut bacon
- 1 Medium onion, diced
- 2 Pound fresh Brussels sprouts
- 2 Tablespoon olive oil
- salt and pepper

Directions:
1. Supply your smoker with wood pellets and follow the start-up procedure. Preheat the grill, with the lid closed, to 350° F.
2. Place bacon directly on grill grate and cook for 15-20 minutes, or until lightly browned. Remove from grill and set aside on paper towel lined plate.
3. Slice onion in half and then slice into 1/4 inch moons and add to large mixing bowl. Slice brussels sprouts in half lengthwise and add to bowl.

4. Cut reserved bacon into 1⁄2 inch pieces and add to bowl. Drizzle with olive oil and sprinkle with salt and pepper. Toss to coat and pour into baking pan.

5. Turn the temperature on grill to 375 and place baking pan on grill. Roast for 30 minutes mixing halfway through cooking. Grill: 375 °F

Grilled Ratatouille Salad

Servings: 4
Cooking Time: 25 Minutes

Ingredients:
- 1 Whole sweet potatoes
- 1 Whole red onion, diced
- 1 Whole zucchini
- 1 Whole Squash
- 1 Large Tomato, diced
- vegetable oil
- salt and pepper

Directions:
1. Supply your smoker with wood pellets and follow the start-up procedure. Preheat the grill, with the lid closed, to High heat.

2. Slice all vegetables to a ¼ inch thickness.

3. Lightly brush each vegetable with oil and season with Traeger's Veggie Shake or salt and pepper.

4. Place sweet potato, onion, zucchini, and squash on grill grate and grill for 20 minutes or until tender, turn halfway through.

5. Add tomato slices to the grill during the last 5 minutes of cooking time.

6. For presentation, alternate vegetables while layering them vertically. Enjoy!

Roasted Fall Vegetables

Servings: 6
Cooking Time: 30 Minutes

Ingredients:
- 1/2 Pound Potatoes, new
- 2 Tablespoon olive oil
- salt and pepper
- 1/2 Pound Butternut Squash, diced
- 1/2 Pound fresh Brussels sprouts

- 1 Pint mushrooms, sliced

Directions:
1. Supply your smoker with wood pellets and follow the start-up procedure. Preheat the grill, with the lid closed, to 200° F.

2. Toss potatoes and squash with olive oil, salt and pepper and spread out on a sheet tray.

3. Place directly on the grill grate and cook for 15 minutes. Add brussels sprouts and mushrooms and toss to coat.

4. Cook another 15-20 minutes until veggies are lightly browned and cooked through.

5. Adjust seasoning as needed. Enjoy!

Butter Braised Green Beans

Servings: 6
Cooking Time: 60 Minutes

Ingredients:
- 24 Ounce thin fresh green beans, trimmed or whole frozen green beans, thawed
- 8 Tablespoon butter, melted
- Veggie Rub or coarse salt
- freshly ground black pepper

Directions:
1. Supply your smoker with wood pellets and follow the start-up procedure. Preheat the grill, with the lid closed, to 325° F.

2. Put the green beans in a pile on a rimmed baking sheet and pour the melted butter over them. Using tongs, spread the beans out in the pan and season with Traeger Veggie Rub and black pepper.

3. Roast the beans for about 1 hour, stirring and lifting with tongs every 20 minutes or so. The beans should be very tender, shriveled, and lightly browned in places. Transfer to a serving bowl and serve while hot. Enjoy!

Bacon Wrapped Corn On The Cob

Servings: 4
Cooking Time: 21 Minutes

Ingredients:
- 4 Whole Corn, ears
- 8 Slices bacon

- 1 Teaspoon freshly ground black pepper
- 1 Teaspoon chili powder
- 1 To Taste Parmesan cheese, grated

Directions:
1. Peel back the corn husks, remove silk strings and rinse corn under cold water.
2. Wrap 2 pieces of bacon around each ear of corn, securing with toothpicks.
3. Dust each ear of corn with some chili powder and cracked black pepper.
4. Supply your smoker with wood pellets and follow the start-up procedure. Preheat the grill, with the lid closed, to 375° F.
5. Place the ears of corn directly on the Traeger and grill for approximately 20 minutes or until the bacon is cooked crisp. Grill: 375 °F
6. Take the corn off the Traeger. Carefully remove the toothpicks and season with a little more chili powder and a grating of parmesan cheese, if desired. Serve & enjoy!

Roasted Garlic Herb Fries

Servings: 4
Cooking Time: 45 Minutes

Ingredients:
- 4 Whole russet potatoes
- 1 Teaspoon salt
- 2 Tablespoon avocado oil
- 1 Teaspoon fresh chopped rosemary
- 1 Teaspoon fresh chopped thyme
- 2 Clove garlic, minced
- 2 Teaspoon flake salt
- 1 Teaspoon chopped parsley, for garnish

Directions:
1. Supply your smoker with wood pellets and follow the start-up procedure. Preheat the grill, with the lid closed, to 425° F.
2. Chop potatoes into fries, (a mandolin works great for this) and place directly into an ice water bath with 1 teaspoon salt for 15 to 30 minutes.
3. Combine oil, rosemary, thyme and garlic in a big bowl. Remove potatoes from ice water and dry thoroughly with paper towels.

4. Toss potatoes in the oil mixture and place them on 2 to 3 parchment-lined baking sheets in a single layer. Sprinkle the flake salt over the fries.
5. Place baking sheets on the grill and roast for 30 minutes, flip the fries, then cook for an additional 15 minutes until golden and crispy. Dust with parsley. Grill: 425 °F
6. Serve with your favorite dipping sauce, side dish or as a nacho base.

Grilled Asparagus & Honey-glazed Carrots

Servings: 4
Cooking Time: 35 Minutes

Ingredients:
- 1 Bunch asparagus, woody ends removed
- 1 Pound Carrots, peeled
- 2 Tablespoon olive oil
- sea salt
- 2 Tablespoon honey
- lemon zest

Directions:
1. Rinse all vegetables under cold water. Drizzle asparagus with olive oil and a generous sprinkling of sea salt. Generously drizzle carrots with honey and lightly sprinkle with sea salt.
2. Supply your smoker with wood pellets and follow the start-up procedure. Preheat the grill, with the lid closed, to 350° F.
3. Place carrots on the grill first and cook for 10-15 minutes, then add asparagus and cook both for another 15 to 20 minutes, or until they're done to your liking. Grill: 350 °F
4. Top the asparagus with some fresh lemon zest. Enjoy!

Potluck Salad With Smoked Cornbread

Servings: 6
Cooking Time: 45 Minutes

Ingredients:

- 1 cup all-purpose flour
- 1 cup yellow cornmeal
- 1 tablespoon sugar
- 2 teaspoons baking powder
- 1 teaspoon salt
- 1 cup milk
- 1 egg, beaten, at room temperature
- 4 tablespoons (½ stick) unsalted butter, melted and cooled
- Nonstick cooking spray or butter, for greasing
- ½ cup milk
- ½ cup sour cream
- 2 tablespoons dry ranch dressing mix
- 1 pound bacon, cooked and crumbled
- 3 tomatoes, chopped
- 1 bell pepper, chopped
- 1 cucumber, seeded and chopped
- 2 stalks celery, chopped (about 1 cup)
- ½ cup chopped scallions

Directions:

1. For the cornbread:
2. In a medium bowl, combine the flour, cornmeal, sugar, baking powder, and salt.
3. In a small bowl, whisk together the milk and egg. Pour in the butter, then slowly fold this mixture into the dry ingredients.
4. Supply your smoker with wood pellets and follow the start-up procedure. Preheat, with the lid closed, to 375°F.
5. Coat a cast iron skillet with cooking spray or butter.
6. Pour the batter into the skillet, place on the grill grate, close the lid, and smoke for 35 to 45 minutes, or until the cornbread is browned and pulls away from the side of the skillet.
7. Remove the cornbread from the grill and let cool, then coarsely crumble.
8. For the salad:
9. In a small bowl, whisk together the milk, sour cream, and ranch dressing mix.
10. In a medium bowl, combine the crumbled bacon, tomatoes, bell pepper, cucumber, celery, and scallions.
11. In a large serving bowl, layer half of the crumbled cornbread, half of the bacon-veggie mixture, and half of the dressing. Toss lightly.
12. Repeat the layering with the remaining cornbread, bacon-veggie mixture, and dressing. Toss again.
13. Refrigerate the salad for at least 1 hour. Serve cold.

Baked Breakfast Mini Quiches

Servings: 8
Cooking Time: 15 Minutes

Ingredients:

- cooking spray
- 1 Tablespoon extra-virgin olive oil
- 1/2 yellow onion, diced
- 3 Cup Spinach, fresh
- 10 eggs
- 4 Ounce shredded cheddar, mozzarella or Swiss cheese
- 1/4 Cup fresh basil
- 1 Teaspoon kosher salt
- 1/2 Teaspoon black pepper

Directions:

1. Spray a 12-cup muffin tin generously with cooking spray.
2. In a small skillet over medium heat, warm the oil. Add the onion and cook, stirring frequently, until softened, about 7 minutes. Add the spinach and cook until wilted, about 1 minute longer.
3. Transfer to a cutting board to cool, then chop the mixture so the spinach if broken up a little.
4. Supply your smoker with wood pellets and follow the start-up procedure. Preheat the grill, with the lid closed, to 350° F.
5. In a large bowl, whisk the eggs until frothy. Add the cooled onions and spinach, cheese, basil, 1 tsp salt and 1/2 tsp pepper. Stir to combine. Divide egg mixture evenly among the muffin cups.

6. Place tray on the grill and bake until the eggs have puffed up, are set, and are beginning to brown, about 18 to 20 minutes. Grill: 350 °F

7. Serve immediately, or allow to cool on a wire rack, then refrigerate in an air tight container for up to 4 days. Enjoy!

Smoked Jalapeño Poppers

Servings: 4
Cooking Time: 60 Minutes

Ingredients:

- 12 Medium jalapeño
- 6 Slices bacon, cut in half
- 8 Ounce cream cheese
- 2 Tablespoon Pork & Poultry Rub
- 1 Cup grated cheese

Directions:

1. Supply your smoker with wood pellets and follow the start-up procedure. Preheat the grill, with the lid closed, to 180° F. For optimal flavor, use Super Smoke if available.

2. Slice the jalapeños in half lengthwise. Scrape out any seeds and ribs with a small spoon or paring knife. Mix softened cream cheese with Traeger Pork & Poultry rub and grated cheese. Spoon mixture onto each jalapeño half. Wrap with bacon and secure with a toothpick.

3. Place the jalapeños on a rimmed baking sheet. Place on grill and smoke for 30 minutes. Grill: 180 °F

4. Increase the grill temperature to 375°F and cook an additional 30 minutes or until bacon is cooked to desired doneness. Serve warm, enjoy! Grill: 375 °F

Traeger Grilled Whole Corn

Servings: 4
Cooking Time: 25 Minutes

Ingredients:

- 3 green onions
- 6 Tablespoon butter, softened
- 1 Teaspoon chile powder
- 1 Teaspoon toasted sesame seeds
- 4 ears corn, in husk

Directions:

1. Supply your smoker with wood pellets and follow the start-up procedure. Preheat the grill, with the lid closed, to 325° F.

2. Place green onions directly on the grill grate and cook 15 minutes until lightly charred. Remove from grill and set aside.

3. Sesame-Chile Butter: Take butter out of fridge and let soften. Chop up charred green onions and add to butter along with chile powder and sesame seeds. Mash all ingredients together.

4. Grill corn, rotating occasionally, until husks are blackened (some will flake and fall off) and kernels are tender with some browned and charred spots, about 25 to 35 minutes. Grill: 325 °F

5. Let corn cool slightly, then shuck. Serve with the Sesame-Chile Butter. Enjoy

Smoked Mashed Potatoes

Servings: 6
Cooking Time: 45 Minutes

Ingredients:

- 2 Pound red bliss potatoes, washed and diced medium
- chicken stock or water
- 1/2 Stick salted butter
- 1 Cup whole milk
- 1/2 Cup sour cream
- 1/2 Cup shredded or grated Parmesan cheese
- kosher salt
- freshly ground black pepper
- 1/2 Cup fresh sliced green onions

Directions:

1. Place the diced red potatoes into a small saucepan or stockpot and cover with chicken stock or water.

2. Bring to a boil and cook on a simmer until fork tender, then cook 4 to 5 minutes past that until soft.

3. Supply your smoker with wood pellets and follow the start-up procedure. Preheat the grill, with the lid closed, to 400° F.

4. In a separate ovenproof pan, such as a cast iron skillet, add butter and milk and place in the Traeger

during start up, until melted (approximately 7 to 10 minutes). Grill: 400 °F

5. Carefully remove the butter/milk mixture from the Traeger using heatproof gloves.

6. Drain the potatoes and place into a large bowl. Add the melted butter/milk mixture and slowly mash.

7. Add sour cream, cheese and green onions, then season to taste with salt and pepper.

8. Place into the cast iron skillet, then place the skillet back into the Traeger and cook until the potatoes have a slight crust and are bubbling, about 15 minutes. Grill: 400 °F

9. Carefully remove the mashed potatoes from the Traeger using heatproof gloves. Allow to cool for 5 minutes. Scoop and enjoy!

Grilled Beer Cabbage

Servings: 4
Cooking Time: 50 Minutes

Ingredients:

- 2 Cabbage, head
- 1 Tablespoon extra-virgin olive oil
- 1 Teaspoon salt
- 1 Teaspoon freshly ground black pepper
- 14 Fluid Ounce Guinness Extra Stout

Directions:

1. Clean and core cabbages. Drizzle with olive oil and salt and pepper. Rub into the cabbage.

2. Supply your smoker with wood pellets and follow the start-up procedure. Preheat the grill, with the lid closed, to 180° F.

3. Place cabbages directly on grill grate; smoke for 15 to 20 minutes. Remove from grill and thickly slice cabbage. Grill: 180 °F

4. Place sliced cabbage in cast-iron skillet. Pour beer over cabbage and return to grill.

5. Increase temperature to 375°F and cook for 30 minutes, or until cabbage has reached desired softness. Grill: 375 °F

6. Serve with corned beef. Enjoy!

Tater Tot Bake

Servings: 4
Cooking Time: 15 Minutes

Ingredients:

- 1 Whole frozen tater tots
- salt and pepper
- 1 Cup sour cream
- 1 Cup shredded cheddar cheese, divided
- 1/2 Cup bacon, chopped
- 1/4 Cup green onion, diced

Directions:

1. Supply your smoker with wood pellets and follow the start-up procedure. Preheat the grill, with the lid closed, to 375° F.

2. Line a baking sheet with aluminum foil for easy clean up and spread frozen tater tots onto sheet.

3. Sprinkle with Veggie Shake or salt and pepper to taste.

4. Place the baking sheet on the preheated grill grate and cook the tater tots for 10 minutes.

5. Drizzle sour cream over cooked tater tots.

6. Sprinkle the cheese, bacon bits and green onions on top of the tater tots.

7. Turn heat up to High heat and cook for 5 more minutes until the cheese melts and serve immediately. Enjoy!

Salt Crusted Baked Potatoes

Servings: 4
Cooking Time: 60 Minutes

Ingredients:

- 6 russet potatoes, scrubbed and dried
- 3 Tablespoon canola oil
- 1 Tablespoon kosher salt
- butter
- sour cream
- Chives, fresh
- Bacon Bits
- cheddar cheese

Directions:

1. In a large bowl, coat the potatoes in canola oil and sprinkle heavily with salt.
2. Supply your smoker with wood pellets and follow the start-up procedure. Preheat the grill, with the lid closed, to 450° F.
3. Place the potatoes directly on the grill grate and bake for 30-40 minutes, or until soft in the middle when pricked with a fork. Serve loaded with your favorite toppings. Enjoy! Grill: 450 °F

Roasted Hasselback Potatoes By Doug Scheiding

Servings: 6
Cooking Time: 120 Minutes

Ingredients:
- 6 Large russet potatoes
- 1 Pound bacon
- 1/2 Cup butter
- salt
- black pepper
- 1 Cup cheddar cheese
- 3 Whole scallions

Directions:
1. To cut potatoes, place two wooden spoons on either side of the potato (this prevents your knife from going all the way through). Slice potato into thin chips leaving about 1/4" attached on the bottom.
2. Freeze bacon slices for about 30 minutes then cut into small pieces about the size of a stamp. Place these in the cracks between every other slice.
3. Place the potato in a large cast iron skillet. Top the potato with slices of hard butter (you can also place thin slivers of cold butter between the potato slices with the bacon if desired). Season with salt and pepper.
4. Supply your smoker with wood pellets and follow the start-up procedure. Preheat the grill, with the lid closed, to 350° F.
5. Place the cast iron directly on the grill grate and cook for two hours. Top potatoes with more butter and baste with melted butter every 30 minutes.
6. In the last 10 minutes of cooking, sprinkle with cheddar and return to grill to melt.
7. To finish, top with chives or scallions. Enjoy!

Roasted Jalapeño Poppers

Servings: 2
Cooking Time: 30 Minutes

Ingredients:
- 8 Slices Bacon, Center Cut
- 2 Cup cream cheese
- 2 Ounce Cheese, sharp cheddar
- 1/2 Cup green onions, minced
- 2 Teaspoon fresh squeezed lime juice
- 4 Tablespoon Seeded Tomato, Chopped
- 4 Tablespoon cilantro, chopped
- 1/2 Teaspoon kosher salt
- 2 Small garlic clove, minced
- 12 Whole Jalapeños

Directions:
1. Supply your smoker with wood pellets and follow the start-up procedure. Preheat the grill, with the lid closed, to 350° F.
2. Place 2 bacon slices directly on the grill grate and cook 10-15 minutes until cooked through and crispy flipping halfway through. Remove from grill, but leave the grill on. When cool enough to handle, coarsely chop the bacon and reserve. Grill: 350 °F
3. In the bowl of a stand mixer, combine cream cheese, cheddar cheese, green onions, chopped bacon, lime juice, tomatoes, cilantro, salt and garlic. Mix on medium speed with a paddle until combined. Transfer mixture to a piping bag.
4. Cut the tops off the jalapeños and remove the seeds and ribs with a small paring knife.
5. Pipe the filling into each pepper so that the filling comes up a 1/4" over the top of the pepper. Place the tops back on each pepper.
6. With a rolling pin, flatten out the remaining six slices of bacon until they are 1/8" thick. Cut each slice in half. Wrap 1/2 a bacon slice around each pepper and secure with a toothpick.
7. Place the peppers in the Traeger Jalapeno Popper Tray. Place the tray directly on the grill grate and cook for 30-40 minutes until the peppers are tender, bacon is crispy, and cheese is melted. Enjoy! Grill: 350 °F

Red Potato Grilled Lollipops

Servings: 4
Cooking Time: 25 Minutes

Ingredients:

- 8 Large red bliss potatoes, halved
- 2 Clove garlic, minced
- 2 Sprig rosemary, minced
- 2 Tablespoon olive oil
- 1 Teaspoon salt
- 1/2 Teaspoon black pepper
- 5 Wooden Skewers, soaked in water
- 1/4 Cup Parmesan cheese, grated

Directions:

1. Supply your smoker with wood pellets and follow the start-up procedure. Preheat the grill, with the lid closed, to 450° F.
2. Halve potatoes and poke each several times with a fork.
3. Put the potatoes in a large bowl and toss with the minced garlic, rosemary leaves, a few tablespoons of olive oil, kosher salt, and pepper. Microwave the potatoes for 4 minutes. Gently toss potatoes and microwave for another 3 minutes.
4. Skewer potato halves threading about 4 or 5 potato halves on each skewer. Brush potatoes with olive oil.
5. Place the potato skewers on the Traeger, cut side down, and grill until the sides begin to brown (4-7 minutes).
6. Flip and grill skin side down for another 7-10 minutes.
7. They are done when a sharp knife tip easily penetrates the sides. Remove potatoes from grill and top with grated parmesan cheese. Enjoy!

Blt Pasta Salad

Servings: 6
Cooking Time: 45 Minutes

Ingredients:

- 1 pound thick-cut bacon
- 16 ounces bowtie pasta, cooked according to package directions and drained
- 2 tomatoes, chopped
- ½ cup chopped scallions
- ½ cup Italian dressing
- ½ cup ranch dressing
- 1 tablespoon chopped fresh basil
- 1 teaspoon salt
- 1 teaspoon freshly ground black pepper
- 1 teaspoon garlic powder
- 1 head lettuce, cored and torn

Directions:

1. Supply your smoker with wood pellets and follow the start-up procedure. Preheat, with the lid closed, to 225°F.
2. Arrange the bacon slices on the grill grate, close the lid, and cook for 30 to 45 minutes, flipping after 20 minutes, until crisp.
3. Remove the bacon from the grill and chop.
4. In a large bowl, combine the chopped bacon with the cooked pasta, tomatoes, scallions, Italian dressing, ranch dressing, basil, salt, pepper, and garlic powder. Refrigerate until ready to serve.
5. Toss in the lettuce just before serving to keep it from wilting.

Sweet Potato Marshmallow Casserole

Servings: 6
Cooking Time: 60 Minutes

Ingredients:

- 5 Yams
- 1 1/2 Stick butter
- 1/2 Cup brown sugar
- 1 Teaspoon vanilla
- 1 Teaspoon kosher salt
- 1 Teaspoon cracked black pepper
- 1 Marshmallows, miniature
- 1/4 Unsalted Butter, Softened

Directions:

1. Supply your smoker with wood pellets and follow the start-up procedure. Preheat the grill, with the lid closed, to 375° F.
2. Pierce the skin of the yams with a fork a few times. Place on a baking sheet or foil tin inside the grill and let

roast for 50 minutes or until extremely softened. Grill: 375 °F

3. Remove yams from the grill and set aside until cool enough to handle. While the potatoes cool, with a stiff whisk, whip together 1/2 cup softened butter, the brown sugar, vanilla, salt and pepper.

4. Remove and discard skins from sweet potatoes and mash until smooth. Fold in the butter mixture and transfer to a cast iron pan.

5. Place cast iron on the grill and bake for 15-20 minutes. Remove from the grill, top with marshmallows and dot with remaining 1/4 cup butter.

6. Place back in the grill for 15 minutes until warm and the marshmallows are golden. Enjoy! Grill: 375 °F

Grilled Street Corn

Servings: 6
Cooking Time: 10 Minutes

Ingredients:
- 6 ears corn, husked
- 1 As Needed extra-virgin olive oil
- 1/4 Cup mayonnaise
- 1 Tablespoon ancho or guajillo chile powder
- 1/2 Cup chopped cilantro, plus more for serving
- 1 lime, zested and juiced
- salt
- 1/2 Cup Cotija cheese
- 1 As Needed cilantro, finely chopped

Directions:
1. Supply your smoker with wood pellets and follow the start-up procedure. Preheat the grill, with the lid closed, to 450° F.
2. Brush corn with oil and place on grill, turning occasionally.
3. While corn is on the grill, mix mayonnaise with chile powder, cilantro, lime juice and zest in a bowl. Season with salt.
4. After about 10 minutes corn should be cooked through and slightly charred on the outside. Remove from grill.
5. Top corn with chile mayonnaise then sprinkle on the Cotija cheese and chopped cilantro. Enjoy!

Smoked Parmesan Herb Popcorn

Servings: 2
Cooking Time: 15 Minutes

Ingredients:
- 4 Tablespoon butter
- 2 Teaspoon Italian Seasoning
- 1 Teaspoon garlic powder
- 1 Teaspoon salt
- 1/4 Cup popcorn kernels
- 1/2 Cup Parmesan cheese, grated

Directions:
1. Supply your smoker with wood pellets and follow the start-up procedure. Preheat the grill, with the lid closed, to 250° F.
2. In a small saucepan, melt the butter over medium heat. Add Italian seasoning, garlic powder, and salt and stir to combine. Remove from heat and set aside.
3. Add 1/4 cup of popcorn to a brown paper lunch bag. Fold the top of the bag over twice to close. Place the bag in the microwave and microwave on high for 1 to 2 minutes, or until there are about 5 seconds between pops. Open the bag with care and dump into a large mixing bowl.
4. Pour butter mixture of popcorn in a bowl and toss to combine. Dump popcorn onto a baking sheet and place in grill.
5. Smoke for 10 minutes; remove from grill. Toss with parmesan cheese to serve. Enjoy! Grill: 250 °F

Traeger Baked Potato Torte

Servings: 6
Cooking Time: 25 Minutes

Ingredients:
- 6 Yukon Gold potatoes, sliced 1/4 inch thick
- 2 Stick butter, melted
- 3 Clove garlic, crushed
- 2 Tablespoon rosemary, chopped
- 1 Cup Parmesan cheese, grated
- salt and pepper

Directions:

1. Supply your smoker with wood pellets and follow the start-up procedure. Preheat the grill, with the lid closed, to 375° F.

2. While the Traeger is heating up, peel and slice the potatoes (make sure to put them in water so they will not oxidize). Melt the butter and combine it with the crushed garlic.

3. Grease a 12" cast iron pan with butter and start to layer the torte. The layers should go as follows, potatoes, butter garlic mixture, rosemary, parmesan, continue layering to the top of the pan, about 4 to 5 layers.

4. Place the pan in the Traeger and bake for 20 to 25 minutes, or until the potatoes are fully cooked. If the top of the torte starts to darken before it is finished cooking, reduce the heat to 325°F. Serve hot and enjoy! Grill: 375 °F

Roasted Pickled Beets

Servings: 8
Cooking Time: 60 Minutes

Ingredients:
- 6 Medium Red Beets, scrubbed and trimmed
- 1 Cup red wine vinegar
- 1/2 Cup sugar
- 10 Whole peppercorns
- 1 Cup water
- 1 1/2 Teaspoon coarse salt
- 8 whole cloves
- 2 Pieces Star Anise, Broken
- 1 cinnamon stick, broken in half

Directions:
1. Make a foil pouch large enough to enclose the beets. Poke a few holes in the top to allow steam to escape.

2. Supply your smoker with wood pellets and follow the start-up procedure. Preheat the grill, with the lid closed, to 350° F.

3. Roast the beets until they are tender, 50 to 60 minutes. Carefully remove the foil and allow the beets to cool until they can be comfortably handled. Grill: 350 °F

4. Slip the skins off with your fingers. (You may wish to wear latex gloves to avoid staining your hands.) Cut the beets into quarters or slices. (Candy cane beets are especially pretty when sliced.)

5. In the meantime, make the brine: Bring the vinegar, sugar, salt, and water to a boil in a small saucepan over high heat.

6. Put the cloves, peppercorns, star anise, and cinnamon in a clean lidded jar, such as a canning jar

7. Add the beets to the jar. Pour the hot brine over the beets. Put the lid on the jar. Cool the beets to room temperature, then refrigerate for 3 to 5 days before serving. Enjoy!

Cast Iron Potatoes

Servings: 4
Cooking Time: 60 Minutes

Ingredients:
- 4 Tablespoon butter, cut into cubes
- 2 1/2 Pound potatoes, peeled and cut into 1/8 inch slices
- 1/2 Large sweet onion, thinly sliced
- salt
- black pepper
- 1 1/2 Cup grated mild cheddar or jack cheese
- 2 Cup milk
- paprika

Directions:
1. Butter the inside of a cast iron skillet and layer half the potato slices on the bottom. Top with half the onions. Season with salt and pepper.

2. Sprinkle 1 cup of the cheese over the potatoes and onions and dot with half the butter. Layer the remaining potatoes and onions on top. Dot with remaining butter.

3. Pour the milk into the skillet. Cover the skillet tightly with aluminum foil.

4. Supply your smoker with wood pellets and follow the start-up procedure. Preheat the grill, with the lid closed, to 350° F.

5. Bake for 1 hour, or until the potatoes are very tender. Grill: 350 °F

6. Remove the foil and top with the remaining 1/2 cup of cheese. Bake for 30 minutes more (uncovered) until the cheese is lightly browned. Dust the top with paprika and serve immediately.

Roasted Potato Poutine

Servings: 5
Cooking Time: 40 Minutes

Ingredients:

- 4 Large russet potatoes
- Tablespoon olive oil or vegetable oil
- Prime Rib Rub
- Cup chicken or beef gravy (homemade or jarred)
- 1 1/2 Cup white or yellow cheddar cheese curds
- freshly ground black pepper
- 2 Tablespoon scallions

Directions:

1. Supply your smoker with wood pellets and follow the start-up procedure. Preheat the grill, with the lid closed, to 500° F.
2. Scrub the potatoes and slice into fries, wedges or preferred shape.
3. Put potatoes into a large mixing bowl and coat with oil. Season generously with Traeger Prime Rib rub.
4. Tip the potatoes onto a rimmed baking sheet and spread in a single layer, cut sides down.
5. Roast for 20 minutes, then using a spatula, turn the potatoes to the other cut side. Continue to roast until the potatoes are tender and golden brown, about 15 to 20 minutes more.
6. While potatoes cook, warm the gravy on the stovetop or in a heat-proof saucepan on your Traeger.
7. To assemble the poutine, arrange the potatoes in a large shallow bowl or on a serving platter. Distribute the cheese curds on top. Pour the hot gravy evenly over the potatoes and cheese curds.
8. Season with black pepper and garnish with thinly sliced scallions. Serve immediately. Enjoy!

Baked Garlic Duchess Potatoes

Servings: 8
Cooking Time: 60 Minutes

Ingredients:

- 12 Medium Potatoes, Yukon gold
- salt
- 5 Large Egg Yolk
- 2 Clove garlic, minced

- 1.24 Cup heavy cream
- 3/4 Cup sour cream
- 10 Tablespoon butter, melted
- black pepper

Directions:

1. Place potatoes in a large pot and fill with water. Season with salt. Bring to a boil over medium-high heat.
2. Reduce heat and simmer until a paring knife easily slides through potatoes, about 25 to 35 minutes. Drain and let cool slightly.
3. Supply your smoker with wood pellets and follow the start-up procedure. Preheat the grill, with the lid closed, to 450° F.
4. Whisk together egg yolks, garlic, cream, sour cream, butter, and pepper in a large bowl. Season with salt.
5. Peel potatoes and push flesh through a ricer or a food mill directly into bowl with egg mixture. Fold in the egg mixture being careful not to overmix.
6. Transfer to a 3-quart baking dish and bake until golden brown and slightly puffed, about 30–40 minutes. Enjoy! Grill: 450 °F

Roasted Olives

Servings: 4
Cooking Time: 45 Minutes

Ingredients:

- 2 Cup mixed olives
- 3 Sprig fresh rosemary
- 2 Clove garlic, minced
- 2 Tablespoon orange zest
- 1/3 Cup extra-virgin olive oil
- 2 Tablespoon orange juice
- 1/2 Teaspoon red pepper flakes

Directions:

1. Combine the olives, rosemary, garlic, orange zest, red pepper flakes, olive oil, and orange juice in a glass oven-safe pie plate or baking dish. Cover with foil.
2. Supply your smoker with wood pellets and follow the start-up procedure. Preheat the grill, with the lid closed, to 300° F.
3. Roast the olives for 45 minutes, stirring once or twice. Serve warm in an attractive bowl. Enjoy! Grill: 300 °F

Mashed Red Potatoes

Servings: 4
Cooking Time: 40 Minutes

Ingredients:

- 8 Large red potatoes
- salt
- black pepper
- 1/2 Cup heavy cream
- 1/4 Cup butter

Directions:

1. Supply your smoker with wood pellets and follow the start-up procedure. Preheat the grill, with the lid closed, to 180° F.
2. Slice red potatoes in half, lengthwise then cut in half again to make quarters. Season potatoes with salt and pepper.
3. Increase the heat to High and preheat. Once the grill is hot, set potatoes directly on the grill grate. Grill: 450 °F
4. Every 15 minutes flip potatoes to ensure all sides get color. Continue to do this until potatoes are fork tender.
5. When tender, mash potatoes with cream, butter, salt, and pepper to taste. Serve warm, enjoy!

Smoked Bbq Onion Brussels Sprout

Servings: 4
Cooking Time: 110 Minutes

Ingredients:

- 4 strip bacon
- 1 onion minced
- 2 cloves garlic minced
- 1 lb brussels sprouts stems trimmed and cut in half
- 1 tbsp BBQ Spice Blend
- 1/2 cup Apple Habanero Bar-B-Que Sauce (or other BBQ sauce)

Directions:

1. Supply your smoker with wood pellets and follow the start-up procedure. Preheat the grill, with the lid closed, to High heat. Place a cast iron skillet over the highest heat spot and cook the bacon until crisp.
2. Remove the bacon from pan and drain, reserving the bacon fat in the pan.
3. Reduce the heat on your smoker to 250°F.
4. Add the onions, garlic, and brussels to the pan and toss to coat in the bacon drippings. Sprinkle the BBQ spice blend over top.
5. Cover the lid and allow to smoke for 1 to 1 1/2 hours, until the sprouts are fork tender.
6. For the last 20 minutes of smoking, toss the brussels sprouts in half of the barbecue sauce.
7. Remove the sprouts from the smoker.
8. Chop the bacon and add it and the remaining barbecue sauce to the pan of sprouts, tossing to coat.
9. Serve hot.

Roasted Tomatoes

Servings: 2
Cooking Time: 180 Minutes

Ingredients:

- 3 Large ripe tomatoes
- 1/2 Tablespoon kosher salt
- 1 Teaspoon coarse ground black pepper
- 1/4 Teaspoon sugar
- 1/4 Teaspoon thyme or basil
- olive oil

Directions:

1. Line a rimmed baking sheet with parchment paper.
2. Supply your smoker with wood pellets and follow the start-up procedure. Preheat the grill, with the lid closed, to 225° F.
3. Remove the stem end from each tomato and cut the tomatoes into 1/2 inch thick slices.
4. Combine the salt, pepper, sugar and thyme or basil in a small bowl and mix.
5. Pour olive oil into the well of a dinner plate.
6. Dip one side of each tomato slice in the olive oil and arrange on the baking sheet. Dust the tomato slices with the seasoning mixture.
7. Arrange the pan directly on the grill grate and roast the tomatoes until the juices stop running and the edges have contracted, about 3 hours. Remove from grill and enjoy!

Baked Sweet And Savory Yams By Bennie Kendrick

Servings: 6
Cooking Time: 60 Minutes

Ingredients:
- 3 Medium Yams
- 3 Tablespoon extra-virgin olive oil
- honey
- Goat Cheese
- 1/2 Cup brown sugar
- 1/2 Cup Pecans, pieces

Directions:
1. Supply your smoker with wood pellets and follow the start-up procedure. Preheat the grill, with the lid closed, to 350° F.
2. While Traeger comes to temperature, wash yams and poke a few holes all over. Wrap yams in foil.
3. Bake for 45-60 minutes or until knife tender. You don't want to overcook and get the yams too soft because you want to be able to cut each yam into rounds.
4. Once yams have cooled to the touch, cut each into 1/4" rounds. Lightly coat each round with oil olive and place on sheet tray.
5. Sprinkle each top with brown sugar. Using a teaspoon, place desired amount of goat cheese on each round. Next top with chopped pecans. Finally, drizzle Bee Local honey over each round.
6. Based on how sweet you like your yams, you can add more brown sugar and honey.
7. After complete, place your sheet tray back in the grill and cook, lid closed, for another 20 minutes. Enjoy!

Roasted Asparagus

Servings: 4
Cooking Time: 30 Minutes

Ingredients:
- 1 Bunch asparagus
- 2 Tablespoon olive oil, plus more as needed
- Veggie Rub

Directions:

1. Coat asparagus with olive oil and Veggie Rub, stirring to coat all pieces.
2. Supply your smoker with wood pellets and follow the start-up procedure. Preheat the grill, with the lid closed, to 350° F.
3. Place asparagus directly on the grill grate for 15-20 minutes.
4. Remove from grill and enjoy!

Roasted Pumpkin Seeds

Servings: 8
Cooking Time: 40 Minutes

Ingredients:
- 1 Whole Pumpkin, seeds
- olive oil or vegetable oil
- Jacobsen Salt Co. Pure Kosher Sea Salt

Directions:
1. As soon as possible after removing the seeds from the pumpkin, rinse pumpkin seeds under cold water in a colander and pick out the pulp and strings.
2. Place the pumpkin seeds in a single layer on an oiled baking sheet, stirring to coat. Supply your smoker with wood pellets and follow the start-up procedure. Preheat the grill, with the lid closed, to 180° F.
3. Place the baking sheet with the seeds on the grill grate, close the lid, and smoke for 20 minutes. Grill: 180 °F
4. Sprinkle your seeds with salt and turn the temperature on your grill up to 325°F. Roast the seeds until toasted, about 20 minutes. Check and stir seeds after the first 10 minutes. Grill: 325 °F
5. Seeds will be brown because they were smoked before being roasted. Enjoy!

Smoked Asparagus Soup

Servings: 4
Cooking Time: 40 Minutes

Ingredients:
- Pound Asparagus Spears
- 1 Tablespoon olive oil
- salt and pepper
- 1/2 yellow onion, diced

- 1 Tablespoon butter
- 2 Clove garlic, minced
- 1 1/2 Cup chicken stock
- 1 1/2 Cup cream
- 2 Stalk Raw Asparagus, Shaved

Directions:

1. Supply your smoker with wood pellets and follow the start-up procedure. Preheat the grill, with the lid closed, to 180° F.

2. Drizzle 1 pound of asparagus with olive oil and season with salt and pepper. Place directly on the grill grate and smoke for 20-30 minutes. Taste along the way to assess smoke level pulling earlier if needed. Grill: 180 °F

3. Place 1 Tbsp butter in a saucepan and melt over medium heat. Add onion and garlic and saute for 2-3 minutes or until onion is translucent.

4. Remove asparagus from the grill and cut into 1" pieces. Place asparagus in the pan with the onions and add stock and cream. Bring to a simmer.

5. Remove from heat and puree using a blender or immersion blender until smooth.

6. Season with salt and pepper and serve. Top with fresh shaved asparagus, sprinkle with salt, pepper, and smoked paprika if desired. Enjoy!

Roasted Red Pepper White Bean Dip

Servings: 4
Cooking Time: 40 Minutes

Ingredients:

- 4 Whole garlic
- 4 Tablespoon extra-virgin olive oil
- 2 Bell Pepper, Red
- 3 Tablespoon Dill Weed, fresh
- 3 Tablespoon chopped flat-leaf parsley
- 2 Can cannellini beans, mashed
- 4 Teaspoon lemon juice
- 1 1/2 Teaspoon salt

Directions:

1. Roasting the garlic and red peppers:

2. Supply your smoker with wood pellets and follow the start-up procedure. Preheat the grill, with the lid closed, to 400° F.

3. Peel away the outside layers of the garlic husk. Cut off the top of the garlic bulb, exposing each of the individual cloves. Drizzle olive oil over the top of the head of garlic and rub it in. Wrap the garlic in foil, completely covering it. Put the head of garlic and the two red peppers (washed and dried) on the Traeger.

4. Roast the garlic for 25-30 minutes and the peppers for about 40 minutes. Rotate the peppers a quarter-turn every 10 minutes until the exterior is blistered and blackened. Grill: 400 °F

5. Pull the peppers off the grill and put them in a bowl. Cover the bowl with plastic wrap and leave them for 15 minutes. The steam will loosen the skins so that they slip off like a drumstick covered in barbecue sauce.

6. Peel off the pepper skin. Cut off the stems and scrape out the seeds and they're ready to use.

7. As for the garlic, let it cool and then pull out the individual cloves as needed.

8. The dip:

9. In a blender put the roasted red peppers, 4 cloves of roasted garlic, dill, parsley, drained and rinsed beans, olive oil, lemon juice and salt.

10. Blend until the dip is smooth and creamy. You may need to scrape down the sides of the blender a couple of times. If it's having difficulty blending or looks too thick add more olive oil or lemon juice. (Add more lemon juice if it tastes like it needs more acid or brightness.) Enjoy!

Skillet Potato Cake

Servings: 4
Cooking Time: 40 Minutes

Ingredients:

- 8 Tablespoon butter, melted
- 2 Pound russet potatoes, peeled and thinly sliced
- 3 Tablespoon kosher salt
- 2 Tablespoon freshly ground black pepper
- thyme

Directions:

1. Supply your smoker with wood pellets and follow the start-up procedure. Preheat the grill, with the lid closed, to 375° F.

2. Brush the bottom of a cast iron skillet with part of the melted butter. Place potato slices vertically around the outer edges then fill in the middle in the same fashion.

3. Pour additional melted butter over the top of the layers and sprinkle with salt and pepper.

4. Place skillet in grill and cook for 35 to 40 minutes or until potatoes are fork tender and golden brown.

5. Garnish with a sprinkle of fresh thyme over the top of the potatoes. Enjoy!

BAKING RECIPES

Baked Cast Iron Berry Cobbler

Servings: 6
Cooking Time: 35 Minutes

Ingredients:
- 4 Cup Berries
- 12 Tablespoon sugar
- Cup orange juice
- 2/3 Cup Flour
- 3/4 Teaspoon baking powder
- 1 Pinch salt
- 1/2 Cup butter
- 1 Tablespoon Sugar, raw

Directions:
1. Supply your smoker with wood pellets and follow the start-up procedure. Preheat the grill, with the lid closed, to 350° F.
2. In a 10-inch (25-cm) cast iron or other baking pan, mix together the berries, 4 Tbsp sugar and the orange juice.
3. In a small bowl, mix together the flour, baking powder and salt. Set aside.
4. In a separate bowl, cream together the butter and granulated sugar. Add the egg and vanilla extract and mix to combine. Gradually fold in the flour mixture.
5. Spoon the batter on top of the berries and sprinkle raw sugar on top.
6. Bake the cobbler for approximately 35-45 minutes. Cool slightly and serve with whipped cream. Enjoy! Grill: 350 °F

Double Chocolate Chip Brownie Pie

Servings: 8-12
Cooking Time: 45 Minutes

Ingredients:
- 1/2 Cup Semisweet Chocolate Chips
- 1 Cup butter
- 1 Cup brown sugar
- 1 Cup sugar
- 4 Whole eggs
- 2 Teaspoon vanilla extract
- 2 Cup all-purpose flour
- 333/500 Cup Cocoa Powder, Unsweetened
- 1 Teaspoon baking soda
- 1 Teaspoon salt
- 1 Cup Semisweet Chocolate Chips
- 3/4 Cup White Chocolate Chips
- 3/4 Cup Nuts (optional)
- 1 Whole Hot Fudge Sauce, 8oz
- 2 Tablespoon Guinness Beer

Directions:
1. Coat the inside of a 10-inch (25 cm) pie plate with non-stick cooking spray.
2. When ready to cook, set the grill temperature to 350°F (180 C)and preheat, lid closed for 15 minutes.
3. Melt 1/2 cup (100 g) of the semi sweet chocolate chips in the microwave. Cream together butter, brown sugar and granulated sugar. Beat in the eggs, adding one at a time and mixing after each egg, and the vanilla. Add in the melted chocolate chips.
4. On a large piece of wax paper, sift together the cocoa powder, flour, baking soda and salt. Lift up the corners of the paper and pour slowly into the butter mixture.
5. Beat until the dry ingredients are just incorporated. Stir in the remaining semi sweet chocolate chips, white chocolate chips, and the nuts. Press the dough into the prepared pie pan.
6. Place the brownie pie on the grill and bake for 45-50 minutes or until the pie is set in the middle. Rotate the pan halfway through cooking. If the top or edges begin to brown, cover the top with a piece of aluminum foil.
7. In a microwave-safe measuring cup, heat the fudge sauce in the microwave. Stir in the Guinness.
8. Once the brownie pie is done, allow to sit for 20 minutes. Slice into wedges and top with the fudge sauce. Enjoy.

Vanilla Chocolate Bacon Cupcakes

Servings: 12
Cooking Time: 120 Minutes

Ingredients:

- 1 Lb Bacon
- 1 1/2 Tsp Baking Powder
- 1 1/2 Tsp Baking Soda
- 1 Cup Cocoa, Powder
- 2 Egg
- 1 3/4 Cups Flour
- 1 Cup Milk, Whole
- 1/2 Cup Oil
- 1 Tsp Salt
- 2 Cups Sugar
- 2 Tsp Vanilla

Directions:

1. Supply your smoker with wood pellets and follow the start-up procedure. Preheat the grill, with the lid closed, to 250° F.
2. Once your grill is preheated, place bacon strips on the grates. Smoke for 1hr-1 ½ hours or until desired crispiness is achieved.
3. Remove the bacon from the grill and set aside.
4. Increase set the temperature to 350°F and preheat.
5. Mix the rest of the ingredients in a bowl with an electric mixer until it is nice and smooth.
6. Pour the mixture into a cupcake tin.
7. Transfer the tin to your grill and bake for about 20 - 25 minutes.
8. Allow the cupcakes to cool on a wire rack. Once cooled, top with your favorite premade icing and a half of strip of the bacon. Serve and enjoy!

Baked Cheesy Parmesan Grits

Servings: 4
Cooking Time: 60 Minutes

Ingredients:

- 4 Cup chicken stock
- 3 Tablespoon butter
- 3/4 Teaspoon salt
- 1 Cup quick grits
- 1 Cup shredded cheddar cheese

- pepper
- 1/2 Cup Monterey Jack cheese, shredded
- 1/2 Cup whole milk
- 2 Large eggs

Directions:

1. Supply your smoker with wood pellets and follow the start-up procedure. Preheat the grill, with the lid closed, to 350° F.
2. Butter an 8" baking dish or a 10" cast iron pan.
3. Bring the chicken stock, butter, and salt to boil in medium saucepan. Gradually whisk in grits.
4. Reduce heat to medium and cook until mixture thickens slightly, stirring often about 8 minutes. Remove from heat.
5. Add cheeses and stir until melted. Season with pepper and salt to taste.
6. Whisk together milk and eggs in small bowl. Gradually whisk mixture into grits.
7. Pour the cheese grits into the buttered cast iron pan. Bake until grits feel firm to touch, about 1 hour. Grill: 350 °F
8. Remove from grill and let stand 10 minutes before serving. Enjoy!

Smoked Sweet Beer Bread

Servings: 6
Cooking Time: 60 Minutes

Ingredients:

- 3 cups all-purpose flour, sifted
- 2 tbsp. sugar
- 1 tbsp. baking powder
- 1 tsp. salt
- 1 (12 oz) can or bottle beer (not too dark or bitter)
- 2 tbsp. honey or agave, warmed
- 6 tbsp. butter, melted

Directions:

1. Supply your smoker with wood pellets and follow the start-up procedure. Preheat the grill, with the lid closed, to 350° F.
2. Lightly grease a 9 ×5 inch loaf pan.
3. In a large mixing bowl, put in the flour, sugar, baking powder, and salt. Whisk to combine and aerate,

using a wire whisk. Add the beer and honey and stir with a wooden spoon until the batter is properly mixed (Do not over-mix).

4. Pour half of the melted butter into the prepared loaf pan and pour in the batter. Pour the remaining butter over the top of the loaf.

5. Place the loaf pan on the grill grate and bake for 50 to 60 minutes or until the bread is golden brown.

6. Allow the loaf to cool slightly in the pan before removing it from the pan. Leftovers make great toast.

Smoked Lemon Cheesecake

Servings: 16
Cooking Time: 130 Minutes

Ingredients:

*   For the crust
*   Vegetable oil, for oiling the pan
*   12 ounces gingersnaps (about 36) or chocolate icebox cookies (about 36)
*   3 tablespoons light brown sugar
*   8 tablespoons (1 stick) unsalted butter, melted
*   For the filling
*   4 packages (8 ounces each) cream cheese, at room temperature
*   1 cup firmly packed light brown sugar
*   2 teaspoons pure vanilla extract
*   2 teaspoons finely grated lemon zest
*   1 tablespoon fresh lemon juice
*   2 tablespoons (1/4 stick) unsalted butter, melted
*   5 large eggs
*   Burnt Sugar Sauce (recipes follows, optional)

Directions:

1. Supply your smoker with wood pellets and follow the start-up procedure. Preheat the grill, with the lid closed, to 400° F. Lightly oil the springform pan with vegetable oil and wrap a sheet of aluminum foil around the outside.

2. Make the crust: Break the cookies into pieces and grind with the brown sugar to a fine powder in a food processor. You'll want about 1 3/4 cups of crumbs. Add the melted butter and run the processor in short bursts to obtain a crumbly dough. Press the mixture evenly across the bottom and halfway up the sides of the springform pan. Indirect-grill or bake the crust until lightly browned, 5 to 8 minutes. Transfer the pan to a wire rack and let cool.

3. Make the filling: Wipe out the food processor bowl. Add the cream cheese, brown sugar, vanilla, lemon zest, lemon juice, and butter, and process until smooth. Work in the eggs one by one, processing until smooth after each addition. (You can also use a stand mixer, beating the cream cheese mixture until smooth and beating in the eggs one at a time.) Pour the filling into the crust. Gently tap the pan on the countertop a few times to knock out any air bubbles.

4. Supply your smoker with wood pellets and follow the start-up procedure. Preheat the grill, with the lid closed, to 225 °F-250 °F.

5. Place the cheesecake in the smoker. Smoke until the top is bronzed with smoke and the filling is set, 1 1/2 to 2 hours. To test for doneness, gently poke the side of the pan—the filling will jiggle, not ripple. Alternatively, insert a slender metal skewer in the center of the cake; it should come out clean.

6. Transfer the cheesecake in its pan to a wire rack to cool to room temperature. Refrigerate until serving; the cheesecake can be made up to 8 hours ahead. Run a slender knife around the inside of the springform pan. Unclasp and remove the ring. (You'll serve the cheesecake off the bottom of the pan.) Let the cheesecake warm slightly at room temperature before serving.

7. If serving with the sauce, pour some of it over the cheesecake and the rest into a pitcher. Cut into wedges and pass the remaining sauce.

Smoked, Salted Caramel Apple Pie

Servings: 4
Cooking Time: 60 Minutes

Ingredients:

*   1 Cup cream
*   1 Cup brown sugar
*   3/4 Cup Light Corn Syrup
*   6 Tablespoon butter

- 1 Teaspoon sea salt
- 1 Pastry for Double-Crust Pie
- 6 Granny Smith Apples, Cut Into Wedges

Directions:

1. Supply your smoker with wood pellets and follow the start-up procedure. Preheat the grill, with the lid closed, to 180° F.

2. Fill a large pan with ice and water. Pour the cream into a smaller, shallow pan. Place the pan with the cream in the ice bath and place them both on the Traeger to smoke for 15-20 minutes. Grill: 180 °F

3. To make the caramel, combine the sugar and corn syrup in a saucepan and cook over medium heat, stirring constantly until it coats the back of your spoon and starts to turn a copper color, then stir in butter, salt, and smoked cream.

4. To assemble the pie, gather the pie crust, salted caramel, and apples. Place one of the pie crusts into the pie plate and fill with apple slices. Pour caramel over the apples. Lay the top crust over the filling, then crimp the top and bottom crusts together.

5. Make slits in the top crust to release the steam and finish by brushing with egg or cream. Sprinkle with raw sugar and sea salt.

6. When ready to bake, set the Traeger to 375°F and preheat, lid closed for 15 minutes.

7. Place the pie on the grill and bake for 20 minutes. Grill: 375 °F

8. Reduce heat to 325°F and cook for 25 more minutes. When ready, the crust should be golden brown and the filling, bubbly. Grill: 325 °F

9. Remove the pie from the grill and let cool. Serve with vanilla ice cream. Enjoy!

Green Bean Casserole Circa 1955

Servings: 6
Cooking Time: 30 Minutes

Ingredients:

- 1 1/2 Pound Green Beans, fresh
- 1 Can cream of mushroom soup
- 1/2 Cup milk
- 2 Teaspoon soy sauce

- 1/2 Teaspoon Worcestershire sauce
- 1/2 Teaspoon black pepper
- 1.334 Cup French's Original Crispy Fried Onions
- 1/4 Cup red bell pepper, diced

Directions:

1. In a mixing bowl, combine the beans (trimmed and cooked until tender, or may use 2 16 oz. cans), soup, milk, soy sauce, Worcestershire sauce, black pepper, 2/3 cup of the onion rings, and red pepper, if using. Transfer to a 1-1/2 quart casserole dish.

2. Supply your smoker with wood pellets and follow the start-up procedure. Preheat the grill, with the lid closed, to 375° F.

3. Cook the casserole until the filling is hot and bubbling, 25 to 30 minutes. Top with the remaining onions and cook for 5 to 10 minutes more, or until the onions are crisp and beginning to brown. Grill: 375 °F

Blueberry Pancakes

Servings: 4
Cooking Time: 10 Minutes

Ingredients:

- 2 Cups Blueberries, Fresh
- 1 Cup Pancake Mix
- 1/2 Cup Sugar
- 3/4 Cup Water, Warm

Directions:

1. Supply your smoker with wood pellets and follow the start-up procedure. Preheat the grill, with the lid closed, to 350° F.

2. Place the cast iron griddle on the grates of your grill.

3. In a large bowl, pour water, pancake mix and 1/2 cup of the blueberries and mix until combined.

4. Pour the batter onto the griddle in 4 equal parts. Cook with the lid closed for about 6 minutes, or until the edges of the pancakes are slightly cooked. Flip each pancake and continue cooking for another 4 minutes.

5. Pour the hot blueberry sauce over your freshly cooked pancakes and enjoy!

Pull-apart Dinner Rolls

Servings: 8
Cooking Time: 10 Minutes

Ingredients:

- 1/4 Cup warm water (110°F to 115°F)
- 1/3 Cup vegetable oil
- 2 Tablespoon active dry yeast
- 1/4 Cup sugar
- 1/2 Teaspoon salt
- 1 egg
- 3 1/2 Cup all-purpose flour
- cooking spray

Directions:

1. Supply your smoker with wood pellets and follow the start-up procedure. Preheat the grill, with the lid closed, to 400° F.
2. In the bowl of a stand mixer, combine warm water, oil, yeast and sugar. Let mixture rest for 5 to 10 minutes, or until frothy and bubbly.
3. With a dough hook, mix in salt, egg and 2 cups of flour until combined. Add remaining flour 1/2 cup at a time (dough will be sticky).
4. Prepare a cast iron pan with cooking spray and set aside.
5. Spray your hands with cooking spray and shape the dough into 12 balls.
6. After shaped, place in the prepared cast iron pan and let rest for 10 minutes. Bake in Traeger for about 10 to 12 minutes, or until tops are lightly golden. Enjoy! Grill: 400 °F

Savory Beaver Tails

Servings: 8
Cooking Time: 2 Minutes

Ingredients:

- 2 Tbsp Butter, Melted
- 1 Tbsp Cinnamon, Ground
- 1 Egg
- 2 1/2 Cups Flour, All-Purpose
- 1/2 Cup Milk, Warm
- 1/2 Tsp Salt
- 1 Tsp Sugar

- 1/2 Tsp Vanilla
- 1 L Vegetable Oil
- 1/4 Cup Water, Warm
- 2 1/2 Tsp Active Yeast, Instant

Directions:

1. In a small bowl, combine water, milk, yeast, and sugar. Let it sit for about 10 minutes or until frothy.
2. In another bowl, pour in the flour and make a well in the middle. Pour in butter, sugar, salt, vanilla and egg. Mix everything together until the dough is smooth. Knead for about 5 minutes and set the dough in a greased bowl. Cover with a towel and set aside for about an hour, or until the dough has doubled in size.
3. After one hour, supply your smoker with wood pellets and follow the start-up procedure. Preheat the grill, with the lid open, to 450° F.Pour 1L of vegetable oil into a cast iron pan and place on the grates of your Grill. Keep your flame broiler closed so as to prevent grease flareups. Preheat the oil so that it is 350 degrees F.
4. While you"re waiting for the oil to heat up, punch down the dough and separate into 8 small balls. Shape each piece of dough into a flat circle. Fry the dough in the preheated oil for about 1 minute per side, or until the dough is golden brown.
5. Sprinkle with cinnamon sugar immediately, or top with your desired toppings. Enjoy!

Smoked Blackberry Pie

Servings: 4-6
Cooking Time: 25 Minutes

Ingredients:

- Nonstick cooking spray or butter, for greasing
- 1 box (2 sheets) refrigerated piecrusts
- 8 tablespoons (1 stick) unsalted butter, melted, plus 8 tablespoons (1 stick) cut into pieces
- ½ cup all-purpose flour
- 2 cups sugar, divided
- 2 pints blackberries
- ½ cup milk
- Vanilla ice cream, for serving

Directions:

1. Supply your smoker with wood pellets and follow the start-up procedure. Preheat, with the lid closed, to 375°F.

2. Coat a cast iron skillet with cooking spray.

3. Unroll 1 refrigerated piecrust and place in the bottom and up the side of the skillet. Using a fork, poke holes in the crust in several places.

4. Set the skillet on the grill grate, close the lid, and smoke for 5 minutes, or until lightly browned. Remove from the grill and set aside.

5. In a large bowl, combine the stick of melted butter with the flour and 1½ cups of sugar.

6. Add the blackberries to the flour-sugar mixture and toss until well coated.

7. Spread the berry mixture evenly in the skillet and sprinkle the milk on top. Scatter half of the cut pieces of butter randomly over the mixture.

8. Unroll the remaining piecrust and place it over the top of skillet or slice the dough into even strips and weave it into a lattice. Scatter the remaining pieces of butter along the top of the crust.

9. Sprinkle the remaining ½ cup of sugar on top of the crust and return the skillet to the smoker.

10. Close the lid and smoke for 15 to 20 minutes, or until bubbly and brown on top. It may be necessary to use some aluminum foil around the edges near the end of the cooking time to prevent the crust from burning.

11. Serve the pie hot with vanilla ice cream.

Pizza Bites

Servings: 6
Cooking Time: 20 Minutes

Ingredients:
- 4 1/2 Cup Bread Flour
- 1 1/2 Tablespoon sugar
- 2 Teaspoon Instant Yeast
- 2 Teaspoon kosher salt
- 3 Tablespoon extra-virgin olive oil
- 15 Fluid Ounce Water, Lukewarm
- 8 Ounce Pepperoni, sliced
- 1 Cup pizza sauce
- 1 Cup mozzarella cheese
- 1 Whole egg, for egg wash
- 1 As Needed salt

Directions:
1. For the Pizza Dough: Combine flour, sugar, salt, and yeast in food processor. Pulse 3 to 4 times until incorporated evenly. Add olive oil and water. Run food processor until mixture forms ball that rides around the bowl above the blade, about 15 seconds. Continue processing 15 seconds longer.

2. Transfer dough ball to lightly floured surface and knead once or twice by hand until smooth ball is formed. Divide dough into three even parts and place each into a 1 gallon zip top bag. Place in refrigerator and allow to rise at least one day.

3. At least two hours before baking, remove dough from refrigerator and shape into balls by gathering dough towards bottom and pinching shut. Flour well and place each one in a separate medium mixing bowl. Cover tightly with plastic wrap and allow to rise at warm room temperature until roughly doubled in volume.

4. When ready to cook, set the grill temperature to 350°F and preheat, lid closed for 15 minutes.

5. After the first rise remove the dough from the fridge and let come to room temperature. Roll dough on a flat surface. Cut dough into long strips 3" wide by 18" long.

6. Slice pepperoni into strips.

7. In a medium bowl combine the pizza sauce, mozzarella and pepperoni.

8. Spoon 1 TBSP of the pizza filling onto the pizza dough every two inches, about halfway down the length of the dough. Dip a pastry brush into the egg wash and brush around pizza filling. Fold the half side of the dough (without the pizza filling) over the other the half that contains the pizza filling.

9. Press down between each pizza bite slightly with your fingers. With a ravioli or pizza cutter, cut around each filling- creating a rectangle shape and sealing the crust in.

10. Transfer each pizza bite onto a parchment lined cookie sheet. Cover with a kitchen towel and let them rise for 30 minutes.

11. When ready to cook, preheat the grill to 350°F with the lid closed for 10-15 minutes.

12. Brush the bites with remaining egg wash, sprinkle with salt and place directly on the sheet tray. Bake 10-15 minutes until the exterior is golden brown.

13. Remove from grill and transfer to a serving dish. Serve with extra pizza sauce for dipping and enjoy!

Savory Cheesecake With Bourbon Pecan Topping

Servings: 6
Cooking Time: 75 Minutes

Ingredients:
- Crust
- 12 ounce Oreos
- 6 ounce melted butter
- Filling
- 24 ounces cream cheese - room temperature
- 1 cup granulated sugar
- 3 tbs cornstarch
- 2 large eggs
- 2/3 cup heavy cream
- 1 tbs vanilla
- 1 1/2 tbs bourbon
- Topping
- 3 large eggs beaten
- 1/3 cup granulated sugar
- 1/3 cup brown sugar
- 8 tbsp corn syrup dark corn syrup recommended
- 2 tbsp bourbon
- 1/2 tbsp vanilla
- 1/8 tbsp salt
- 3/4 cup rough chopped pecans (smoked pecans recommended)

Directions:
1. Supply your smoker with wood pellets and follow the start-up procedure. Preheat the grill, with the lid closed, to 350 °F.
2. Wrap foil on the bottom and up the sides of a 9" spring-form pan (outside of pan).
3. Butter the bottom & insides of the pan.
4. Crust
5. Throw ingredients in a food processor until they are finely ground.

6. Spread in 9" cheesecake pan on bottom & about ½ way upsides.
7. Filling
8. Place 8 oz of cream cheese in mixer bowl with 1/3 of sugar & cornstarch.Mix until smooth andcreamy.
9. Add another 8 oz cream cheese andbeat until smooth, then add remaining cream cheese,beating until smooth.
10. Then mix in the rest of the sugar, bourbon & vanilla.
11. Add eggs one at a time beating well after each one.
12. Add the heavy cream and mix just until smooth. Reminder: Do not over mix.
13. Pour batter into the prepared crust.
14. Topping
15. Mix all together except pecans.
16. Sprinkle pecans on top of cheesecake batter.
17. Pour topping over cheesecake batter.
18. Place in a pan big enough to hold a spring-form pan. Pour boiling water in the roasting pan to come up about ½ way up the spring-form pan.
19. Bake at 350 °F for 75 minutes until the top just barely jiggles. Carefully take the pan out of water-bath and put on cooling rack.
20. Let cool for 2 hours in pan. After 2 hours put in fridge until totally chilled then serve.

Baked Chocolate Brownie Cookies With Egg Nog

Servings: 6
Cooking Time: 12 Minutes

Ingredients:
- 16 Ounce Bar bittersweet chocolate, finely chopped
- 4 Tablespoon unsalted butter, room temperature
- 4 eggs
- 1 1/3 Cup granulated sugar
- 1 Teaspoon vanilla extract
- 1 1/2 Cup all-purpose flour
- 1/2 Teaspoon baking powder
- 1 Cup semisweet chocolate chips

Directions:

1. Supply your smoker with wood pellets and follow the start-up procedure. Preheat the grill, with the lid closed, to 350° F.
2. Line two baking sheets with parchment paper.
3. Put the finely chopped chocolate and butter in a heatproof bowl and set over a saucepan of barely simmering water; stir occasionally until chocolate is completely melted and smooth. Set aside and allow to cool to room temperature.
4. Whisk together eggs, sugar and vanilla extract in a medium bowl. Set aside.
5. Sift together the flour and baking powder in a small bowl. Add the melted chocolate mixture to the egg mixture and stir with a rubber spatula until completely combined.
6. Add the flour mixture in three batches, folding gently into the batter with a spatula. Once all of the flour has been incorporated, stir in the chocolate chips.
7. Scoop 1-1/2 tablespoons of dough onto prepared baking sheets. Bake for 10 to 12 minutes or until they are firm on the outside. Do not over bake. Grill:350° F
8. Leave to cool completely on the baking sheets. Enjoy!

Basil Margherita Pizza

Servings: 6
Cooking Time: 25 Minutes

Ingredients:
- Basil, Chopped
- 2 Cups Flour, All-Purpose
- Mozzarella Cheese, Sliced Rounds
- 1 Cup Pizza Sauce
- 1 Teaspoon Salt
- 1 Teaspoon Sugar
- 1 Tomato, Sliced
- 1 Cup Water, Warm
- 1 Teaspoon Yeast, Instant

Directions:
1. Combine the water, yeast, and sugar in a small bowl and let sit for about 5 minutes.
2. In a large bowl, stir together the flour and salt. Pour in the yeast mixture and mix until a soft dough forms.

Knead for about 2 minutes. Place in an oiled bowl and cover with a cloth. Let the dough sit and rise for about 45 minutes or until the dough has doubled in size.
3. Roll out on a flat, floured surface (or on a pizza stone) until you"ve reached your desired shape and thickness.
4. Supply your smoker with wood pellets and follow the start-up procedure. Preheat the grill, with the lid closed, to 350° F.
5. On the rolled out dough, pour on the pizza sauce, cheese, and then tomatoes and basil. Place in your Grill and bake for about 25 minutes, or until the cheese is melted and slightly golden brown.

Grilled Beer Cheese Dip

Servings: 6
Cooking Time: 20 Minutes

Ingredients:
- 6 Oz Beer, Can
- 8 Oz Cream Cheese
- 1 Tsp Onion Powder
- ½ Tsp Pepper
- ½ Tsp Salt
- 2 Cups Shredded Cheese

Directions:
1. Supply your smoker with wood pellets and follow the start-up procedure. Preheat the grill, with the lid closed, to 350° F. If you're using a gas or charcoal grill, set it up for medium high heat. Preheat with lid closed for 10-15 minutes.
2. In the cast iron pan add cream cheese, shredded cheese, beer, onion powder, salt and pepper. Once grill is at 350°F place cast iron skillet onto the grill and cook for about 10 minutes, stir and cook for another 5-10 minutes.
3. Top with more shredded cheese and fresh parsley. Serve with fresh baked pretzels as well.

Quick Baked Dinner Rolls

Servings: 8
Cooking Time: 30 Minutes

Ingredients:

- 2 Tablespoon quick-rise yeast
- 1 Teaspoon salt
- 1/4 Cup sugar
- 3 1/3 Cup flour
- 1/4 Cup unsalted butter, softened
- 1 egg
- cooking spray
- 1 egg, for egg wash

Directions:

1. Combine yeast and warm water in a small bowl to activate the yeast. Let sit until foamy, about 5-10 minutes.
2. Combine salt, sugar, and flour in the bowl of a stand mixer fitted with the dough hook. Pour water and yeast into the dry ingredients with the machine running on low.
3. Add butter and egg and mix for 10 minutes gradually increasing the speed from low to high.
4. Form the dough into a ball and place in a buttered bowl. Cover with a cloth and let the dough rise for approximately 40 minutes.
5. Transfer the risen dough to a lightly floured surface and divide into 8 pieces forming a ball with each.
6. Lightly spray a cast iron pan with cooking spray and arrange balls in the pan. Cover with a cloth and let rise 20 minutes.
7. Supply your smoker with wood pellets and follow the start-up procedure. Preheat the grill, with the lid closed, to 375° F.
8. Brush rolls with egg wash and then bake for 30 minutes until lightly browned. Serve hot. Enjoy! Grill: 375 °F

Smoked Vanilla Apple Pie

Servings: 6
Cooking Time: 45 Minutes

Ingredients:

- 1 1/2 cups of self-raising flour
- 3/4 cup of sugar
- 0.3 lbs of butter melted
- 1 tsp of vanilla extract
- 1 egg
- 0.9-lb tin of pie apples
- sugar & cinnamon for dusting

Directions:

1. Supply your smoker with wood pellets and follow the start-up procedure. Preheat the grill, with the lid closed, to 350° F.
2. Combine the self-raising flour, sugar, melted butter, vanilla, and egg in a large bowl until a golden dough texture is formed.
3. Spread half the mixture in a pie dish and press the bottoms and up the sides of the dish.
4. Pour pie apple tin into the pie and spread out evenly.
5. Sprinkle the remaining mixture over the top of the apple evenly and place in the smoker.
6. Leave for 45 minutes or until the golden crust forms on the top.
7. Dust with cinnamon and a little sugar if desired.
8. Serve warm with custard, ice cream, or both.

Chocolate Almond Cake

Servings: 8
Cooking Time: 50 Minutes

Ingredients:

- 7 oz good quality dark chocolate; melted
- 5 eggs; separated
- Pinch salt
- 6.5 oz caster sugar
- 7 oz butter; cubed at room temperature
- 7 oz ground almonds
- 1 oz cocoa powder
- 1 tsp. baking powder
- Icing sugar; for dusting

Directions:

1. Supply your smoker with wood pellets and follow the start-up procedure. Preheat the grill, with the lid closed, to 347 °F.
2. Beat together the butter and sugar until light and fluffy. Then beat in the yolks, one at a time.

3. Gently fold in the almonds.

4. Add the melted chocolate and mix well.

5. Beat the egg whites with a pinch of salt in a separate bowl until stiff.

6. Sift the baking powder and cocoa powder into the cake mix and fold in gently, then fold in the egg whites.

7. Pour the mix into an 8.5" round spring form cake tin (greased and lined), smooth over, and bake in the center of the grill for about 50 minutes. If the top starts to dry out after 25-30 minutes, cover with foil.

Marbled Brownies With Amaretto & Ricotta

Servings: 4
Cooking Time: 30 Minutes

Ingredients:
- 1 Cup Ricotta Cheese
- 1 eggs
- 1 Tablespoon Amaretto Liqueur
- 1/4 Cup sugar
- 2 Teaspoon cornstarch
- 1/2 Teaspoon vanilla extract
- 1 Brownie Mix

Directions:

1. Coat a 9- by 13-inch nonstick baking pan with cooking spray or softened butter and set aside. (If you do not have a nonstick pan, line a regular one with buttered foil or parchment paper.)

2. In a medium bowl, combine the ricotta, egg, amaretto, sugar, cornstarch, and vanilla and whisk together thoroughly. Set aside.

3. Prepare the brownie mix according to the package directions. Spread the brownie batter evenly in the prepared pan. Randomly drop dollops of the ricotta mixture over the batter. Run a plastic knife through the ricotta mixture to give the brownies a marbled look. (A plastic knife is less likely to scratch your pan's nonstick surface.)

4. Supply your smoker with wood pellets and follow the start-up procedure. Preheat the grill, with the lid closed, to 350° F.

5. Put the pan with the brownie mixture directly on the grill grate and bake, about 25 to 30 minutes. Insert a bamboo skewer or toothpick in the center of the brownies to determine if they are done: the batter should not be wet. Grill: 350 °F

6. Transfer the brownies to a wire cooling rack to cool completely. Cut into squares.

Baked Peach Cobbler Cupcakes

Servings: 8
Cooking Time: 30 Minutes

Ingredients:
- 2 Large Peaches, fresh
- 3/4 Cup sugar
- 2 Teaspoon lemon juice
- 1/2 Teaspoon ground cinnamon
- Yellow Cake Mix, Boxed
- 1 Can vanilla icing

Directions:

1. Bring a pot of water to a boil. Turn peaches upside down and cut a small shallow X across the bottom. Put peaches in boiling water and boil for 1 minute to help loosen the skin.

2. Drain the peaches into a colander and rinse off with cold water. Peel skin off peaches.

3. Filling: Dice peaches and place into a large pan. Cook peaches over medium heat. As it starts to sizzle, add sugar, lemon and cinnamon. Cook mixture on medium heat for 10-15 minutes until a majority of the juice from the peaches evaporates leaving a thick syrup.

4. Transfer to a bowl to cool.

5. Supply your smoker with wood pellets and follow the start-up procedure. Preheat the grill, with the lid closed, to 350° F.

6. Cupcakes: Follow the directions on box cake mix and put the mixture into cupcake pan with liners.

7. When grill has preheated, bake cupcakes for 13-16 minutes, until a light golden brown. Grill: 350 °F

8. When cupcakes have cooled, use a piping bag to pipe the peach cobbler mixture into the middle of the cupcake.

9. Ice with your favorite vanilla icing. Enjoy!

Carrot Cake

Servings: 4-6
Cooking Time: 60 Minutes

Ingredients:

- 8 carrots, peeled and grated
- 4 eggs, at room temperature
- 1 cup vegetable oil
- ½ cup milk
- 1 teaspoon vanilla extract
- 2 cups sugar
- 2 cups self-rising or cake flour
- 2 teaspoons baking soda
- 1 teaspoon salt
- 1 cup finely chopped pecans
- Nonstick cooking spray or butter, for greasing
- 8 ounces cream cheese
- 1 cup confectioners' sugar
- 8 tablespoons (1 stick) unsalted butter, at room temperature
- 1 teaspoon vanilla extract
- ½ teaspoon salt
- 2 tablespoons to ¼ cup milk

Directions:

1. For the cake:
2. Supply your smoker with wood pellets and follow the start-up procedure. Preheat, with the lid closed, to 350°F.
3. In a food processor or blender, combine the grated carrots, eggs, oil, milk, and vanilla, and process until the carrots are finely minced.
4. In a large mixing bowl, combine the sugar, flour, baking soda, and salt.
5. Add the carrot mixture to the flour mixture and stir until well incorporated. Fold in the chopped pecans.
6. Coat a 9-by-13-inch baking pan with cooking spray.
7. Pour the batter into prepared pan and place on the grill grate. Close the lid and smoke for about 1 hour, or until a toothpick inserted in the center comes out clean.
8. Remove the cake from the grill and let cool completely.
9. For the frosting:
10. Using an electric mixer on low speed, beat the cream cheese, confectioners' sugar, butter, vanilla, and salt, adding 2 tablespoons to ¼ cup of milk to thin the frosting as needed.
11. Frost the cooled cake and slice to serve.

Delicious Pellet Grill Cornbread

Servings: 6
Cooking Time: 35 Minutes

Ingredients:

- 1 cup flour
- 1 cup cornmeal
- 2 teaspoons baking powder
- 2 teaspoons salt
- 3/4 cup sugar
- 2 tablespoons honey
- 1/2 cup butter
- 1 cup sour cream
- 3 eggs
- 1 cup milk

Directions:

1. Supply your smoker with wood pellets and follow the start-up procedure. Preheat the grill, with the lid closed, to 350° F.
2. Grease a 12-inch cast iron skillet or an equivalent baking pan.
3. Add flour, cornmeal, baking powder, salt, sugar, honey, butter, sour cream, eggs, and milk into a mixing bowl.
4. Mix well then pour into pan and bake on the grill for 30-35 minutes or until the cornbread is baked through in the center.

Garlic Lemon Pepper Chicken Wings

Servings: 4
Cooking Time: 30 Minutes

Ingredients:

- 1/4 Cup Black Peppercorns, Ground
- 4 Pounds Chicken, Wing
- 2 Tsp Coriander, Ground
- 2 Tsp Garlic Powder
- 2-3 Tbsp Lemon, Zest

- 1 Tsp Salt, Kosher
- 3 Tsp Dried Thyme, Fresh Sprigs

Directions:

1. Supply your smoker with wood pellets and follow the start-up procedure. Preheat the grill, with the lid closed, to 400° F.
2. In a bowl, begin to mix the ground pepper and zest of the lemon together, then add the rest of the ingredients.
3. Place the wings in a bowl and toss with a little olive oil, add a few tablespoons of the seasoning, toss with your hands, then repeat until the wings are well seasoned to your liking.
4. Place the wings on the grill, and cook them for about 15 minutes, then flip and grill for another 15 minutes.
5. Continue to flip the wings, until they are done and crispy. Remove the wings from the grill, and serve.

Beer Bread

Servings: 4
Cooking Time: 60 Minutes

Ingredients:

- 400 g all-purpose flour
- 2 Tablespoon sugar
- 1 Tablespoon baking powder
- 1 Teaspoon salt
- 12 Ounce beer
- 2 Tablespoon honey
- 6 Tablespoon butter, melted

Directions:

1. Supply your smoker with wood pellets and follow the start-up procedure. Preheat the grill, with the lid closed, to 350° F.
2. Spray a loaf pan (9x5x3 inches) (55x12x20 cm) with nonstick cooking spray and set aside.
3. Put the flour, sugar, baking powder, and salt in a large mixing bowl. Whisk with a wire whisk to combine and aerate. Add the beer and honey and stir with a wooden spoon until the batter is just mixed. (Do not overmix.) If desired, gently stir in one or more of the optional add-ins.

4. Pour half of the melted butter in the prepared loaf pan and spoon in the batter. Pour the remainder of the butter over the top of the loaf.
5. Put the loaf pan directly on the grill grate and bake until a wooden skewer or toothpick inserted in the center of the loaf comes out clean, 50 to 60 minutes, and the bread is golden-brown. (Note: If using a glass loaf pan, the baking time might be shorter.)
6. Let the loaf cool slightly in the pan before removing from the pan. Leftovers make great toast.
7. Optional Add-ins: Bacon, cooked and crumbled, 1 cup (100 g) Grated Cheese, Red Bell Pepper and Onion, diced and sauted in Butter (1/4 cup each), Green Onions, minced, Dried Herbs such as Dill, Rosemary, Mixed Italian Herbs, etc,.Cracked Black Pepper, Your favorite Barbecue Rub, such as Traeger's Pork and Poultry Shake, Ground Cinnamon, Dry Ranch Dressing Mix, Coarse-grained Mustard.

Sourdough Pizza

Servings: 4
Cooking Time: 12 Minutes

Ingredients:

- 1 1/2 Cup Fresh Sourdough Starter
- 1 Tablespoon olive oil
- 1 Teaspoon Jacobsen Salt Co. Pure Kosher Sea Salt
- 1 1/4 Cup all-purpose flour

Directions:

1. Supply your smoker with wood pellets and follow the start-up procedure. Preheat the grill, with the lid closed, to 450° F.
2. Mix together the fresh sourdough starter, one tablespoon of oil, Jacobsen salt and 1-1/4 cups of flour. Add more flour, a little at a time, as needed to form a pizza dough consistency.
3. Allow the dough to rest for 30 minutes, to allow for easier rolling. Roll the dough out into a circle, using a small amount of flour to prevent sticking.
4. Place on a pizza stone. Bake the crust for approximately 7 minutes Grill: 450 °F
5. Remove the crust from the grill; brush on remaining oil to prevent toppings from soaking into the crust. Add the desired toppings and return pizza to grill; bake until the crust browns and the cheese melts.

Baked Molten Chocolate Cake

Servings: 4
Cooking Time: 20 Minutes

Ingredients:
- all-purpose flour
- butter
- 4 Ounce butter
- 6 Ounce Chocolate, Bittersweet
- 2 eggs
- 2 egg yolk
- 1/2 Cup sugar
- 1 Pinch salt

Directions:

1. Supply your smoker with wood pellets and follow the start-up procedure. Preheat the grill, with the lid closed, to 450° F.

2. Butter and flour four (6oz) ramekins. Tap out excess flour. Place ramekins on a baking sheet and reserve.

3. Melt butter and chocolate in a double boiler over simmering water. In a medium bowl, beat eggs and yolks with sugar and salt on high until thick and pale.

4. Whisk in chocolate until smooth and quickly fold into the egg mixture along with flour.

5. Spoon the batter into prepared ramekins and bake for 20 minutes or until sides are firm but centers are soft. Grill: 450 °F

6. Let cool for 1 minute, then cover each with an inverted dessert plate. Carefully turn each over, let stand 10 seconds, then unmold.

7. Serve immediately with Maple Ice Cream with Candied Bacon. Enjoy!

Easy Smoked Cornbread

Servings: 4
Cooking Time: 75 Minutes

Ingredients:
- 2 cups self rising flour
- 1 1/2 cups white corn meal
- 2 cups sharp cheddar cheese
- 1/2 cup sour cream
- 1/2 cup sugar
- 1 Tbsp baking powder

- 1 teaspoon sea salt
- 1 12 oz can of evaporated milk
- 1/2 cup vegetable oil
- 2 large eggs beaten

Directions:

1. Mix all ingredients together well and fold into a greased baking pan (such as a round cake Pan).

2. Supply your smoker with wood pellets and follow the start-up procedure. Preheat the grill, with the lid closed, to 375° F. Smoke on 375 °F for 1 hour and 15 minutes or until toothpick comes clean and edges look brown.

3. Rub some butter on top and sprinkle a little Fred's Butt Rub on top before serving.

4. Enjoy!

Smoky Pimento Cheese Cornbread

Servings: 4
Cooking Time: 30 Minutes

Ingredients:
- 2 Tsp Baking Powder
- 2 Cups Buttermilk, Low Fat
- 1/2 Cup Cornmeal, Yellow
- 2 Egg
- 1 1/2 Cups Flour, All-Purpose
- 16 Oz Pimento Cheese Spread
- 2 Tbsp Bacon Cheddar Seasoning
- 1/4 Cup Sugar

Directions:

1. Supply your smoker with wood pellets and follow the start-up procedure. Preheat the grill, with the lid closed, to 350° F. Place a cast iron skillet in the grill to preheat.

2. In a bowl, mix together the eggs, buttermilk, Bacon Cheddar Seasoning, and pimento cheese spread. Add in the sugar, baking powder, cornmeal and flour. Mix until well combined.

3. With cooking gloves, carefully remove the cast iron skillet from the grill, grease it, and add the cornbread batter.

4. Grill for 25-30 minutes, or until the cornbread is golden and pulling away from the edges of the skillet.

220

Chicken Pot Pie

Servings: 6
Cooking Time: 60 Minutes

Ingredients:

- 2 Chicken, Boneless/Skinless
- 1 Cream Of Chicken Soup, Can
- 1 Tsp Curry Powder
- 1/2 Cup Mayo
- 1 1/2 Cups Mixed Frozen Vegetables
- 1 Onion, Sliced
- 2 Frozen Pie Shell, Deep
- 1/2 Cup Sour Cream

Directions:

1. Supply your smoker with wood pellets and follow the start-up procedure. Preheat the grill, with the lid closed, to 425° F.
2. Cut the onion in half and place on the grates of the grill. If you"re using fresh chicken breasts, barbecue the chicken at the same time as the onions. The chicken is fully cooked when the internal temperature reached 170F. While the onion and chicken are cooking, prepare the pie crust by putting one crust in a pie plate. When the chicken and onions are done, shred chicken and chop onion into small pieces and place in the prepared pie plate along with the mixed vegetables.
3. Combine cream of chicken soup, mayo, sour cream, and curry powder in a bowl. Pour into the pie crust with the chicken and mix to combine. Wet the sides of the bottom crust with a small amount of water and top with the second pie crust. Push gently along the sides of the crust to seal the two pie crusts together.
4. Place in the and bake for 40 minutes, or until the crust is golden brown. Serve hot.

Butternut Squash Macaroni And Cheese

Servings: 2
Cooking Time: 50 Minutes

Ingredients:

- 1 Medium butternut squash
- 2 Cup macaroni, uncooked
- 1 Small yellow onion
- 1/2 Cup chicken broth
- 1 Cup milk
- salt
- pepper
- 1 Cup cheese, grated

Directions:

1. Supply your smoker with wood pellets and follow the start-up procedure. Preheat the grill, with the lid closed, to 225° F.
2. Puncture butternut squash with a fork several times and place on grill grate. Cook until tender, about 40 minutes to an hour. When cooked, scoop out meat and discard seeds. Grill: 225 °F
3. Cook elbow macaroni according to package instructions. Drain and set aside.
4. In a medium skillet, sauté chopped onion until fragrant and golden. Add broth, milk, salt, onions and butternut squash to a food processor. Puree until smooth and creamy. Add salt and pepper to taste.
5. Pour pureed sauce over cooked noodles and add the shredded cheese. Stir to melt the cheese and add milk to reach desired consistency. Serve warm. Enjoy!

Smokin' Lemon Bars

Servings: 8-12
Cooking Time: 60 Minutes

Ingredients:

- 3/4 Cup lemon juice
- 1 1/2 Cup sugar
- 2 eggs
- 3 Egg Yolk
- 1 1/2 Teaspoon cornstarch
- Pinch sea salt
- 4 Tablespoon unsalted butter
- 1/4 Cup olive oil
- 1/2 Tablespoon lemon zest
- 1 1/4 Cup flour
- 1/4 Cup granulated sugar
- 3 Tablespoon Confectioner's Sugar
- 1 Teaspoon lemon zest
- 1/4 Teaspoon Sea Salt, Fine

- 10 Tablespoon Unsalted Butter, Cut Into Cubes

Directions:

1. When ready to cook, set grill temperature to 180℉ and preheat, lid closed for 15 minutes.

2. In a small mixing bowl, whisk together lemon juice, sugar, eggs and yolks, cornstarch and fine sea salt. Pour into a sheet tray or cake pan and place on grill. Smoke for 30 minutes whisking mixture halfway through smoking. Remove from grill and set aside.

3. Pour mixture into a small saucepan. Place on stove top set to medium heat until boiling. Once boiling, boil for 60 seconds. Remove from heat and strain through a mesh strainer into a bowl. Whisk in cold butter, olive oil, and lemon zest.

4. To make a crust, pulse together the flour, granulated sugar, confectioners' sugar, lemon zest and salt in a food processor. Add butter and pulse until just mixed into a crumbly dough. Press dough into a prepared 9" by 9" baking dish lined with parchment paper that is long enough to hang over 2 of the sides.

5. When ready to cook, set the smoker to 350℉ and preheat, lid closed for 15 minutes.

6. Bake until crust is very lightly golden brown, about 30 to 35 minutes.

7. Remove from grill and pour the lemon filling over the crust. Return to grill and continue to bake until filling is just set about 15 to 20 minutes.

8. Allow to cool at room temperature, then refrigerate until chilled before slicing into bars. Sprinkle with confectioners' sugar and flaky sea salt right before serving. Enjoy!

Spiced Lemon Cherry Pie

Servings: 6-8
Cooking Time: 60 Minutes

Ingredients:

- 1/2 Teaspoon Cinnamon, Ground
- 1/2 Teaspoon Cloves, Ground
- 1/2 Cup Cornstarch
- 1 Pound Frozen Sweet Dark Cherries, Thawed
- 1 Teaspoon Water (Beaten With Egg) 1 Egg
- 1 Lemon, Juice

- 1 Lemon, Zest
- 2 Prepared Store Bought Or Homemade Pie Crust
- 1 Teaspoon Hickory Honey Sea Salt Seasoning
- 1 Cup Sugar, Granulated
- 1 Teaspoon Vanilla Extract

Directions:

1. In a large bowl, mix together the thawed cherries and their juices, sugar, cornstarch, lemon zest, lemon juice, cinnamon, clove, vanilla extract and Hickory Honey Sea Salt. Allow to sit for 30 minutes.

2. Flour a work surface and roll out one of the prepared pie crusts so that it fits a 9 inch pie tin. Fill with the cherry pie filling and refrigerate. When the pie is chilled, roll out the second pie crust, brush the edge of the first pie crust with the egg mixture, top with the second pie crust, crimp the edge with a fork, and chill. Alternatively, cut the second pie crust into strips and form a lattice pattern, attaching the strips with the egg mixture. Chill the pie for 15-30 minutes, or until the dough is very cold and firm. Brush the top of the pie with the remaining egg mixture.

3. Supply your smoker with wood pellets and follow the start-up procedure. Preheat the grill, with the lid closed, to 350° F and grill for 45 minutes to 1 hour, or until the pie crust is golden and firm and the filling is bubbly. Remove from the grill and allow to cool at room temperature for at least 4 hours to set the filling, then serve and enjoy!

Donut Bread Pudding

Servings: 8
Cooking Time: 40 Minutes

Ingredients:

- 16 Cake Donuts
- 1/2 Cup Raisins, seedless
- 5 eggs
- 3/4 Cup sugar
- 2 Cup heavy cream
- 2 Teaspoon vanilla extract
- 1 Teaspoon ground cinnamon
- 3/4 Cup Butter, melted, cooled slightly
- Ice Cream

Directions:

1. Lightly butter a 9- by 13-inch baking pan. Layer the donuts in an even thickness in the pan. Distribute the raisins over the top, if using. Drizzle evenly with the butter.

2. Make the custard: In a medium bowl, whisk together the sugar, eggs, cream, vanilla, and cinnamon. Whisk in the butter. Pour over the donuts. Let sit for 10 to 15 minutes, periodically pushing the donuts down into the custard. Cover with foil.

3. Supply your smoker with wood pellets and follow the start-up procedure. Preheat the grill, with the lid closed, to 350° F.

4. Bake the bread pudding for 30 to 40 minutes, or until the custard is set. Remove the foil and continue to bake for 10 additional minutes to lightly brown the top. Grill: 350 °F

5. Let cool slightly before cutting into squares. Drizzle with melted ice cream, if desired. Enjoy!

Baked Pumpkin Pie

Servings: 6
Cooking Time: 50 Minutes

Ingredients:

- 4 Ounce cream cheese
- 15 Ounce pumpkin puree
- 1/3 Cup Cream, whipping
- 1/2 Cup brown sugar
- 1 Teaspoon pumpkin pie spice
- 3 Large eggs
- 1 frozen pie crust, thawed

Directions:

1. Supply your smoker with wood pellets and follow the start-up procedure. Preheat the grill, with the lid closed, to 325° F.

2. Mix cream cheese, puree, milk, sugar, and spice. One at a time, incorporate an egg to the mixture. Pour mixture into pie shell.

3. Bake for 50 minutes, edges should be golden and pie should be firm around edges with slight movement in middle. Let cool before whip cream is applied. Serve and enjoy! Grill: 325 °F

Baked Green Chile Mac & Cheese By Doug Scheiding

Servings: 8
Cooking Time: 120 Minutes

Ingredients:

- 24 Ounce shredded cheddar cheese, divided
- 8 Ounce mozzarella cheese, shredded
- 6 Tablespoon unsalted butter
- 16 Ounce large dry elbow macaroni noodles
- 2 1/2 Cup half-and-half
- 2 Cup heavy whipping cream
- 8 Ounce cream cheese
- 16 Ounce 505 Southwestern Hatch Valley Flame Roasted Green Chile
- 2 Tablespoon Prime Rib Rub

Directions:

1. Supply your smoker with wood pellets and follow the start-up procedure. Preheat the grill, with the lid closed, to 165° F.

2. Place 16 ounces of the shredded cheddar and the 8 ounces of shredded mozzarella cheese into a shallow pan or cookie sheet and place the pan directly on the grill grate. Smoke for 30 to 40 minutes. Remove from grill and set aside. Grill: 165 °F

3. Increase the grill temperature to 300°F and place a large disposable aluminum half pan in the Traeger with the butter. Remove the pan from the grill after the butter has fully melted. Grill: 300 °F

4. Add the noodles to the pan, along with half-and-half, heavy whipping cream, 16 ounces of the cold smoked cheddar, all of the smoked mozzarella cheese and cream cheese broken into small pieces. Add the green chiles to taste (12 ounces for mild and 16 ounces for spicy) and stir to combine.

5. Place the pan in the grill and bake for 2 hours, stirring every 20 minutes. If macaroni and cheese looks like it is getting dry, add a little more half-and-half and stir to combine. Grill: 300 °F

6. During the last 20 minutes of cooking, sprinkle the remaining (unsmoked) cheddar cheese on top and add a light dusting of Traeger Prime Rib Rub. Serve hot. Enjoy!

Dark Chocolate Brownies With Bacon-salted Caramel

Servings: 8
Cooking Time: 40 Minutes

Ingredients:
- 8 Strips bacon
- 1/2 Cup kosher salt
- 1 Whole Brownie Mix
- 1 Jar caramel sauce

Directions:

1. For the bacon salt: Cook a few strips of bacon (6 to 8) until very crisp: 350 degrees for about 25 minutes should do it. Let cool, then pulse in a food processor until finely chopped. Mix with 1/2 cup kosher salt. Store in the refrigerator until ready to use.

2. Supply your smoker with wood pellets and follow the start-up procedure. Preheat the grill, with the lid closed, to 350° F.

3. Mix the brownies according to package directions and pour into a greased pan. Drizzle approximately 2 tablespoons of the caramel sauce over the brownie batter. Sprinkle with approximately 1 teaspoon of the bacon salt. Place directly on the grill grate of your preheated Traeger.

4. Bake the brownies for 20-25 minutes, until the batter has started to set up. Remove from the grill and drizzle with 2 more tablespoons of caramel sauce and sprinkle with more bacon salt. Return to the grill for 20-25 more minutes, or until a toothpick inserted in the middle of the brownies comes out clean.

5. If you like extra caramel, drizzle another layer of caramel on the hot brownies and sprinkle with a final bit of bacon salt. Allow the brownies to cool completely before cutting them into squares. Clean your knife in between each slice to prevent the brownies from sticking to the knife. Enjoy!

Onion Cheese Nachos

Servings: 6
Cooking Time: 10 Minutes

Ingredients:
- 1 Pound Beef, Ground
- 3 Cups Cheddar Cheese, Shredded
- 1 Green Bell Pepper, Diced
- 1/2 Cup Green Onion
- 1/2 Cup Red Onion, Diced
- 1 Large Bag Tortilla Chip

Directions:

1. Supply your smoker with wood pellets and follow the start-up procedure. Preheat the grill, with the lid closed, to 350° F.

2. While you're waiting, empty a large bag of nacho chips evenly onto a cast iron pan. Start loading up with toppings - cooked ground beef, red onion, red pepper, cheese, green onions. These are just the toppings we had on hand, so feel free to add anything you like! Make sure you do a couple layers of chips so everyone gets a good serving of nachos. And don't be skimpy with the cheese - lay it on heavy!

3. Place your loaded nachos on the grill and let the hot smoke melt your toppings into one cheesy creation. Heat at 350°F for 10 minutes or until the cheese has fully melted. Remove and serve with sour-cream and salsa.

Smoked Lemon Tea

Servings: 6 - 8
Cooking Time: 60 Minutes

Ingredients:
- 8 Black Tea Bags
- 4 Cups Boiling Water
- 2 Cups Ice
- 8 Lemons
- 2 Cups Sugar
- 2 Cups Water

Directions:

1. Place the tea bags in a heat-safe pitcher. Bring 4 Cups of water to a boil and pour over tea bags. Let steep for 5-10 minutes. Remove tea bags and set pitcher aside to cool.

2. Turn on your grill and set to smoke mode. Combine 2 cups of sugar and 2 cups water in a small aluminum pan. Smoke for about 45 minutes, stirring occasionally, or until the mixture reduces to a thick, simple syrup. Remove from the grill and let it cool.

3. Supply your smoker with wood pellets and follow the start-up procedure. Preheat the grill, with the lid closed, to 450° F. If using a charcoal or gas grill, set heat to high.

4. Cut the lemons in half and sear over the flame broiler until charred, about 7 minutes. Remove from grill and set aside to cool.

5. Juice the lemons into a medium bowl. Pour lemon juice through a metal strainer into the tea pitcher to remove seeds and pulp.

6. Pour the cooled simple syrup into pitcher and stir until fully incorporated with tea and lemons. Add 2 cups of ice and refrigerate until serving.

Eyeball Cookies

Servings: 20
Cooking Time: 35 Minutes

Ingredients:
- 2 Packages Candy Eyeballs
- Green, Blue And Purple Food Coloring
- 1 Box Of Yellow Gluten Free Cake Mix
- 1/2 Cup (Optional) Granulated Sugar
- 2 Large Eggs
- 1/3 Cup Powdered Sugar
- 1 Teaspoon Pure Vanilla Extract
- 6 Tablespoon Melted Vegan Butter (Unsalted)

Directions:
1. Supply your smoker with wood pellets and follow the start-up procedure. Preheat the grill, with the lid closed, to 350° F.

2. Line two large baking sheets with parchment paper. In a large bowl, combine cake mix, melted butter, eggs (or egg substitute), powdered sugar, sugar (optional), and vanilla and stir until combined. (substitute 2 flax eggs for Vegan – 1 tbsp flax seed meal and 5 tbsp water per egg).

3. Divide dough between 3 bowls and dye each bowl a different color.(We used green, blue and purple).

4. Roll dough into tablespoon-sized balls.

5. Place about 2" apart on the baking sheet and grill until tops have cracked and the tops look set, 8 to 10 minutes. – Turn half way through baking, after 4-5 minutes.

6. Immediately, while the cookies are still warm, stick candy eyeballs all over the cookies.

7. Let cool completely before serving.

Baked Irish Creme Cake

Servings: 4
Cooking Time: 60 Minutes

Ingredients:
- 1 Cup Pecans, pieces
- 1 Yellow Cake Mix, Boxed
- 1 Vanilla Pudding Mix, Instant Package (3.4oz)
- 4 Large eggs
- 1/2 Cup water
- 1/2 Cup vegetable oil
- 1 Cup Irish Cream Liquor
- 1/2 Cup butter
- 1 Cup sugar

Directions:
1. Grease and flour a 10" (25 cm) Bundt pan. Sprinkle pecans along the bottom.

2. In a large bowl, with a mixer, combine yellow cake mix, pudding mix, eggs, water, oil, and Irish Cream liquor. Pour batter over nuts in the pan.

3. Supply your smoker with wood pellets and follow the start-up procedure. Preheat the grill, with the lid closed, to 325° F.

4. Place Bundt pan on the Traeger and bake for 1 hour, or until a toothpick comes out clean. Remove from heat, cool for 10 minutes. Grill: 325 °F

5. While the cake is cooling, combine the butter, water and sugar and bring to a boil. Boil for 5 minutes, stirring constantly. Remove from heat and add Irish cream liquor.

6. Use a bamboo skewer to poke holes in the cooled cake. Spoon glaze over the cake. Allow cake to absorb the glaze. Enjoy!

Cake With Smoked Berry Sauce

Servings: 12
Cooking Time: 90 Minutes

Ingredients:
- 12 Oz Blackberries
- 18 Oz Blueberries, Fresh

- 1/4 Cup Brown Sugar
- 2 Tsp Cinnamon, Ground
- 4 Eggs
- 2 Tbsp Flour
- 1 3/4 Cup Granulated Sugar
- 1 Lemon, Juice & Zest
- 1/2 Cup Unsalted Butter
- 3.4 Ounce Box Vanilla Instant Pudding Mix
- 3/4 Cup Vegetable Oil
- 3/4 Cup Water
- 1 Cup White Wine
- 1 Box Yellow Cake Mix

Directions:

1. Fire up your Grill and set to Smoke mode. If using a gas or charcoal grill, set it up for low, indirect heat. Supply your smoker with wood pellets and follow the start-up procedure. Preheat the grill, with the lid closed, to 450° F.

2. Place blueberries and blackberries on a sheet tray, then transfer to upper shelf of smoking cabinet. Make sure that the sear slide and side dampers are open, then preheat the grill, with the lid closed, to 375° F, to ensure the cabinet maintains temperature between 225° F and 250° F. Smoke for 30 to 45 minutes.

3. Place cast iron skillet on grill grate. Add sugar, lemon juice and zest, and wine to skillet. Stir with a wooden spoon until sugar dissolves, then add berries from smoking cabinet.

4. Simmer berries for 15 minutes, then remove sauce from grill to cool.

5. While berries are smoking, prepare cake pans and batter. Grease and flour 2 - 9-inch round cake pans. Set aside.

6. In a large mixing bowl, combine cake mix, brown sugar, granulated sugar, pudding mix, cinnamon, eggs, water, oil, and white wine. Using a hand mixer, mix on low speed for 1 minute, then slowly increase mixing speed to high, and beat an additional 2 to 3 minutes, or until batter is smooth.

7. Evenly distribute batter among cake pans, then place pans on grill shelf and bake at 350° F, for 25 to 30 minutes, or until a toothpick inserted comes out clean. Remove from grill and set aside to cool slightly.

8. While cake is cooling, prepare glaze. Melt butter with sugar in a sauce pot on the grill. Stir for 3 minutes, then add wine. Remove from grill and set aside.

9. Turn out cake onto a sheet tray lined with parchment. Use a toothpick to poke holes in the cake, then slowly pour hot glaze over cake.

10. Spread half of smoked berry sauce on top of one layer, then place second cake layer on top. Pour additional sauce on top of cake and dust with powdered sugar, if desired. Serve warm, or room temperature.

Delicious Peanut Butter Cookies

Servings: 24
Cooking Time: 15 Minutes

Ingredients:
- 1 Egg
- 1 Cup Peanut Butter
- 1 Cup Sugar

Directions:

1. Supply your smoker with wood pellets and follow the start-up procedure. Preheat the grill, with the lid closed, to High heat.

2. Combine all ingredients in a bowl. Drop tablespoon amounts of dough on a prepared baking sheet and bake in your Grill for 15-20 minutes. Allow cookies to cool for 5 minutes on the baking sheet before you enjoy!

Crème Brûlée

Servings: 2
Cooking Time: 45minutes

Ingredients:
- 1 Quart heavy whipping cream
- 1 Pieces Vanilla Bean, split and scraped
- 6 Large egg yolk
- 1 Cup sugar

Directions:

1. Supply your smoker with wood pellets and follow the start-up procedure. Preheat the grill, with the lid closed, to 325° F.

2. Pour the cream into a saucepan over medium-high heat, add the vanilla bean and the scraped seeds. Bring to a boil. Remove from the heat and allow to steep (about

15 minutes). Remove the vanilla bean from saucepan and discard.

3. In a bowl, whisk together egg yolks and 1/2 cup (100 g) of the sugar until the mix starts to lighten in color. Add the cream a little at a time, stirring continually.

4. Pour the mixture into 6 (8 oz) ramekins and place the ramekins into a large roasting pan. Pour hot water into the pan so that it comes halfway up the sides of the ramekins.

5. Place water bath pan on the grill and bake until the Crème Brûlées still jiggle in the center, about 40 to 45 minutes. Grill: 325 °F

6. Remove the ramekins from the roasting pan and refrigerate for at least 2 hours and up to 2 days.

7. To serve, let the Crème Brûlée come to temperature (about 20 minutes) before torching the tops.

8. Sprinkle the remaining 1/2 cup (100 g) sugar equally on top of each ramekin. Using a torch in a circular motion, melt the sugar until it caramelizes and forms a crispy top.

9. Allow the Crème Brûlée to sit for a few minutes before serving. Enjoy!

Pretzel Rolls

Servings: 6
Cooking Time: 20 Minutes

Ingredients:
- 2 3/4 Cup Bread Flour
- 1 Quick-Rising Yeast, envelope
- 1 Teaspoon salt
- 1 Teaspoon sugar
- 1/2 Teaspoon celery seed
- 1/2 Teaspoon Caraway Seeds
- 1 Cup hot water
- As Needed Cornmeal
- 8 Cup water
- 1/4 Cup baking soda
- 2 Tablespoon sugar
- 1 Whole Egg White
- Coarse salt

Directions:

1. Combine bread flour, 1 envelope yeast, salt, 1 teaspoon sugar, caraway seeds and celery seeds in food processor or standing mixer with dough hook and blend.

2. With machine running, gradually pour hot water, adding enough water to form smooth elastic dough. Process 1 minute to knead. (You could also knead it by hand for a few minutes.)

3. Grease medium bowl. Add dough to bowl, turning to coat. Cover bowl with plastic wrap, then towel; let dough rise in warm draft-free area until doubled in volume, about 35 minutes.

4. Flour a large baking sheet. Punch dough down and knead on lightly floured surface until smooth. Divide into 8 pieces. Form each dough piece into a ball.

5. Place dough balls on prepared sheet, flattening each slightly. Using serrated knife, cut X in top center of each dough ball. Cover with towel and let dough balls rise until almost doubled in volume, about 20 minutes.

6. When ready to cook, start the smoker on Smoke with the lid open until a fire is established (4-5 minutes). Turn temperature to 375 F (190 C) and preheat, lid closed, for 10 to 15 minutes.

7. Grease another baking sheet and sprinkle with cornmeal. Bring water to boil in large saucepan. Add baking soda and sugar (water will foam up). Add 3 rolls (or however many will fit comfortably in the pot) and cook 30 seconds per side.

8. Using slotted spoon, transfer rolls to prepared sheet, arranging X side up. Repeat with remaining rolls. Brush rolls with egg white glaze. Sprinkle rolls generously with coarse salt.

9. Bake rolls until brown, about 20 to 25 minutes. Transfer to racks and cool 10 minutes. Serve rolls warm or at room temperature. Enjoy!

Baked Bourbon Monkey Bread

Servings: 6
Cooking Time: 40 Minutes

Ingredients:
- 3 Can Pillsbury Grands Buttermilk Biscuits
- 1 Cup sugar
- 3 Teaspoon ground cinnamon

- 1 Cup Butter, unsalted
- 1 Cup dark brown sugar
- Tablespoon bourbon

Directions:

1. Supply your smoker with wood pellets and follow the start-up procedure. Preheat the grill, with the lid closed, to 350° F.

2. Cut each biscuit into quarters. In a Ziploc bag, combine sugar and cinnamon and add quartered biscuits. Toss to coat in cinnamon sugar.

3. Dump coated biscuit dough into a bundt pan coated with non-stick spray.

4. In a small saucepan, combine the brown sugar, butter, and bourbon. Cook over medium heat until the sugar has dissolved.

5. Pour the butter mixture over the biscuits in the bundt pan.

6. Place in the center of the grill and cook for 40 minutes or until dark golden brown.

7. Let cool on the counter for 5-10 minutes, then flip out onto a serving plate. Enjoy!

Crescent Rolls

Servings: 8
Cooking Time: 12 Minutes

Ingredients:
- 1 Crescent Dough, Can

Directions:

1. Supply your smoker with wood pellets and follow the start-up procedure. Preheat the grill, with the lid closed, to 375° F.

2. Unroll the dough and separate into triangles. Roll up the triangles and place on an ungreased nonstick cookie sheet. Bake for 10 -12 minutes on your Grill. You will know that they are finished when the rolls are golden brown.

Bananas Rum Foster

Servings: 4
Cooking Time: 10 Minutes

Ingredients:
- 1/3 Cup Banana Nectar

- 4 Bananas, Quartered
- 3/4 Cup Brown Sugar
- 1/4 Cup Butter
- 1/2 Tsp Cinnamon, Ground
- 1/3 Cup Dark Rum
- Vanilla Ice Cream

Directions:

1. Supply your smoker with wood pellets and follow the start-up procedure. Preheat the grill, with the lid closed, to medium heat. If using a gas or charcoal grill, preheat a cast iron skillet.

2. Place a large skillet on the griddle, then melt butter in the skillet. Whisk in brown sugar and cinnamon, stirring until sugar dissolves.

3. Add the banana nectar and bananas. Stir to coat

4. Once the bananas begin to soften and turn brown, add the rum. Stir, then ignite the sauce with a stick lighter. After the flames subside, simmer the sauce for 2 minutes.

5. Divide the bananas among 4 scoops/bowls of vanilla ice cream, then spoon the warm sauce over the top of the ice cream. Serve immediately.

Zucchini Bread

Servings: 6
Cooking Time: 50 Minutes

Ingredients:
- 1 Cup Walnuts, Chopped
- 2 Large zucchini
- 1 Teaspoon salt
- 1 Teaspoon ground cinnamon
- 1/4 Teaspoon ground cloves
- 1/4 Teaspoon baking powder
- 3 Cup all-purpose flour
- 1 eggs
- 2 Cup sugar
- 1/2 Cup vegetable oil
- 1/2 Cup Yogurt
- 1 1/2 Teaspoon vanilla extract

Directions:

1. Grease and flour two 9- by 5-inch bread pans, preferably nonstick.

2. When ready to cook, set the temperature to 350°F and preheat, lid closed for 15 minutes.

3. Spread the walnuts on a pie plate and toast for 10 minutes, stirring once. Let cool, then coarsely chop. Set aside.

4. Trim the ends off the zucchini, then coarsely grate into a colander set over the sink on a box grater (or use the shredding disk on a food processor). You'll need 2 cups.

5. Sprinkle with the salt and let drain for 30 minutes. Press on the zucchini with paper towels to expel excess water.

6. Sift the flour, baking powder, cinnamon, and cloves in a mixing bowl or on a large sheet of parchment or wax paper.

7. Combine the eggs, sugar, oil, yogurt, and vanilla in a large mixing bowl and mix on medium speed. (You can mix the batter by hand, if desired.) Add half the dry ingredients and mix on low speed; add the remaining dry ingredients and mix until just combined.

8. Stir in the walnuts and zucchini by hand.

9. Divide the batter between the prepared baking pans.

10. Arrange the pans directly on the grill grate and bake for 50 minutes, or until a bamboo skewer inserted in the center of the breads comes out clean.

11. Transfer to a wire rack and let cool for 10 minutes, then remove the breads from the pans. For best results, let the breads cool completely before slicing.

Maple Syrup Pancake Casserole

Servings: 6
Cooking Time: 60 Minutes

Ingredients:
- 2 Tbsp Butter
- 1/2 Cup Chocolate Chips
- 4 Egg
- Maple Syrup
- 12 - 14 Pancakes
- Powdered Sugar
- 1/4 Cup Sugar, Granulated
- 1 Tsp Vanilla Extract
- 1 1/2 Cup Whole Milk

Directions:

1. In a mixing bowl, whisk together flour, baking powder, sugar, and salt. Then pour in the milk, egg and melted butter; mix until smooth.

2. Supply your smoker with wood pellets and follow the start-up procedure. Preheat the grill, with the lid closed, to medium-low heat. If using a gas or charcoal grill, preheat a large cast iron skillet over medium-low heat.

3. Lightly oil the griddle, then scoop the batter onto the griddle, using approximately ¼ cup for each pancake. Cook 1 to 2 minutes per side, until golden brown. Set aside to cool for 15 minutes, then assemble the casserole.

Chicken Pizza On The Grill

Servings: 4
Cooking Time: 10 Minutes

Ingredients:
- 3 Boneless, Skinless Chicken Breast
- 5 Cups Flour, Strong
- 3 Cups Georgia Style Bbq Sauce
- 3 Cups Mozzarella Cheese, Shredded
- 1 Tsp Olive Oil
- 3 Cups Georgia Style BBQ Sauce
- 1 1/2 Cups Red Bell Peppers, Diced
- 1 1/2 Cups Red Onion, Diced
- 1 Tsp Sugar
- 1/2 Cup Water, Hot
- 1 1/4 Cup Water, Warm
- 2 Tsb Active Yeast, Instant

Directions:

1. Roll your pizza dough so it forms a base about a 1/2 inch thick. To impress your friends and family, you'll want to aim for a nice, pizza like shape. HINT: use a sprinkle of cornmeal on the countertop to aid in moving the dough.

2. Now for the toppings! Start by spreading 1 cup of Georgia Style BBQ sauce onto each base. Make sure to leave a small portion for the crust! Next, load up with sliced, cooked chicken breasts, diced red onions and red bell peppers before finishing off with a two cups of shredded mozzarella cheese.

3. Supply your smoker with wood pellets and follow the start-up procedure. Preheat the grill, with the lid closed, to 500° F. Place the pizza stone in your grill. Pick up your pizza using a flat surface like a chopping board and slide the pizza carefully onto the hot stone. Close the lid and let your homemade wood-fired pizza bake for 10 - 12 minutes. Remove once your pizza has a golden crust and the cheese is bubbling. Cut and serve for pizza you'll hardly want to share.

Sweet And Spicy Baked Pork Beans

Servings: 20
Cooking Time: 120 Minutes

Ingredients:
- 1 - 21 Oz Apple Pie Filling, Can
- 1 Gallon Baked Beans
- 1 Tbs Chilli, Powder
- 1 Green Bell Pepper, Diced
- 1 10 Oz Drained Jalapeno, Can Diced
- 1 Cup Maple Syrup
- 1 Onion, Diced
- 1 Lb Pork, Pulled

Directions:
1. Supply your smoker with wood pellets and follow the start-up procedure. Preheat the grill, with the lid closed, to 350° F.
2. Place all ingredients in mixing bowl and mix well.
3. Pour bean mixture into foil pans.
4. Bake in grill till bubbling throughout – about 2 hours.
5. Rest at least 15 minutes before serving.

Eggs Ham Benedict

Servings: 6
Cooking Time: 15 Minutes

Ingredients:
- 1 Biscuit Dough, Tube
- 6 Egg
- 16 Ham, Sliced
- 1 Packet Hollandaise Sauce, Package

Directions:

1. Supply your smoker with wood pellets and follow the start-up procedure. Preheat the grill, with the lid closed, to 350° F.
2. Grease a muffin tin and crack an egg in each cup. Place on the grate of the for about 10 minutes or until the whites are fully cooked.
3. At the same time, place your biscuit dough on a greased pan. Follow the directions on the packaging but bake on the . Place 2 slices of ham per biscuit on the pan as well.
4. While the ham, eggs, and biscuits are cooking, prepare the Hollandaise Sauce according to the directions on the packet.
5. When everything is fully cooked, cut a biscuit in half, and stack one or two slices of ham, 1 egg and a dollop of Hollandaise sauce. Repeat for each half biscuit. Serve with fresh fruit.

Cinnamon Pull-aparts

Servings: 6
Cooking Time: 20 Minutes

Ingredients:
- 16.3 Ounce Biscuits, Homestyle, Canned
- 1 Cup packed brown sugar
- 1/2 Cup butter
- 1/4 Cup water
- 1 Teaspoon ground cinnamon
- 1/2 Cup Nuts (optional)

Directions:
1. Cut each biscuit into 4 pieces and peel each piece in half; set aside.
2. Combine brown sugar, butter and water in a large saucepan and bring to a boil; reduce heat and simmer for 1 minute. Stir in cinnamon and nuts; add biscuit quarters and mix to coat. Pour into greased 13 by 9 inch casserole dish and spread evenly in the dish.
3. Supply your smoker with wood pellets and follow the start-up procedure. Preheat the grill, with the lid closed, to 350° F.
4. Place the casserole dish on the grill; close lid and cook for 20 to 25 minutes or until the biscuits are done. Grill: 350 °F
5. Remove from the grill and transfer to a serving platter making sure to get all the gooey syrup onto the biscuits. Serve warm. Enjoy!

Pumpkin Bread

Servings: 6
Cooking Time: 60 Minutes

Ingredients:

- 1 Cup Pumpkin, canned
- 2 eggs
- 2/3 Cup vegetable oil
- 1/2 Cup sour cream
- 1 Teaspoon vanilla extract
- 2 1/2 Cup flour
- 1 1/2 Teaspoon baking soda
- 1 Teaspoon salt
- 1/2 Teaspoon ground cinnamon
- 1/4 Teaspoon ground nutmeg
- 1/4 Teaspoon ground cloves
- 1/4 Teaspoon ground ginger
- As Needed butter

Directions:

1. In a large mixing bowl, combine the pumpkin, eggs, vegetable oil, sour cream, and vanilla and whisk to blend.
2. In a separate bowl, combine the flour, baking soda, salt, cinnamon, nutmeg, cloves, and ginger. Add the dry ingredients to the wet ingredients and stir to combine. Do not overmix.
3. If desired, stir in one or more of the optional ingredients (walnuts, dried cranberries, raisins, or chocolate chips). Butter the interiors of two loaf pans.
4. Sprinkle with flour to coat the buttered surfaces, and tap out any excess. Divide the batter evenly between the two pans.
5. When ready to cook, set the smoker to 350°F and preheat, lid closed for 15 minutes.
6. Arrange the loaf pans directly on the grill grate. Bake for 45 to 50 minutes, or until a skewer or toothpick inserted in the center comes out clean. Also, the top of the loaf should spring back when pressed gently with a finger.
7. Transfer the loaf pans to a cooling rack and let cool for 10 minutes before carefully turning out the pumpkin bread. Let the loaves cool thoroughly before slicing. Wrap in aluminum foil or plastic wrap if not eating right away. Serve and enjoy!

Baked Buttermilk Biscuits

Servings: 4
Cooking Time: 15 Minutes

Ingredients:

- 2 Cup all-purpose flour
- 1/4 Cup butter
- 3/4 Cup buttermilk

Directions:

1. Supply your smoker with wood pellets and follow the start-up procedure. Preheat the grill, with the lid closed, to High heat. Spoon the flour into a measuring cup and level with a knife.
2. Put the flour into a mixing bowl. Using a pastry blender, cut the butter into the flour until the mixture resembles coarse crumbs.
3. With a fork, gently stir in just enough of the buttermilk so the dough leaves the sides of the bowl. (You may not need all the buttermilk.) For the most tender biscuits, do not overmix.
4. Lightly flour a work surface as well as your hands. Tip the dough onto the floured surface and gently bring together using your fingertips. (Re-flour your hands or the board if the dough is too sticky.) Knead two or three times, just to bring the dough together.
5. With a floured rolling pin, lightly and quickly roll the dough out to a thickness of about 1/2". Using a 1-1/2" floured cutter, cut out as many biscuits as you can. (Do not twist the cutter; push it straight down.) You can reroll the scraps if desired, but the "second string" biscuits will be tougher.
6. Transfer the biscuits to an ungreased baking sheet. Using a pastry brush, brush the tops with melted butter. Bake until golden brown, 10 to 15 minutes. Enjoy! Grill: 500 °F

Sopapilla Cheesecake By Doug Scheiding

Servings: 8
Cooking Time: 45 Minutes

Ingredients:

- 2 Tablespoon softened butter
- 24 Ounce cream cheese
- 2 Cup granulated sugar, divided
- 2 Teaspoon vanilla
- 2 Can Pillsbury Butter Flake Crescent Rolls
- 1/2 Cup butter, melted
- cinnamon

Directions:

1. Coat a 9x13 inch baking dish with 2 tablespoons softened butter and set aside.
2. Supply your smoker with wood pellets and follow the start-up procedure. Preheat the grill, with the lid closed, to 350° F.
3. In a mixer, combine cream cheese, 1 to 1-1/2 cups of sugar and vanilla. Mix for 60 to 90 seconds on high with paddle attachment.
4. Take crescents out of the refrigerator. Open one can and place into the buttered 9x13 inch rectangular metal pan or glass dish. Make sure to fill in the gaps in this bottom layer of crescents.
5. Put the cream cheese mixture on the top of the crescent layer using a spatula to make it level.
6. Open the second can of crescents and put on top of the cream cheese layer, again filling in the gaps in the crescents to cover middle.
7. Pour 1/2 cup of melted butter on the top of the last layer of crescent. Start on sides first then middle.
8. Then sprinkle 1/4 cup to 1/2 cup of sugar over the entire pan followed by a light, even dusting of cinnamon.
9. Place pan directly on the grill grate and bake for 40 to 50 minutes until top is brown and starting to get crusty. Grill: 350 ˚F
10. Remove from grill and let cool 5 to 10 minutes. This allows the cheesecake to set which makes portioning easier. This dessert can be served warm or cold. Enjoy!

Mexican Black Bean Cornbread Casserole

Servings: 6
Cooking Time: 30 Minutes

Ingredients:

- 1 Lb Beef, Ground
- 1 15Oz Drained Black Beans, Can
- 1 Box Corn Muffin Mix
- 1 15Oz Enchilada Sauce, Can
- 1 Onion, Chopped
- 1 15Oz Drained Pinto Beans, Can

Directions:

1. Supply your smoker with wood pellets and follow the start-up procedure. Preheat the grill, with the lid closed, to 300° F.
2. Mix corn muffin mix according to directions.
3. Place cast iron skillet over flame broiler and heat for a few minutes, leaving Grill lid open.
4. Add onion and ground beef/sausage to skillet and break up
5. Cook until meat is done about 5 to 10 minutes.
6. Add both cans of beans, and enchilada sauce, stir to combine.
7. Bring mixture to a simmer.
8. Carefully close flame broiler and turn Grill up to 400 degrees.
9. Spread prepared corn muffin mix over top of meat and bean mixture and bake for 15 minutes until cornbread mixture is lightly browned.
10. Let sit 15 minutes before serving.

Skillet Buttermilk Cornbread

Servings: 6
Cooking Time: 25 Minutes

Ingredients:

- 1 Cup Cornmeal
- 1 Cup all-purpose flour
- 1/3 Cup granulated sugar
- 1 Teaspoon salt
- 1 Teaspoon baking powder
- 1 1/2 Cup buttermilk

- 2 Whole eggs
- 8 Tablespoon butter, melted

Directions:

1. Grease a cast iron skillet or 9-inch square baking pan with bacon fat. Put a 10-inch well-seasoned cast iron skillet on the grill grate. If using a regular baking pan, do not preheat.

2. Supply your smoker with wood pellets and follow the start-up procedure. Preheat the grill, with the lid closed, to 400° F.

3. In a large mixing bowl, combine the cornmeal, flour, sugar, salt, and baking powder and whisk to mix thoroughly. Make a well in the center of the dry ingredients.

4. In a separate mixing bowl, whisk together the buttermilk and eggs until well-combined. Add the melted butter. Pour into the dry ingredients and mix until the batter is fairly smooth. Do not overmix.

5. Carefully pour the batter into the preheated skillet. Bake for 20 to 25 minutes, or until the top is firm and a tester inserted in the center of the cornbread comes out clean. Be careful when removing the skillet from the grill as it will be very hot. Let the cornbread cool slightly on a trivet or cooling rack before slicing into wedges or squares.

Vanilla Chocolate Chip Cookies

Servings: 12
Cooking Time: 20 Minutes

Ingredients:
- 3/4 cup brown sugar
- 3/4 cup white sugar
- 1 stick butter, room temp
- 2 eggs
- 1 tsp vanilla
- 2 1/2 cups flour
- 1/2 tsp salt
- 1 tsp baking soda
- 1 cup Chocolate Chips

Directions:

1. Cream your butter and sugar together in a mixing bowl using a hand mixer or stand mixer on medium speed for about 4-5 minutes.

2. Once the butter is creamed, add the eggs and vanilla. Continue mixing for an additional minute.

3. Put flour, salt, and baking soda in a sifter. Sift it into your creamed butter mixture.

4. Scrape the sides of your mixing bowl with a rubber spatula, and then turn your mixer on to low speed.

5. Let it mix a little, and then scrape the sides again. Stop mixing when there are one or two streaks of flour left in the cookie dough.

6. Scrape the sides of your bowl and pour in a cup of chocolate chips, and turn the mixer to low again to mix the chocolate. It should take just a few turns for the chocolate pieces to be well incorporated.

7. Line a large baking sheet with parchment paper. Using a medium cookie scoop (about 1.5 tbsp), drop evenly spaced dollops of cookie dough onto the cookie sheet.

8. Supply your smoker with wood pellets and follow the start-up procedure. Preheat the grill, with the lid closed, to 350° F. Place the cookie sheet in your smoker, and let them cook for about 12 minutes.

9. Let them sit on a cooling rack while you continue to cook the additional cookies.

10. Cool for a few minutes to let cookies set.

11. Enjoy!

Chili Cheese Fries

Servings: 6
Cooking Time: 10 Minutes

Ingredients:
- 1 Cup Cheddar Cheese, Shredded
- 1 Cup Chili Con Carne, Prepared
- 1 Bag French Fries
- 1 Tablespoon Olive Oil
- 1 Tablespoon Sweet Heat Rub

Directions:

1. Supply your smoker with wood pellets and follow the start-up procedure. Preheat the grill, with the lid

closed, to 350° F. If you're using charcoal or gas, set it up for medium high heat.

2. Bake the fries according to manufacturer's instructions. Once the fries are done, place them in a large bowl and add the olive oil and Sweet Heat Rub. Toss the fries to coat. Once everything is well coated with the oil and seasoning, spread the fries on a baking sheet.

3. Top the fries with the chili and the shredded cheddar cheese. Place the baking sheet on the grill and grill for 7-10 minutes, or until the cheese is melted and bubbly, and the chili is warm all the way through.

4. Remove the baking sheet from the grill and serve the fries immediately.

Italian Herb & Parmesan Scones

Servings: 8
Cooking Time: 20 Minutes

Ingredients:
- 2 1/2 Cup all-purpose flour
- 2 Teaspoon baking powder
- 1 Teaspoon baking soda
- 1/2 Teaspoon garlic salt
- 1 Tablespoon Italian Seasoning
- 1 Cup Parmesan cheese, grated
- 2 Large eggs
- 1 1/2 Cup buttermilk
- 1/4 Cup olive oil

Directions:
1. In a large mixing bowl, combine flour, baking powder, baking powder, soda, garlic salt, Italian seasoning, and 1/2 cup of the cheese. Make a well in the center.

2. In a smaller bowl, whisk together eggs, buttermilk, and olive oil.

3. Pour into the well in the dry ingredients, and stir batter just until it's combined. It will appear lumpy.

4. Oil 12 muffin cups, spray with cooking spray, or line with disposable paper liners.

5. Divide the batter evenly between the cups. Sprinkle the tops of the muffins with the remaining Parmesan cheese.

6. Supply your smoker with wood pellets and follow the start-up procedure. Preheat the grill, with the lid closed, to 400° F.

7. Arrange the muffin tin directly on the grill grate and bake the muffins for 20 to 25 minutes, or until a toothpick inserted in the center of the muffin comes out clean.

8. Cool for several minutes before removing from the muffin tin. Serve warm with butter or olive oil. Enjoy!

Cornbread Chicken Stuffing

Servings: 6 - 8
Cooking Time: 95 Minutes

Ingredients:
- 2 Tbsp Butter
- 1 Cup Chicken Stock
- 6 Cups Cornbread, Cubed
- ½ Cup Dried Cranberries
- 1 Egg
- ½ Cup Heavy Whipping Cream
- 1 Lb. Italian Sausage
- 1 Diced Onion
- 1 ½ Tsp Pulled Pork Rub
- 2 Tbsp Sage, Fresh
- ½ Tsp Fresh Thyme

Directions:
1. Supply your smoker with wood pellets and follow the start-up procedure. Preheat the grill, with the lid closed, to 250° F. If using a gas or charcoal grill, set the temp to low heat.

2. Portion sausage into quarter-size pieces and place on mesh grate. Place grate on the grill and cook for 1 hour. Sausage pieces will have a smoky deep brown color. Move the mesh tray of sausage to the side of the grill with indirect heat.

3. Open the Flame Broiler Plate and increase the temperature to 350°F. Place a large cast iron skillet on the grill, over direct flame. Add butter and onions and cook until the onions caramelize lightly, stirring often. Add the sage and thyme and stir to combine.

4. Gently fold in the dried cranberries and cubed cornbread, then add sausage directly from mesh grate.

5. In a small mixing bowl, whisk together the heavy cream, chicken stock, egg, and Pulled Pork Rub. Pour mixture over the cornbread stuffing mix.

6. Cover grill and cook 30 minutes or until heated through and crispy on top.

Blueberry Sour Cream Muffins

Servings: 8
Cooking Time: 25 Minutes

Ingredients:
- 2 Cup flour
- 1/2 Teaspoon salt
- 1/2 Teaspoon baking soda
- 1/2 Cup butter
- 3/4 Cup sugar, plus more for muffin tops
- 2 Large eggs
- 3/4 Cup sour cream
- 1 1/2 Teaspoon vanilla extract
- 1 1/2 Cup blueberries, fresh or thawed

Directions:
1. In a small mixing bowl, whisk together the flour, salt and baking soda.
2. In another bowl, using a wooden spoon or a mixer, beat the butter and sugar until light-colored and fluffy. Beat in the eggs, one at a time. Stir in sour cream and vanilla.
3. Add the flour mixture gradually and mix just until incorporated. Using a rubber spatula, gently fold in the blueberries.
4. Line a 12-cup muffin tin with the cupcake liners. Using an ice cream scoop or spoon, fill each muffin cup two-thirds full with the batter. Sprinkle sugar evenly over the top of each muffin.
5. Supply your smoker with wood pellets and follow the start-up procedure. Preheat the grill, with the lid closed, to 375° F.
6. Bake the muffins 25 to 30 minutes, or until a toothpick inserted comes out clean. Served warm and with butter. Grill: 375 °F

Smoky Apple Crepes

Servings: 6

Cooking Time: 60 Minutes

Ingredients:
- 1/2 Cup Apple Juice
- 2 Lbs Apples
- 2 Tbsp Brown Sugar
- 5 Tbsp Butter
- 3 Tbsp Butter, Melted
- Tt Caramel
- 3/4 Tsp Cinnamon, Ground
- Tt Cinnamon-Sugar
- 3/4 Tsp Cornstarch
- 2 Eggs
- 1 Cup Flour
- 2 Tsp Lemon Juice
- Tennessee Apple Butter Seasoning
- 1/2 Cup Water
- 3/4 Cup Milk

Directions:
1. Supply your smoker with wood pellets and follow the start-up procedure. Preheat the grill, with the lid closed, to 225° F. If using a gas or charcoal grill, set it up for low, indirect heat.
2. Peel, halve, and core apples.
3. Season apples with Tennessee Apple Butter then place directly on the grill grate, and smoke for 1 hour.
4. Meanwhile, prepare crêpe batter: combine eggs, milk, water, flour, and 3 tbsp of melted butter in a blender, and blend until smooth.
5. Refrigerate for 30 minutes.
6. Remove apples from grill, cool slightly, then slice thin.
7. Place a cast iron skillet on the grill and melt 3 tbsp butter with brown sugar, cinnamon, cornstarch, apple and lemon juices. Cook for 5 minutes until thick.
8. Add apples and cook for another 3 to 5 minutes, stirring to coat apples in sauce.
9. Remove from grill and set aside.
10. Preheat griddle to medium-low. If using a standard grill, preheat a cast iron skillet on medium-low heat.
11. Melt 1 teaspoon of butter on the griddle.

12. Then add ½ cup of batter, and spread with the bottom of a metal spatula, working quickly, as the batter cooks fast.

13. Cook one minute per side, until edges begin to brown. Remove from griddle, set aside, and repeat with remaining batter.

14. Spoon ¼ cup of apple filling into the center of each crêpe, then quarter-fold into a triangle.

15. Serve warm with additional apple filling, drizzle of warm caramel, and a dusting of cinnamon-sugar.

Traeger Baked Protein Bars

Servings: 6
Cooking Time: 25 Minutes

Ingredients:

- 2 Cup Frozen Sweet Cherries
- 1 Cup Apricots, Frozen
- 1 Scoop Vanilla Protein Powder
- 2 Tablespoon honey
- 1 Teaspoon vanilla extract
- 1 Cup rolled oats

Directions:

1. Supply your smoker with wood pellets and follow the start-up procedure. Preheat the grill, with the lid closed, to 350° F.

2. In the bowl of a food processor, add cherries, apricots (revived in hot water for 5 minutes and drained), vanilla protein powder, honey, and vanilla. Pulse about 10 to 15 times, to break the fruit into smaller pieces and to mix all ingredients.

3. In a separate bowl, fold together oats and fruit mixture. Transfer mixture to a loaf pan or silicone mold and place in grill.

4. Bake for approximately 20 to 25 minutes. Grill: 350 °F

5. Let cool completely and cut into 8 pieces. Enjoy!

Baked Brie

Servings: 6
Cooking Time: 8 Minutes

Ingredients:

- 16 Ounce (16 oz) brie wheel

- 1/3 Cup honey
- 1/4 Cup pecans
- Crackers
- apple, sliced

Directions:

1. Supply your smoker with wood pellets and follow the start-up procedure. Preheat the grill, with the lid closed, to 350° F.

2. Line a rimmed baking sheet with a piece of parchment or aluminum foil. Using a sharp serrated knife, slice top—the white rind—off the brie. (Le the ave the rind on the sides and bottom intact.)

3. Put the brie, cut side up, on the prepared baking sheet and drizzle with the honey. Sprinkle nuts on top.

4. Bake the brie until it is soft and oozing, but not melting, 8 to 10 minutes. Let it cool for a couple of minutes and transfer to a serving plate. Grill: 350 °F

5. Serve with crackers and sliced apple wedges. Drizzle with more honey, if desired. Enjoy!

Baked Wood-fired Pizza

Servings: 6
Cooking Time: 12 Minutes

Ingredients:

- 2/3 Cup warm water (110°F to 115°F)
- 2 1/2 Teaspoon active dry yeast
- 1/2 Teaspoon granulated sugar
- 1 Teaspoon kosher salt
- 1 Tablespoon oil
- 2 Cup all-purpose flour
- 1/4 Cup fine cornmeal
- 1 Large grilled portobello mushroom, sliced
- 1 Jar pickled artichoke hearts, drained and chopped
- 1 Cup shredded fontina cheese
- 1/2 Cup shaved Parmigiano-Reggiano cheese, divided
- To Taste Roasted Garlic, minced
- 1/4 Cup extra-virgin olive oil
- To Taste banana peppers

Directions:

1. In a glass bowl, stir together the warm water, yeast and sugar. Let stand until the mixture starts to foam,

about 10 minutes. In a mixer, combine 1-3/4 cup flour, sugar and salt. Stir oil into the yeast mixture. Slowly add the liquid to the dry ingredients while slowly increasing the mixers speed until fully combined. The dough should be smooth and not sticky.

2. Knead the dough on a floured surface, gradually adding the remaining flour as needed to prevent the dough from sticking, until smooth, about 5 to 10 minutes.

3. Form the dough into a ball. Apply a thin layer of olive oil to a large bowl. Place the dough into the bowl and coat the dough ball with a small amount of olive oil. Cover and let rise in a warm place for about 1 hour or until doubled in size.

4. When ready to cook, set smoker temperature to 450°F and preheat, lid closed for 15 minutes.

5. Place a pizza stone in the grill while it preheats.

6. Punch the dough down and roll it out into a 12-inch circle on a floured surface.

7. Spread the cornmeal evenly on the pizza peel. Place the dough on the pizza peel and assemble the toppings evenly in the following order: olive oil, roasted garlic, fontina, portobello, artichoke hearts, Parmigiano-Reggiano and banana peppers.

8. Carefully slide the assembled pizza from the pizza peel to the preheated pizza stone and bake until the crust is golden brown, about 10 to 12 minutes. Enjoy!

Anzac Coconut Biscuits

Servings: 4
Cooking Time: 30 Minutes

Ingredients:

- This recipe makes a dozen biscuits.
- 1 cup rolled oats
- 3/4 cup raw sugar
- 3/4 cup desiccated coconut
- 1 cup plain flour, sifted
- 125 g butter, melted
- 2 tablespoons Golden Syrup
- 1/2 tsp bicarb soda
- 3 tablespoons boiling water

Directions:

1. Combine and mix thoroughly sifted flour, oats, sugar and coconut in a large bowl.

2. Melt the butter and Golden Syrup over low heat.

3. Add boiling water to the bicarb soda, once dissolved add into the butter/syrup mix, it will bubble/fizz up a bit.

4. Add the liquid into the dry ingredients and mix throughly.

5. Rolls the mix into golf ball size balls and layout on grease proof paper on baking tray and flatten the tops just slightly.

6. Space the balls with about 3 fingers between each ball as they will flatten to about triple the diameter as they cook.

7. Supply your smoker with wood pellets and follow the start-up procedure. Preheat the grill, with the lid closed, to 350° F. Cook for 25-30 minutes until golden brown.

8. Rest on cooling rack until at room temperature then store in air-tight container.

Blueberry Bread Pudding

Servings: 4
Cooking Time: 60 Minutes

Ingredients:

- 5 eggs
- 3 Cup sugar
- 2 1/2 Cup milk
- 1 1/2 Teaspoon vanilla
- 1 Teaspoon cinnamon
- 1 Pinch salt
- 5 Cup Bread
- 3 Cup blueberries

Directions:

1. Beat the eggs in a large mixing bowl. Whisk in the sugar, milk, vanilla, cinnamon, and salt.

2. In another large bowl, combine the bread and 2 cups (200 g) of the blueberries.

3. Pour the egg mixture over the bread-blueberry mixture and let sit for 30 minutes. Meanwhile, place muffin liners in a muffin tin.

4. Supply your smoker with wood pellets and follow the start-up procedure. Preheat the grill, with the lid open.

5. Spoon the bread-blueberry mixture into the prepared cups; evenly top each with the remaining cup of blueberries, pressing them gently into the pudding with the back of a spoon.

6. Dust the top with sugar.

7. Arrange the pan directly on the grill grate and smoke for 30 minutes. Grill:180°F

8. Increase the temperature to 350F (180 C), and bake until the pudding is set and golden brown on top, about 25 minutes. Grill:350°F

9. Let cool slightly, then sift powdered sugar on top. Serve warm with sweetened whipped cream or vanilla ice cream, if desired.

Mint Butter Chocolate Chip Cookies

Servings: 24
Cooking Time: 12 Minutes

Ingredients:

- 1/2 Cup Butter, Melted
- 1 Package Chocolate Chip Cookie Mix
- 8-10 Drop Food Coloring
- 1/2 Tsp Mint, Extract

Directions:

1. Supply your smoker with wood pellets and follow the start-up procedure. Preheat the grill, with the lid closed, to 350° F.

2. Follow the directions on the back of the Chocolate Chip Cookie mix and also add the mint extract and green food coloring. Mix until combined.

3. On a baking sheet lined with parchment paper, drop balls of dough about 2 tbsp in size onto the pan.

4. Place in your Grill and bake for 10-12 minutes. Let cool for a couple minutes before removing from the pan. Enjoy!

The Dan Patrick Show Pull-apart Pesto Bread

Servings: 8
Cooking Time: 25 Minutes

Ingredients:

- 1 Sourdough Bread, loaf
- 1/2 Cup butter, melted
- 1 Cup Pesto Sauce
- 1 1/2 Cup Italian Cheese Blend

Directions:

1. Supply your smoker with wood pellets and follow the start-up procedure. Preheat the grill, with the lid closed, to 350° F.

2. Using a serrated knife, make 1" diagonal cuts through the bread leaving the bottom crust intact. Turn the bread and make diagonal cuts in the opposite direction, creating diamonds.

3. Place the bread on a sheet of foil large enough to wrap around the entire loaf. Pour the melted butter into the cracks in the bread. Using a spoon spread the pesto into the cracks then follow with the cheese stuffing it down into each crack.

4. Fold up the edges of the foil to wrap up the loaf and transfer to a baking sheet. Place the baking sheet directly on the grill grate.

5. Bake for 15 minutes then unwrap the foil and cook for an additional 10 minutes. Remove from the grill and serve. Enjoy! Grill: 350 °F

6. Follow along as we give you a recipe each day this week from The Dan Patrick Show Game Day Recipes eBook.

Smoker Wheat Bread

Servings: 6
Cooking Time: 60 Minutes

Ingredients:

- As Needed extra-virgin olive oil
- 2 Cup all-purpose flour
- 1 Cup whole wheat flour
- 1 1/4 Ounce Packet, Active Dry Yeast
- 1 1/4 Teaspoon salt
- 1 1/2 Cup water
- As Needed Cornmeal

Directions:

1. Oil a large mixing bowl and set aside. In a second mixing bowl, combine the flours, yeast, and salt.

2. Push your sleeve up to your elbow and form your fingers into a claw. Mix the dry ingredients until well-combined.

3. Add the water and mix until blended. The dough will be wet, shaggy, and somewhat stringy.

4. Tip the dough into the oiled mixing bowl and cover with plastic wrap.

5. Allow the dough to rise at room temperature-- about 70 degrees-- for 2 hours, or until the surface is bubbled.

6. Turn the dough out onto a lightly floured work surface and lightly flour the top. With floured hands, fold the dough over on itself twice. Cover loosely with plastic wrap and allow the dough to rest for 15 minutes.

7. Dust a clean lint-free cotton towel with cornmeal, wheat bran, or flour. With floured hands, gently form the dough into a ball and place it, seam side down, on the towel.

8. Dust the top of the ball with cornmeal, wheat bran, or flour, and cover the dough with a second towel. Let the dough rise until doubled in size; the dough will not spring back when poked with a finger.

9. In the meantime, start the smoker grill and set temperature to 450 F. Preheat, lid closed, for 10-15 minutes.

10. Put a lidded 6- to 8-quart cast iron Dutch oven - preferably one coated with enamel, on the grill grate.

11. When the dough has risen, remove the top towel, slide your hand under the bottom towel to support the dough, then carefully tip the dough, seam side up, into the preheated pot.

12. Remove the towel. Shake the pot a couple of times if the dough looks lopsided: It will straighten out as it bakes.

13. Cover the pot with the lid and bake the bread for 30 minutes. Remove the lid and continue to bake the bread for 15 to 30 minutes more, or until it is nicely browned and sounds hollow when rapped with your knuckles.

14. Turn onto a wire rack to cool. Slice with a serrated knife. Enjoy!

Focaccia

Servings: 6

Cooking Time: 40 Minutes

Ingredients:
- 1 Cup warm water (110°F to 115°F)
- 1/2 Ounce Yeast, active
- 1 Teaspoon sugar
- 2 1/2 Cup flour
- 1 Teaspoon salt
- 1/4 Cup extra-virgin olive oil
- 1 1/2 Teaspoon Italian herbs, dried
- 1/8 Teaspoon red pepper flakes
- As Needed coarse sea salt

Directions:
1. Measure the water in a glass-measuring cup. Stir in the yeast and sugar. Let rest for in a warm place. After 5 to 10 minutes, the mixture should be foamy, indicating the yeast is "alive." If it does not foam, discard it and start again.

2. Pour the water/yeast mixture in the bowl of a food processor. Add 1 cup of the flour as well as the salt and 1/4 cup of olive oil. Pulse several times to blend. Add the remaining flour, Italian herbs, and hot pepper flakes.

3. Process the dough until it's smooth and elastic and pulls away from the sides of the bowl, adding small amounts of flour or water through the feed tube if the dough is respectively too wet or too dry.

4. Let the dough rise in the covered food processor bowl in a warm place until doubled in bulk, about 1 hour5. Remove the dough from the food processor (it will deflate) and turn onto a lightly floured surface.

5. Oil two 8- to 9-inch round cake pans generously with olive oil. (Just pour a couple of glugs in and tilt the pan to spread the oil.) Divide the dough into two equal pieces, shape into disks, and put one in each prepared cake pan.

6. Oil the top of each disk with olive oil and dimple the dough with your fingertips. Sprinkle lightly with coarse salt, and if desired, additional dried Italian herbs.

7. Cover the focaccia dough with plastic wrap and let the dough rise in a warm place, about 45 minutes to an hour.

8. When ready to cook, start the smoker grill and set the temperature to 400F and preheat, lid closed, for 10 to 15 minutes.

9. Put the pans with the focaccia dough directly on the grill grate. Bake until the focaccia breads are light golden in color and baked through, 35 to 40 minutes, rotating the pans halfway through the baking time.

10. Let cool slightly before removing from the pans. Cut into wedges for serving.

Grilled Apple Pie

Servings: 4
Cooking Time: 40 Minutes

Ingredients:
- 5 Whole Apples
- 1/4 Cup sugar
- 1 Tablespoon cornstarch
- 1 Whole refrigerated pie crust
- 1/4 Cup Peach, preserves

Directions:
1. Supply your smoker with wood pellets and follow the start-up procedure. Preheat the grill, with the lid closed, to 375° F.In a medium bowl, mix the apples, sugar, and cornstarch; set aside.

2. Unroll pie crust. Place in ungreased pie pan. With the back of a spoon, spread preserves evenly on crust. Arrange the apple slices in an even layer in the pie pan. Slightly fold crust over filling.

3. Place a baking sheet upside down on the grill grate to make an elevated surface. Put the pan with pie on top so it is elevated off grill. (This will help prevent the bottom from overcooking.) Cook the pie for 30 to 40 minutes or until crust is golden brown, the filling is bubbly. Grill: 375 ˚F

4. Remove from grill; cool 10 minutes before serving. Enjoy! *Cook times will vary depending on set and ambient temperatures.

Garlic Cheese Pull Apart Bread

Servings: 2
Cooking Time: 20 Minutes

Ingredients:
- 1 Loaf Bread, Sourdough Round
- 2 1/2 Tbsp Butter, Salted
- 8 Oz Fontina Cheese
- 1 Grated Garlic, Roasted
- 1/4 Cup Parsley, Minced Fresh
- 1 Tsp Red Flakes Pepper
- 1 Pinch Salt

Directions:
1. Start your Grill on "smoke" with the lid open until a fire is established in the burn pot (3-7 minutes). Supply your smoker with wood pellets and follow the start-up procedure. Preheat the grill, with the lid closed, to 300° F.

2. In a small bowl, add the soft butter, grated garlic, red pepper flakes, sea salt, and ¼ cup of the chopped parsley, and whisk together. With a bread serrated knife, cut 1-inch slices into the bread, not cutting all the way through the bottom of the load. With a butter knife, spread a thin layer of the butter mixture on each slice of the bread. Take the serrated knife again, and cut across the loaf to form 1 inch squares. Next, slice the cheese into small thin slices, then stuff one slice into each bread opening. Place the bread on a baking sheet, and cover tightly with aluminum foil. Place on the grill for about 10 minutes, remove the foil, and grill for a few more minutes until the top is nicely golden and the cheese is oozing. Remove from the grill, sprinkle with fresh parsley leaves, then serve.

RECIPE INDEX

3-2-1 Bbq Beef Cheeks 107

A

A Smoking Classic Cocktail 168

Alder Smoked Scallops With Citrus & Garlic Butter Sauce 23

Anzac Coconut Biscuits 237

Apple & Bourbon Glazed Ham 58

Apple-smoked Bacon 70

Apple-smoked Pork Tenderloin 58

Apricot Glazed Ham 158

B

Baby Back Ribs With Mustard Slather 78

Bacon Old-fashioned Cocktail 167

Bacon Pork Pinwheels (kansas Lollipops) 117

Bacon Stuffed Onion Rings 78

Bacon Weaved Stuffed Turkey Breast 144

Bacon Wrapped Asparagus 63

Bacon Wrapped Chicken Wings 142

Bacon Wrapped Corn On The Cob 194

Bacon Wrapped Pickles 54

Bacon Wrapped Scallops 15

Bacon Wrapped Shrimp 26

Bacon Wrapped Turkey Legs 157

Bacon-draped Injected Pork Loin Roast 61

Bacon-swiss Cheesesteak Meatloaf 91

Bacon-wrapped Chicken Breasts 154

Bacon-wrapped Jalapeño Poppers 116

Baked Bacon Green Bean Casserole 184

Baked Bourbon Monkey Bread 227

Baked Breakfast Mini Quiches 196

Baked Brie 236

Baked Buttermilk Biscuits 231

Baked Cast Iron Berry Cobbler 208

Baked Cheesy Parmesan Grits 209

Baked Chocolate Brownie Cookies With Egg Nog 214

Baked Garlic Duchess Potatoes 203

Baked German Pork Schnitzel With Grilled Lemons 62

Baked Green Chile Mac & Cheese By Doug Scheiding 223

Baked Heirloom Tomato Tart 183

Baked Honey Glazed Ham 70

Baked Irish Creme Cake 225

Baked Kale Chips 183

Baked Loaded Tater Tots 193

Baked Molten Chocolate Cake 220

Baked Peach Cobbler Cupcakes 217

Baked Prosciutto-wrapped Chicken Breast With Spinach And Boursin 141

Baked Pumpkin Pie 223

Baked Sage & Sausage Stuffing 56

Baked Steelhead 17

Baked Stuffed Avocados 185

Baked Sweet And Savory Yams By Bennie Kendrick 205

Baked Sweet Potato Casserole With Marshmallow Fluff 181

Baked Tuna Noodle Casserole 33

Baked Winter Squash Au Gratin 186

Baked Wood-fired Pizza 236

Balsamic Brussels Sprouts With Bacon 62

Bananas Rum Foster 228

Barbecued Scallops 43

Barbecued Shrimp 38

Barbecued Tenderloin 71

Basil Margherita Pizza 215

Batter Up Cocktail 165

Bayou Wings With Cajun Rémoulade 117

Bbq Bacon Meatballs 94

Bbq Bacon-wrapped Water Chestnuts 79

Bbq Breakfast Sausage 149

Bbq Brisket Tacos 85

Bbq Brown Sugar Bacon Bites 66

Bbq Burnt End Sandwich 108

Bbq Burnt Ends 112

Bbq Chicken Breasts 135

Bbq Chicken Tostada 156

Bbq Oysters 31

Bbq Pork Belly 54

Bbq Pork Chops 79

Bbq Pork Short Ribs 67

Bbq Pork Shoulder Steaks 65

Bbq Pulled Pork Grilled Cheese Sandwich 80

Bbq Pulled Pork With Sweet & Heat Bbq Sauce 63
Bbq Pulled Turkey Sandwiches 138
Bbq Rib Sandwich 73
Bbq Roasted Salmon 27
Bbq Spatchcocked Chicken 137
Beef Brisket With Chophouse Steak Rub 114
Beer Braised Garlic Bbq Pork Butt 67
Beer Bread 219
Beer Chili Bratwurst 82
Beer Pork Belly Chili Con Carne 65
Bistecca Alla Fiorentina With Mushroom Ragout 101
Blt Pasta Salad 200
Blueberry Bread Pudding 237
Blueberry Pancakes 211
Blueberry Sour Cream Muffins 235
Bourbon Chicken Waffles 134
Bourbon-brined Turkey Thighs 151
Braised Creamed Green Beans 178
Braised Onion Chuck Roast Beef Sandwiches 113
Broccoli-cauliflower Salad 188
Buffalo Chicken 126
Buffalo Chicken Wings 131
Butter Braised Green Beans 194
Butternut Squash 180
Butternut Squash Macaroni And Cheese 221

C

Cajun Brined Maple Smoked Turkey Breast 146
Cajun Double-smoked Ham 60
Cajun Spatchcock Turkey 137
Cajun-blackened Shrimp 22
Cake With Smoked Berry Sauce 225
Carne Asada Recipe 84
Carolina Baked Beans 179
Carrot Cake 218
Carrot Celery Chicken Drumsticks 143
Cast Iron Potatoes 202
Cheesy Skillet Shepherd's Pie 86
Chef Curtis' Famous Chimichurri Sauce 188
Chicken Breast Calzones 157
Chicken On A Throne 137
Chicken Parmesan Sliders With Pesto Mayonnaise 150
Chicken Pizza On The Grill 229
Chicken Pot Pie 221

Chicken Tenders 139
Chicken Wings With Teriyaki Glaze 116
Chile Chicken Thighs 129
Chili Cheese Fries 233
Chocolate Almond Cake 216
Chorizo Cheese Stuffed Burgers 90
Chorizo Queso Fundido 118
Christmas Brussel Sprouts 193
Chuckwagon Beef Jerky 122
Cider Hot-smoked Salmon 24
Cider-brined Turkey 155
Cinnamon Pull-aparts 230
Citrus Grilled Lamb Chops 96
Citrus-infused Marinated Olives 118
Citrus-smoked Trout 32
Classic Pulled Pork 61
Cocoa-crusted Pork Tenderloin 77
Cold-smoked Cheese 125
Cold-smoked Salmon Gravlax 36
Competition Style Bbq Pork Ribs 49
Cornbread Chicken Stuffing 234
County Fair Turkey Legs 141
Cran-apple Tequila Punch With Smoked Oranges 168
Cranberry Turkey Breast 135
Crème Brûlée 226
Crescent Rolls 228
Cucumber Beef Kefta 84

D

Dark Chocolate Brownies With Bacon-salted Caramel 224
Delicious Deviled Crab Appetizer 123
Delicious Peanut Butter Cookies 226
Delicious Pellet Grill Cornbread 218
Delicious Smoked Bone-in Pork Chops 77
Delicious Smoked Trout 25
Deviled Eggs With Smoked Paprika 120
Dijon-smoked Halibut 19
Donut Bread Pudding 222
Double Chocolate Chip Brownie Pie 208
Double-decker Pulled Pork Nachos With Smoked Cheese 76
Double-smoked Cheese Potatoes 190
Dry Brine Traeger Turkey 136

Dublin Delight Cocktail 171
Duck Breast With Pomegranate Sauce 128
Duck Fat Fries (confit) 103

E
Easy Grilled Chicken Shawarma 135
Easy Smoked Cornbread 220
Egg Bacon French Toast Panini 72
Eggs Ham Benedict 230
Eyeball Cookies 225

F
Fig Slider Cocktail 167
First-timer's Pulled Pork 59
Flavour Bbq Brisket Burnt Ends 109
Flavour Fire Spiced Shrimp 25
Flavour Reverse Seared T-bone Steak 95
Flavour Smoked Corned Beef Brisket Hash 81
Flavour Texas Smoke Beef 97
Florentine Shrimp Al Cartoccio 40
Focaccia 239
Fried Chicken Sliders 143

G
Garden Gimlet Cocktail 164
Garlic Bacon Wrapped Shrimp 29
Garlic Blackened Catfish 44
Garlic Cheese Pull Apart Bread 240
Garlic Grilled Shrimp Skewers 16
Garlic Lemon Pepper Chicken Wings 218
Garlic Pepper Shrimp Pesto Bruschetta 38
Garlic Sriracha Buffalo Chicken Wings 130
Garlic Standing Rib Roast 101
Greek Leg Of Lamb 99
Green Bean Casserole 189
Green Bean Casserole Circa 1955 211
Green Chile Chicken Enchiladas 153
Grilled Albacore Tuna With Potato-tomato Casserole 17
Grilled Apple Pie 240
Grilled Artichoke Cheese Salmon 28
Grilled Asparagus & Honey-glazed Carrots 195
Grilled Asparagus And Hollandaise Sauce 189
Grilled Asparagus And Spinach Salad 191
Grilled Beer Cabbage 198
Grilled Beer Cheese Dip 215

Grilled Bell Pepper Flank Steak Fajitas 84
Grilled Bison Rib Eye Kabobs 98
Grilled Blackened Saskatchewan Salmon 42
Grilled Blood Orange Mimosa 161
Grilled Broccoli Rabe 183
Grilled Cabbage Steaks With Warm Bacon Vinaigrette 178
Grilled Cheesy Chicken 146
Grilled Chili-lime Corn 185
Grilled Corn On The Cob With Parmesan And Garlic 187
Grilled Dr. Pepper Ribs 60
Grilled Fingerling Potato Salad 191
Grilled Fresh Fish 43
Grilled Frozen Strawberry Lemonade 165
Grilled Garlic Shrimp With Cajun Dip 17
Grilled Garlic Tomahawk Steak 104
Grilled Garlic Tri Tip 111
Grilled German Sausage With A Smoky Traeger Twist 66
Grilled Guacamole 119
Grilled Ham & Egg Cups 78
Grilled Hawaiian Sour 164
Grilled Honey Chicken Wings 158
Grilled Honey Garlic Wings 132
Grilled Lasagna With Cold-smoked Mozzarella 75
Grilled Lemon Salmon 15
Grilled Lemon Skirt Steak 107
Grilled Lemon Steak Pinwheels 115
Grilled Lobster Tails With Smoked Paprika Butter 33
Grilled Loco Moco Burger 108
Grilled Maple Syrup Salmon 26
Grilled Mussels With Lemon Butter 39
Grilled Oysters With Mignonette 44
Grilled Peach Mint Julep 171
Grilled Peach Smash Cocktail 175
Grilled Peach Sour Cocktail 162
Grilled Pepper Lobster Tails 27
Grilled Pork Tacos Al Pastor 57
Grilled Rabbit Tail Cocktail 173
Grilled Ratatouille Salad 194
Grilled Rosemary Rack Of Lamb 103
Grilled Salmon 15
Grilled Skirt Steak Quesadillas 94

Grilled Street Corn 201
Grilled Tilapia With Blistered Cherry Tomatoes 36
Grilled Tomahawk Steak 109
Grilled Trout With Citrus & Basil 20
Grilled Tuna Steaks With Lemon & Caper Butter 31
Grilled Whole Steelhead Fillet 40
Grilled Zucchini Squash Spears 193

H
Hanging St. Louis-style Grilled Ribs 52
Hawaiian Pulled Pig 74
Home-cured Hickory-smoked Bacon 69
Home-cured Picnic Ham With Mustard Caviar 67
Honey Balsamic Salmon 41
Honey Glazed Grapefruit Shandy Cocktail 174
Honey Pork Belly Burnt Ends 47
Hot & Fast Smoked Baby Back Ribs 74
Hot Coffee-rubbed Brisket 85
Hot Turkey Sandwich With Gravy 156
Hot-smoked Salmon 37

I
In Traeger Fashion Cocktail 161
Irish Pasties 100
Italian Beef Pinwheels 105
Italian Grilled Barbecue Chicken Wings 148
Italian Herb & Parmesan Scones 234

J
Jalapeno Pepper Jack Cheese Bacon Burgers 88
Jalapeño Poppers With Chipotle Sour Cream 124
Jamaican Jerk Pork Chops 58

K
Kalbi-style Steak Wraps 110
Kansas City Cheese Brisket Burger 93
Kansas City Hot Fried Chicken 144
Kimi's Simple Grilled Fresh Fish 29
Kodiak Cakes Candied Bacon Crumble Brownies 53
Korean Style Bbq Prime Ribs 109

L
Leftover Pulled Pork With Eggs 73
Lemon Herb Grilled Salmon 43
Lemon Lobster Rolls 34
Lemon Parmesan Chicken Wings 140
Lemon Rosemary Beer Can Chicken 139

Lemon Shrimp Scampi 24
Lemon Tomahawk Steak 89
Lime Mahi Mahi Fillets 32
Loaded Chicken Fries 128
Lobster Tail 24

M
Mango Rice Wine Thai Shrimp 15
Maple Baby Backs 59
Maple Syrup Bacon Wrapped Tenderloin 74
Maple Syrup Pancake Casserole 229
Marbled Brownies With Amaretto & Ricotta 217
Mashed Red Potatoes 204
Mexican Black Bean Cornbread Casserole 232
Mexican Mahi Mahi With Baja Cabbage Slaw 35
Mezcal Shrimp With Salsa De Molcajete 30
Mini Turducken Roulade 147
Mint Butter Chocolate Chip Cookies 238
Moules Marinières With Garlic Butter Sauce 21

N
Nashville Spiced Smoked Chicken 154

O
Oktoberfest Pretzel Mustard Chicken 132
Onion Cheese Nachos 224
Orange & Maple Baked Ham 53
Oysters In The Shell 20

P
Pacific Northwest Salmon 26
Parmesan Roasted Cauliflower 186
Pastrami 114
Perfect Roast Prime Rib 82
Pickle Brined Grilled Pork Chops 47
Pig On A Stick With Buffalo Glaze 71
Pig Pops (sweet-hot Bacon On A Stick) 121
Pigs In A Blanket 120
Pineapple-pepper Pork Kebabs 51
Pizza Bites 213
Planked Trout With Fennel, Bacon & Orange 21
Pork Tenderloin With Bourbon Peaches 72
Portobello Marinated Mushroom 192
Potluck Salad With Smoked Cornbread 196
Pretzel Rolls 227
Prosciutto-wrapped Scallops 38

Pull-apart Dinner Rolls 212
Pulled Beef 98
Pulled Pork Corn Tortillas 61
Pulled Pork Loaded Nachos 118
Pulled Pork Shoulder And Chicken 61
Pulled Pork Sliders Hawaiian Rolls 50
Pulled Pork Stew 54
Pulled Pork Taquitos With Sour Cream 56
Pumpkin Bread 231

Q
Quick Baked Dinner Rolls 216

R
Red Potato Grilled Lollipops 200
Reverse Sear Tomahawk Chop 106
Roasted Asparagus 205
Roasted Bacon Weave Holiday Ham 76
Roasted Beet & Bacon Salad 187
Roasted Chicken With Wild Rice & Mushrooms 136
Roasted Do-ahead Mashed Potatoes 188
Roasted Duck 95
Roasted Duck With Cherry Salsa 127
Roasted Fall Vegetables 194
Roasted Garlic Herb Fries 195
Roasted Green Beans With Bacon 180
Roasted Halibut With Spring Vegetables 29
Roasted Hasselback Potatoes By Doug Scheiding 199
Roasted Honey Bourbon Glazed Turkey 134
Roasted Jalapeno Cheddar Deviled Eggs 180
Roasted Jalapeño Poppers 199
Roasted Mashed Potatoes 188
Roasted New Potatoes 184
Roasted New Potatoes With Compound Butter 180
Roasted Olives 203
Roasted Pickled Beets 202
Roasted Potato Poutine 203
Roasted Pumpkin Seeds 205
Roasted Red Pepper Dip 123
Roasted Red Pepper White Bean Dip 206
Roasted Sheet Pan Vegetables 182
Roasted Stuffed Turkey Breast 142
Roasted Sweet Potato Steak Fries 185
Roasted Tin Foil Dinners 126
Roasted Tomatoes 204

Roasted Vegetable Napoleon 186
Rosemary-smoked Lamb Chops 105
Ryes And Shine Cocktail 162

S
Salmon Cakes With Homemade Tartar Sauce 35
Salt & Pepper Dinosaur Bones 88
Salt Crusted Baked Potatoes 198
Santa Maria Tri-tip 106
Savory Beaver Tails 212
Savory Cajun Bbq Chicken 145
Savory Cheese Steak Rolls With Puff Pastry 92
Savory Cheesecake With Bourbon Pecan Topping 214
Savory Chili Mac And Cheese 87
Savory Smoked Turkey Legs 132
Savory Whiskey Grilled Elk Steaks 100
Savory-sweet Turkey Legs 133
Seared Ahi Tuna Steak With Soy Sauce 41
Seared Bluefin Tuna Steaks 41
Shrimp Cabbage Tacos With Lime Cream 20
Simple Cream Cheese Sausage Balls 120
Simple Glazed Salmon Fillets 23
Simple Smoked Baby Backs 47
Skillet Buttermilk Cornbread 232
Skillet Potato Cake 206
Skinny Smoked Chicken Breasts 148
Slow Smoked Spiced Beef 98
Smoke And Bubz Cocktail 176
Smoke Roasted Chicken With Herb Butter 149
Smoked & Loaded Baked Potato 178
Smoked Apple Cider 161
Smoked Apple Pork Belly 77
Smoked Asparagus Soup 205
Smoked Avocado Turkey Tamale Pie 145
Smoked Baby Back Ribs 47
Smoked Bacon Brisket Flat 113
Smoked Bacon Roses 50
Smoked Barnburner Cocktail 170
Smoked Bbq Onion Brussels Sprout 204
Smoked Beef Back Ribs 81
Smoked Beef Ribs 93
Smoked Beer Brisket 107
Smoked Beer Corned Beef 99
Smoked Beet-pickled Eggs 190

Smoked Berry Cocktail 160
Smoked Black Pepper Beef Back Ribs 90
Smoked Blackberry Pie 212
Smoked Bourbon Jerky 102
Smoked Burgers 107
Smoked Cashews 121
Smoked Cheese 122
Smoked Cheese Beef Burgers 114
Smoked Cheesy Chicken Quesadilla 154
Smoked Chicken Steak Sandwiches 96
Smoked Chicken Vermicelli Noodles 130
Smoked Chicken With Apricot Bbq Glaze 126
Smoked Cold Brew Coffee 169
Smoked Corned Beef & Cabbage 92
Smoked Corned Beef Brisket 113
Smoked Crab Legs 39
Smoked Eggnog 175
Smoked Fish Chowder 45
Smoked Garlic Prime Rib Roast 110
Smoked Grape Lime Rickey 174
Smoked Ham 68
Smoked Hibiscus Sparkler 169
Smoked Honey Chicken Drumsticks 159
Smoked Honey Salmon 34
Smoked Hot Buttered Rum 163
Smoked Ice Mojito Slurpee 165
Smoked Irish Coffee 172
Smoked Jacobsen Salt Margarita 170
Smoked Jalapeño Poppers 197
Smoked Lemon Cheesecake 210
Smoked Lemon Tea 224
Smoked Lobster Scampi 22
Smoked Longhorn Brisket 110
Smoked Macaroni Salad 182
Smoked Mango Shrimp 39
Smoked Maple Syrup Thanksgiving Turkey 140
Smoked Mashed Potatoes 197
Smoked Meatball Egg Sandwiches 95
Smoked Mulled Wine 165
Smoked Mushrooms 192
Smoked New York Steaks 102
Smoked Parmesan Herb Popcorn 201
Smoked Pickled Green Beans 192
Smoked Pineapple Hotel Nacional Cocktail 170

Smoked Plum And Thyme Fizz Cocktail 174
Smoked Pomegranate Lemonade Cocktail 164
Smoked Porchetta 55
Smoked Pork Spare Ribs 63
Smoked Pork Tomato Tamales 50
Smoked Pulled Chicken 140
Smoked Pumpkin Spice Latte 166
Smoked Quarters 156
Smoked Rack Of Pork 64
Smoked Raspberry Bubbler Cocktail 176
Smoked Red Wine Beef Roast 86
Smoked Salmon Candy 18
Smoked Salted Caramel White Russian 167
Smoked Sangria 166
Smoked Spare Ribs 64
Smoked Spiced Pulled Beef Chuck Roast 83
Smoked Sweet Beer Bread 209
Smoked Texas Bbq Brisket 81
Smoked Texas Ranch Water 172
Smoked Thanksgiving Turkey 138
Smoked Traeger Pulled Pork 48
Smoked Trout 34
Smoked Turkey Sandwich 124
Smoked Vanilla Apple Pie 216
Smoked Whiskey Peach Pulled Chicken 133
Smoked Whole Chicken 142
Smoked Wings 150
Smoked, Salted Caramel Apple Pie 210
Smoker Wheat Bread 238
Smoke-roasted Beer-braised Brats 68
Smoke-roasted Chicken Thighs 159
Smoke-roasted Halibut With Mixed Herb Vinaigrette 32
Smokin' Lemon Bars 221
Smoking Gun Cocktail 160
Smoky Apple Crepes 235
Smoky Crab Dip 18
Smoky Mountain Bramble Cocktail 176
Smoky Pimento Cheese Cornbread 220
Smoky Pork Tenderloin 48
Smoky Scotch & Ginger Cocktail 168
Sopapilla Cheesecake By Doug Scheiding 232
Sourdough Pizza 219

Spatchcocked Chicken With Toasted Fennel & Garlic 150

Spatchcocked Chicken With White Barbecue Sauce 152

Spatchcocked Quail With Smoked Fruit 105

Spiced Lemon Cherry Pie 222

Spiced Orange Ribs 55

Spiced Smoked Chicken Quarters 143

Spicy Asian Brussels Sprouts 186

Spicy Bbq Whole Chicken 153

Spicy Beer Beef Jerky 100

Spicy Lime Shrimp 18

Spicy Ribs 49

Spicy Shrimp Skewers 19

Sriracha & Maple Cashews 124

St Louis Style Bbq Ribs With Texas Spicy Bbq Sauce 52

Steak Fries With Horseradish Creme 184

Steak Tips With Mashed Potatoes 87

Strawberry Mule Cocktail 163

Stuffed Jalapenos 179

Stuffed Pork Crown Roast 57

Sunset Margarita 161

Sweet And Spicy Baked Pork Beans 230

Sweet And Spicy Beef Sirloin Tip Roast 91

Sweet Cajun Wings 148

Sweet Mandarin Salmon 36

Sweet Potato Marshmallow Casserole 200

Swordfish With Sicilian Olive Oil Sauce 19

T

Tater Tot Bake 198

Teriyaki Apple Cider Turkey 152

Teriyaki Bbq Beef Skewers 90

Teriyaki Smoked Honey Tilapia 43

Texas-style Smoked Beef Brisket By Doug Scheiding 104

Thai Chicken Satays 129

Thai-style Swordfish Steaks With Peanut Sauce 42

The Boss Beef Burger 89

The Dan Patrick Show Pull-apart Pesto Bread 238

Traditional Tomahawk Steak 93

Traeger Baked Potato Torte 201

Traeger Baked Protein Bars 236

Traeger Baked Rainbow Trout 45

Traeger Bbq Half Chickens 151

Traeger Boulevardier Cocktail 173

Traeger Cajun Broil 75

Traeger Crab Legs 40

Traeger Gin & Tonic 176

Traeger Grilled Whole Corn 197

Traeger Jerk Shrimp 23

Traeger Old Fashioned 172

Traeger Paloma Cocktail 173

Traeger Pulled Pork Sandwiches 51

Traeger Roasted Easter Ham 79

Traeger Smoked Coleslaw 191

Traeger Smoked Daiquiri 160

Traeger Smoked Salmon 28

Turkey & Bacon Kebabs With Ranch-style Dressing 147

Tuscan Cheesesteaks 112

U

Unique Carolina Mustard Ribs 69

V

Vanilla Chocolate Bacon Cupcakes 209

Vanilla Chocolate Chip Cookies 233

Vietnamese Beef Jerky 83

Vodka Brined Smoked Wild Salmon 16

W

Whiskey- & Cider-brined Pork Shoulder 70

Whole Roasted Cauliflower With Garlic Parmesan Butter 182

Whole Roasted Chicken 131

Whole Smoked Honey Chicken 158

Wood-fired Chicken Breasts 131

Wood-fired Halibut 45

Y

Yucatán-spiced Chicken Thighs 139

Z

Zombie Cocktail Recipe 163

Zucchini Bread 228

Printed in the USA
CPSIA information can be obtained
at www.ICGtesting.com
LVHW071500241123
764822LV00012B/537